Statement of Purpose

The YEAR BOOK Service

The YEAR BOOK series was devised in 1901 by practicing health professionals who observed that the literature of medicine and related disciplines had become so voluminous that no one individual could read and place in perspective every potential advance in a major specialty. In the final decade of the 20th century, this recognition is more acutely true than it was in 1901.

More than merely a series of books, YEAR BOOK volumes are the tangible results of a unique service designed to accomplish the following:

- to *survey* a wide range of journals of proven value
- to *select* from those journals papers representing significant advances and statements of important clinical principles
- to provide *abstracts* of those articles that are readable, convenient summaries of their key points
- to provide *commentary* about those articles to place them in perspective

These publications grow out of a unique process that calls on the talents of outstanding authorities in clinical and fundamental disciplines, trained literature specialists, and professional writers, all supported by the resources of Mosby, the world's preeminent publisher for the health professions.

The Literature Base

Mosby and its editors survey approximately 500 journals published worldwide, covering the full range of the health professions. On an annual basis, the publisher examines usage patterns and polls its expert authorities to add new journals to the literature base and to delete journals that are no longer useful as potential YEAR BOOK sources.

The Literature Survey

The publisher's team of literature specialists, all of whom are trained and experienced health professionals, examines every original, peer-reviewed article in each journal issue. More than 250,000 articles per year are scanned systematically, including title, text, illustrations, tables, and references. Each scan is compared, article by article, to the search strategies that the publisher has developed in consultation with the 270 outside experts who form the pool of YEAR BOOK editors. A given article may be reviewed by any number of editors, from one to a dozen or more, regardless of the discipline for which the paper was originally published. In turn, each editor who receives the article reviews it to determine whether the article should be included in the YEAR BOOK. This decision is based on the article's inherent quality, its probable usefulness to readers of that YEAR BOOK, and the editor's goal to represent a balanced picture of a given field in each volume of the YEAR BOOK. In addition, the editor indicates when to include figures and tables from the article to help the YEAR BOOK reader better understand the information.

Of the quarter million articles scanned each year, only 5% are selected for detailed analysis within the YEAR BOOK series, thereby assuring readers of the high value of every selection.

The Abstract

The publisher's abstracting staff is headed by a seasoned medical professional and includes individuals with training in the life sciences, medicine, and other areas, plus extensive experience in writing for the health professions and related industries. Each selected article is assigned to a specific writer on this abstracting staff. The abstractor, guided in many cases by notations supplied by the expert editor, writes a structured, condensed summary designed so that the reader can rapidly acquire the essential information contained in the article.

The Commentary

The YEAR BOOK editorial boards, sometimes assisted by guest commentators, write comments that place each article in perspective for the reader. This provides the reader with the equivalent of a personal consultation with a leading international authority—an opportunity to better understand the value of the article and to benefit from the authority's thought processes in assessing the article.

Additional Editorial Features

The editorial boards of each YEAR BOOK organize the abstracts and comments to provide a logical and satisfying sequence of information. To enhance the organization, editors also provide introductions to sections or individual chapters, comments linking a number of abstracts, citations to additional literature, and other features.

The published YEAR BOOK contains enhanced bibliographic citations for each selected article, including extended listings of multiple authors and identification of author affiliations. Each YEAR BOOK contains a Table of Contents specific to that year's volume. From year to year, the Table of Contents for a given YEAR BOOK will vary depending on developments within the field.

Every YEAR BOOK contains a list of the journals from which papers have been selected. This list represents a subset of approximately 500 journals surveyed by the publisher and occasionally reflects a particularly pertinent article from a journal that is not surveyed on a routine basis.

Finally, each volume contains a comprehensive subject index and an index to authors of each selected paper.

The 1998 Year Book Series

Year Book of Allergy, Asthma, and Clinical Immunology: Drs. Rosenwasser, Borish, Boguniewicz, Nelson, Routes, and Spahn

Year Book of Anesthesiology and Pain Management®: Drs. Tinker, Abram, Chestnut, Roizen, Rothenberg, and Wood

Year Book of Cardiology®: Drs. Schlant, Collins, Gersh, Graham, Kaplan, and Waldo

Year Book of Chiropractic®: Dr. Lawrence

Year Book of Critical Care Medicine®: Drs. Parrillo, Balk, Calvin, Franklin, and Shapiro

Year Book of Dentistry®: Drs. Meskin, Berry, Jeffcoat, Leinfelder, Roser, Summitt, and Zakariasen

Year Book of Dermatologic Surgery®: Drs. Greenway, Barrett, Papadopoulos, and Whitaker

Year Book of Dermatology®: Dr. Thiers

Year Book of Diagnostic Radiology®: Drs. Osborn, Groskin, Dalinka, Maynard, Pentecost, Rebner, Ros, Smirniotopoulos, and Young

Year Book of Drug Therapy®: Drs. Lasagna and Weintraub

Year Book of Emergency Medicine®: Drs. Wagner, Dronen, Davidson, King, Niemann, and Roberts

Year Book of Endocrinology®: Drs. Bagdade, Braverman, Horton, Kannan, Landsberg, Molitch, Morley, Nathan, Odell, Poehlman, Rogol, and Ryan

Year Book of Family Practice®: Drs. Berg, Bowman, Davidson, Dexter, and Scherger

Year Book of Gastroenterology®: Drs. Aliperti and Fleshman

Year Book of Geriatrics and Gerontology®: Drs. Burton, Beck, Ostwald, Rabins, Reuben, Roth, Shapiro, and Whitehouse

Year Book of Hand Surgery®: Drs. Amadio and Hentz

Year Book of Hematology®: Drs. Spivak, Bell, Ness, Quesenberry, Wiernik, and Horowitz

Year Book of Infectious Diseases: Drs. Keusch, Barza, Bennish, Poutsiaka, Skolnik, and Snydman

Year Book of Medicine®: Drs. Cline, Frishman, Jett, Klahr, Malawista, Mandell, McCallum, and Utiger

Year Book of Neonatal and Perinatal Medicine®: Drs. Fanaroff, Maisels, and Stevenson

Year Book of Nephrology, Hypertension, and Mineral Metabolism: Drs. Schwab, Bennett, Emmett, Hostetter, Kumar, and Toto

Year Book of Neurology and Neurosurgery®: Drs. Bradley and Gibbs

Year Book of Nuclear Medicine®: Drs. Gottschalk, Blaufox, Neumann, Strauss, and Zubal

Year Book of Obstetrics, Gynecology, and Women's Health: Drs. Mishell, Herbst, and Kirschbaum

Year Book of Occupational and Environmental Medicine®: Drs. Emmett, Frank, Gochfeld, and Hessl

Year Book of Oncology®: Drs. Ozols, Eisenberg, Glatstein, Loehrer, and Tallman

Year Book of Ophthalmology®: Drs. Wilson, Augsburger, Cohen, Eagle, Grossman, Laibson, Maguire, Nelson, Penne, Rapuano, Sergott, Spaeth, Tipperman, Ms. Gosfield, and Ms. Salmon

Year Book of Orthopedics®: Drs. Morrey, Beauchamp, Currier, Tolo, Trigg, and Swiontkowski

Year Book of Otolaryngology–Head and Neck Surgery®: Drs. Paparella and Holt

Year Book of Pathology and Laboratory Medicine®: Drs. Raab, Cohen, Olson, Sirgi, and Stanley

Year Book of Pediatrics®: Dr. Stockman

Year Book of Plastic, Reconstructive, and Aesthetic Surgery®: Drs. Miller, Bartlett, Garner, McKinney, Ruberg, Salisbury, and Smith

Year Book of Psychiatry and Applied Mental Health®: Drs. Talbott, Ballenger, Frances, Lydiard, Meltzer, Schowalter, and Tasman

Year Book of Pulmonary Disease®: Drs. Jett, Maurer, Ryu, Strollo, and Wenzel

Year Book of Rheumatology®: Drs. Panush, Hadler, LeRoy, Liang, Reichlin, Simon, and Weinblatt

Year Book of Sports Medicine®: Drs. Shephard, Drinkwater, Eichner, Torg, Alexander, and Mr. George

Year Book of Surgery®: Drs. Copeland, Bland, Deitch, Eberlein, Howard, Luce, Seeger, Souba, and Sugarbaker

Year Book of Thoracic and Cardiovascular Surgery®: Drs. Ginsberg, Wechsler, and Williams

Year Book of Urology®: Drs. Andriole and Coplen

Year Book of Vascular Surgery®: Dr. Porter

1998

The Year Book of OPHTHALMOLOGY®

Editor-in-Chief

Richard P. Wilson, M.D.

Attending Surgeon, Glaucoma Service, Wills Eye Hospital; Associate Professor of Ophthalmology, Jefferson Medical College of Thomas Jefferson University, Philadelphia, Pennsylvania

Wills Eye Hospital®

Mosby

St. Louis Baltimore Boston Carlsbad Naples New York Philadelphia Portland London Madrid Mexico City Singapore Sydney Tokyo Toronto Wiesbaden

Mosby
Dedicated to Publishing Excellence

A Times Mirror
Company

Associate Publisher: Susan Patterson
Developmental Editor: Tania Banak
Manager, Periodical Editing: Kirk Swearingen
Production Editor: Stephanie M. Geels
Project Supervisor, Production: Joy Moore
Production Assistant: Karie House
Manager, Literature Services: Idelle L. Winer
Illustrations and Permissions Coordinator: Chidi C. Ukabam

1998 EDITION

Printed in the United States of America
Composition by Reed Technology and Information Services, Inc.
Printing/binding by Maple-Vail

Editorial Office:
Mosby, Inc.
11830 Westline Industrial Drive
St. Louis, MO 63146
Customer Service: customer.support@mosby.com
www.mosby.com/Mosby/CustomerSupport/index.html

International Standard Serial Number: 0084-392X
International Standard Book Number: 0-8151-9713-6

Editorial Board

Table of Contents

Editorial Board ix

Journals Represented xiii

Publisher's Preface xv

Introduction xvii

1. **Cataract** 1
   Cataract Surgery 1997 1
2. **Refractive Surgery** 33
   Managing Corneal Haze After Excimer Laser PRK 33
3. **Glaucoma** 61
   Introduction 61
   Suggested Reading 86
4. **Cornea** 91
   Review of Cornea 91
5. **Retina** 109
   Vitreous Substitutes 109
   Suggested Reading 136
6. **Oculoplastic Surgery** 137
   Adopting New Technology 137
7. **Pediatric Ophthalmology** 165
   Current Issues in Intraocular Lens Implantation in Children 165
8. **Neuro-ophthalmology** 177
   Graves' Ophthalmopathy: What Should We Do Now? . . . 177
9. **Imaging** 191
   Telemedicine: A Trojan Horse 191
10. **Ocular Oncology** 235
    Does Fine-needle Aspiration Biopsy Have a Role in the Diagnostic Evaluation of Small Melanocytic Choroidal Lesions? 235
11. **Pathology** 255
    Ectopia Lentis in Heritable Disorders of Connective Tissue 255
    Suggested Reading 265

12. Social Economics 281
1997—The Year in Review 281
Suggested Reading 301
13. Office Management 303
Practice Management 303
14. Medicolegal Issues in an Era of Health Care Reform 323
Legal Issues for Ophthalmologists: The More Things Change the More They Stay the Same 323
Managed Care and Liability: As the World Turns 325
Private Contracting by Medicare Physicians: The Pit and the Pendulum 335
Stark II Proposed Regulations: Down the Rabbit Hole 346
Subject Index 357
Author Index 383

Journals Represented

Mosby and its editors survey approximately 500 journals for its abstract and commentary publications. From these journals, the editors select the articles to be abstracted. Journals represented in this YEAR BOOK are listed below.

Acta Ophthalmologica Scandinavica
Age and Ageing
American Journal of Human Genetics
American Journal of Managed Care
American Journal of Ophthalmology
Annals of Neurology
Annals of Rheumatic Diseases
Archives of Neurology
Archives of Ophthalmology
Arthritis and Rheumatism
Blood
British Journal of Ophthalmology
Clinical Infectious Diseases
Cornea
Investigative Ophthalmology and Visual Science
Journal of Cataract and Refractive Surgery
Journal of Clinical Chiropractic Pediatrics
Journal of Medical Genetics
Journal of Neuro-Ophthalmology
Journal of Neurosurgery
Journal of Pediatric Ophthalmology and Strabismus
Journal of Refractive Surgery
Journal of the American Medical Association
Medical Economics
MGM Journal
Nature Genetics
Neurology
New England Journal of Medicine
Ophthalmic Plastic and Reconstructive Surgery
Ophthalmic Surgery and Lasers
Ophthalmology
Orbit
Physician's Management
Radiology
Retina
Science
Survey of Ophthalmology

STANDARD ABBREVIATIONS

The following terms are abbreviated in this edition: acquired immunodeficiency syndrome (AIDS), cardiopulmonary resuscitation (CPR), central nervous system (CNS), cerebrospinal fluid (CSF), computed tomography (CT), deoxyribonucleic acid (DNA), diopter (D), electrocardiography (ECG), health maintenance organization (HMO), human immunodeficiency virus (HIV), intensive care unit (ICU), intramuscular (IM), intravenous (IV), magnetic resonance (MR) imaging (MRI), ribonucleic acid (RNA), and ultrasound (US).

Note

The Year Book of Ophthalmology® is a literature survey service providing abstracts of articles published in the professional literature. Every effort is made to assure the accuracy of the information presented in these pages. Neither the editors nor the publisher of the Year Book of Ophthalmology® can be responsible for errors in the original materials. The editors' comments are their own opinions. Mention of specific products within this publication does not constitute endorsement.

To facilitate the use of the Year Book of Ophthalmology® as a reference tool, all illustrations and tables included in this publication are now identified as they appear in the original article. This change is meant to help the reader recognize that any illustration or table appearing in the Year Book of Ophthalmology® may be only one of many in the original article. For this reason, figure and table numbers will often appear to be out of sequence within the Year Book of Ophthalmology®.

Publisher's Preface

The Wills Eye Alumni Society, a professional organization of ophthalmologists committed to providing leadership in research, education, and patient care, has recognized the YEAR BOOK OF OPHTHALMOLOGY® as a major resource contributing to the goal of providing high-quality information to ophthalmologists worldwide through its highlighting of significant clinical and research developments in the area of ophthalmology. We are honored by this recognition and look forward to a long and rewarding relationship with this distinguished group of physicians.

Introduction

This last year has seen a number of significant advances, many of them in the areas of cell biology and genetics. These advances not only further our knowledge of disease processes but should enable us to develop tests that can predict disease in individuals who do not presently exhibit symptoms. Understanding the way genes are involved in a particular disease may enable researchers to develop chemical regulators that disable or slow down the promoter part of the gene causing the disease. Such a basic attack on glaucoma is now taking place in relation to the Trabecular Meshwork Glucocorticoid Responder gene, which offers the basis for a predictive test and possibly a way to turn off the promoter gene. Such intervention might be a boon to the majority of patients with primary open-angle glaucoma.

Keeping up with all the advances in this as well as other areas of ophthalmology is the main thrust of the YEAR BOOK. The commentaries should enable the reader to assign the proper amount of importance (vs. distrust) to each article selected. As in last year's YEAR BOOK, the subjects of practice management and the legal environment we must endure are included to provide a global view of what each ophthalmologist should know to dispense the best medical care in the most efficient manner.

As always, I am interested in your thoughts on how to make the YEAR BOOK more responsive to your needs. Please direct your thoughts and suggestions to:

wilson@wills-glaucoma.org

or

Richard P. Wilson, M.D., Glaucoma Service, Wills Eye Hospital
Ninth and Walnut Streets, Philadelphia, PA 19107.

Your input will be seriously considered, so please take the time to let me know what you like and what you do not, as well as your opinions concerning the section editors.

Richard P. Wilson, M.D.

1 Cataract

Cataract Surgery 1997

by Richard Tipperman, M.D.

Cataract surgery continued to advance in 1997. Perhaps one of the biggest strides was the increasing acceptance of topical anesthesia for cataract surgery. The advantages of topical anesthesia include increased patient comfort, rapid recovery of vision, and avoidance of complications associated with injection anesthetics. Three excellent peer review articles (Abstracts 1–7, 1–8, and 1–9) concerning topical anesthesia are included in this chapter.

Although topical anesthesia is often performed "hand-in-hand" with temporal clear corneal surgery, the topical approach works quite well for superior surgery.* Like topical anesthesia, temporal surgery has significant advantages over traditional techniques. These include improved ergonomics, better red reflex, improved fluid drainage, fewer subconjunctival hemorrhages, avoidance of against-the-rule astigmatism, and rapid recovery of vision (because of the greater distance between the incision site and the center of the visual axis). Disadvantages of temporal surgery include a "learning curve" connected with the transition, less flexibility for dealing with either intraoperative or incisional complications, and an incision which is less forgiving to wound construction errors.

Another area in which cataract surgery advanced in 1997 was in the use of intraocular lenses in pediatric patients. The difficulties with managing aphakia and amblyopia with congenital cataracts are clear. Obviously, if intraocular lenses work as well in pediatric patients as they do in adults, they should have significant advantages. Several articles in this chapter review issues associated with pediatric intraocular lenses including power selection, surgical technique, and outcomes.

One potential highlight of 1997 was the approval of a multi-focal intraocular lens for use in the United States. The possibility of avoiding difficulties with near and intermediate vision in patients is exciting. Surgeons using this intraocular lens are encouraged by the parent company to develop their own "A" constant so their implant power calculations will

*In my own practice, if I am working superiorly, I will leave a cellulose sponge saturated with Tetracaine on the region of the superior limbus for a full minute "by the clock."

be as accurate as possible. In addition, rather than erring on the "myopic side" of plano, it is recommended that the postoperative aim be either plano or slightly hyperopic to maximize the full range of vision given by the intraocular lens.

What does the future hold for the rest of 1998? One exciting development is the use of an endocapsular ring. Although not yet approved in the United States, the ring is being used extensively in other countries. There are significant potential advantages in both pseudoexfoliation and cases of zonular compromise. An excellent article reviewing the use of the endocapsular ring is covered in this chapter (Abstract 1–11). Perhaps later this year we will be able to report its approval in the United States.

Outcomes of Cataract Extraction With Multifocal Intraocular Lens Implantation: Functional Status and Quality of Life

Javitt JC, Wang F, Trentacost DJ, et al (Georgetown Univ, Washington, DC; AMO Surgical Products, Irvine, Calif; Allergan, Inc, Irvine, Calif)

Ophthalmology 104:589–599, 1997 1–1

Background.—The primary objective of intraocular lens implantation has been to correct aphakic vision by obtaining the best distance vision without spectacle correction. An ideal prosthetic lens would reproduce the original function of the crystalline lens at near and distance vision. In patients with cataracts, attempts have been made to correct lens opacity and presbyopia, but initial efforts to fabricate a bifocal intraocular lens were associated with loss of clarity, decreased contrast sensitivity, halos, and glare. One alternative is to use concentric zones of progressive aspheric surfaces to provide repeatable power distributions and obtain multifocal correction rather than bifocal correction.

Methods.—In a retrospective, case-control study, functional status was measured after bilateral implantation of a multifocal intraocular lens in 100 study subjects and bilateral implantation of a monofocal intraocular lens in 103 control subjects. The Cataract TyPE specification was modified, validated, and administered via telephone interview. Vision, functional status, and quality of life of study and control subjects were compared.

Results.—The Cataract TyPE specification had moderate correlation with Snellen acuity. Study subjects who had multifocal implantation were more likely to never wear spectacles than control subjects who had monofocal implantation. Vision without spectacles was rated as being significantly better by study subjects than by control subjects; the most significant difference was for near vision without spectacles. Study subjects reported less limitation in specific visual tasks without spectacles related to distance vision and near vision activities, as well as social activities.

Discussion.—The study subjects who had bilateral multifocal intraocular lens implantation had a better overall functional outcome than control subjects who had monofocal intraocular lens implantation. The study subjects reported better overall vision, less limitation in visual function, and less use of spectacles.

► I thought this was an important article to review because the Allergan Medical Optics multifocal lens has now received Food and Drug Administration approval. This is the first multifocal lens approved for implantation in the United States. The article shows that patients with bilateral multifocal lenses have better overall vision, less limitation in their overall visual function, and less need for spectacles, compared with patients who have monofocal implants.

As "word gets out" regarding multifocal lenses, more and more patients will require them as an option in cataract surgery. Although this article states the patient advantages of multifocal lenses, it does not really discuss the clinical considerations in managing patients with these lenses. The clinical considerations include appropriate patient selection for multifocal lens use and the need for extremely accurate implant power calculations. Obviously, if a patient is not plano for distance, the multifocal near correction will also not be correct. Often, the patients with the highest visual demands who desire the best uncorrected distance and near vision, may also be patients who are the least tolerant of the need for any spectacle correction. Nonetheless, what this article demonstrates is that even when patients are not plano, their improved near vision gives them better overall functional vision.

I have implanted many Allergan Medical Optics SI40 lenses, which are the monofocal equivalent of the Allergan multifocal lens. It is a silicone foldable lens with polymethylmethacrylate haptics. I have personally been quite happy with the performance of this lens. However, I have also implanted a large number of the Alcon Acrysof lens and been very happy with the acrylic lenses as well. There are certainly a number of theoretical considerations that could make a surgeon prefer an acrylic lens over a silicone lens or vice versa. However, I believe the ability to use a multifocal lens will shift a fair number of surgeons back to using a foldable silicone lens.

R. Tipperman, M.D.

The Impact of Cataract Surgery on Low Vision Patients: A Population Based Study

Mönestam E, Wachtmeister L (Umeå Univ, Sweden)

Acta Ophthalmol Scand 75:569–576, 1997 1–2

Background.—From the patient's perspective, a successful cataract operation is one which offers improvement in his specific visual needs. The ability to do visual activities such as reading, sewing, and watching television is more important to the patient than the results of visual acuity testing. A group of low-vision patients were studied to determine how cataract surgery affected their ability to perform specific visual tasks, and how those subjective results were related to visual acuity.

Methods.—Fifty-two low-vision patients undergoing cataract surgery during a 1-year period were studied. The study criterion for low vision was binocular visual acuity of 6/20 or worse, given normal visual fields, or up to 6/12 in the setting of advanced visual field loss. Most patients underwent extracapsular cataract extraction with posterior intraocular lens implantation. The patients were asked about their ability to perform visually demanding tasks before and after their cataract surgery, as well as their satisfaction with cataract surgery. The tasks questioned involved reading, watching television, orientation in unfamiliar surroundings, and near and distance estimation. These and other outcomes were evaluated 5–6 months after surgery, after the patients had received and adapted to their new refractions and visual aids. Measurements of visual acuity were performed as well.

Results.—The characteristics and visual acuity results of patients with age-related maculopathy and glaucoma were similar. Reported reading ability was improved after surgery in 54% of patients, unchanged in 33%, and worse in 13%. Visual acuity was better in patients with subjective improvement in reading than in those with no change, but not significantly different from those with decreased reading performance. The percentage of patients who were unable to read newspaper-size print decreased from 44% to 21%. Overall, 81% of patients felt that surgery improved their ability to perform visually demanding tasks. Patients with greater visual disability had higher expectations of their surgery. Preoperative visual acuity in the better eye was significantly related to patient expectations. After surgery, 50% of patients said they were managing their daily lives better, 38% reported no change, and 10% reported worsening. The improvement of visual acuity in the operated eye was not significantly related to the change in management of daily life. However, satisfaction with the surgical results was significantly related to both subjective and objective visual improvement.

Conclusions.—For most low-vision patients with functionally disturbing cataracts, surgery significantly improves subjective visual ability in vision-dependent activities. Surgery reduces subjective visual problems while improving visual acuity results. Particularly for patients with peripheral visual field loss, surgery seems to improve orientation capacity. Patient satisfaction is related to postoperative subjective improvement and to the visual acuity in the operated eye. The surgeon should seek to address unreasonable expectations about the results of cataract surgery in low-vision patients.

► Cataract surgery in patients with age-related macular disease has always been an interest of mine. There are many patients who have advanced cataracts and advanced retinal problems who will have an improvement in their overall level of visual function if the cataract is removed. Despite this, many patients are quite disappointed with the results of their surgery even with very thorough and careful preoperative counseling. Even after being told they may not obtain an improvement in their overall visual acuity, and will still not be able to read without special magnifiers, many patients with advanced age-related macular disease after surgery come in frustrated saying, "Why can't I read?"

This study demonstrates that in terms of overall functional improvement, patients can significantly benefit from cataract surgery if they have coexisting ocular pathology such as advanced glaucoma or macular disease. It is interesting to speculate why the patients in this article seem to benefit so much more than patients who I see day in and day out. Perhaps this is a cultural phenomenon because all the patients in this study were from Sweden. Interestingly, the authors stress the importance of preoperative counseling of patients to reduce any unreasonable expectations they may have regarding the outcome of their surgery.

R. Tipperman, M.D.

Impact of Cataract Surgery on Car Driving: A Population Based Study in Sweden

Mönestam E, Wachtmeister L (Umeå Univ, Sweden)

Br J Ophthalmol 81:16–22, 1997 1–3

Background.—Visual information is extremely important in the task of driving, particularly for elderly people in whom reaction times have slowed. There has been little research into patients' assessments of their vision before and after cataract surgery. How cataract surgery affects patients' ability to drive, from their own point of view, is unknown.

Methods.—The impact of cataract surgery on patients' estimates of their own visual function during driving was studied prospectively. The study sample comprised 208 consecutive patients with driver's licenses who underwent cataract surgery with intraocular lens implantation. They completed a questionnaire regarding visual problems during driving before and after surgery. Visual problems with other tasks—including reading, watching television, and moving around—were addressed as well.

Results.—Eighty-two percent of patients reported visual problems while driving before surgery. The major problem reported was difficulty in driving in darkness and twilight. Other problems included trouble estimating distances, glare from other cars, and eye fatigue. Only 5% reported such problems after surgery. The percentage of patients driving at a visual acuity below the legal limit decreased from 23% before surgery to 4% afterward. Twenty-five percent of patients who weren't driving before surgery started to drive afterward, and 40% of all drivers reported driving more frequently. The percentage of patients with difficulties estimating distance decreased from 46% to 14%. This problem was more common in patients with visual acuity of less than 20/40 in 1 eye after surgery.

Conclusion.—Visual function during driving is significantly improved by cataract surgery. Visual problems during driving should be regarded as an indication for cataract surgery. Surgery should be performed in the second eye, if appropriate, to achieve good binocular vision and optimize the ability to estimate distances.

► Ophthalmologists always like to describe their results in terms of visual acuities. It is interesting that patients never describe their pleasure or displeasure with their visual function in terms of Snellen acuities. When was the last time you had a patient say, "Doctor, my vision is only 20/50," or "My vision is only 20/100," or "Boy, I'm really happy with my vision. Now I see 20/25." Patients describe their difficulties in terms of functional visual problems: "I can't drive at night," "I can't see the T.V.," or "I can't see my crosswords."

Obviously, one of the greatest and most frequent complaints that patients have is difficulty in driving. Once patients can no longer drive, they often lose their ability to remain independent.

This is the first study I know of that specifically looks just at patients' driving abilities before and after cataract surgery. As most practicing ophthalmologists know, a patient's driving ability is significantly improved after cataract surgery. One of the highlights of this article which should be stressed, however, is the improvement in patients' driving ability once they receive cataract/lens implant surgery on the second eye. It was found that, after cataract surgery in the second eye, patients had marked improvement in their overall visual function. This, along with quality of life studies done on patients after cataract surgery in *both* eyes, is another reason why many patients function better after "second eye" cataract surgery.

R. Tipperman, M.D.

Intraocular Lens Power Prediction in Patients Who Undergo Cataract Surgery Following Previous Radial Keratotomy

Lyle WA, Jin GJC (Eye Inst of Utah, Salt Lake City)

Arch Ophthalmol 115:457–461, 1997 1–4

Introduction.—Radial keratotomy (RK) for correction of myopia has been performed in the United States for 2 decades. Some patients who undergo the procedure will eventually need cataract surgery. Although there should be no technical difficulty in operating on such patients, some studies report problems in intraocular lens (IOL) power selection. Ten cases of phacoemulsification with IOL implantation performed after RK were reviewed for visual and refractive outcome and for the value of different formulas used to calculate IOL power.

Patients and Methods.—The patients were 6 men and 4 women with a median age of 57 years. Radial keratotomy had been performed at an average age of 51.1 years. Cataract surgery was performed at a mean interval of 79.1 months after RK. In all cases, foldable IOLs were implanted by an in-the-bag technique. Postoperative follow-up averaged 27.8 months. The Binkhorst, SRK II, and Holladay formulas were used to retrospectively calculate IOL power. Each patient's final refractive error was used as a criterion to judge the accuracy and predictability for each formula and different variables used in the formula.

Results.—Three eyes underwent IOL exchange and were excluded from IOL power calculation because of relatively short follow-up; mathematical evaluation was impossible in a fourth patient who had extreme refractive changes after surgery. The 7 eyes that did not undergo an IOL exchange showed a hyperopic shift in the early postoperative period, but the shift regressed approximately 3 months later. Five of 7 eyes had a hyperopic error at the final examination, and 2 showed more than 1.00 D. Six eyes (60%) achieved an uncorrected visual acuity of 20/40 or better and all 10 had a 20/25 or better postoperative best-corrected visual acuity. The mean spherical equivalent refraction was −0.78 D preoperatively and 0.45 D postoperatively. The Binkhorst and Holladay formulas were more accurate than the SRK II formula. Most of the eyes would achieve a refraction of −2.00 to +0.50 D with use of an adjusted keratometric value (K) (the current average K minus 1.0 D) in combination with the Binkhorst and Holladay formulas.

Conclusion.—Cataract surgery tends to produce a corneal flattening in patients who have undergone previous RK. Accuracy in IOL power selection may be improved by the use of an average between the Binkhorst and Holladay formulas with adjusted Ks, but an unexpectedly high refractive error cannot always be avoided.

► I wish someone would give me the "right answer" to this problem. I am hoping this article has the best solution. Although I have operated on only a handful of patients in this situation, trying to choose the appropriate strength implant can be extremely difficult. These are also the type of patients who will be most unhappy with even half a diopter implant power error.

It is best to have a lengthy discussion with these patients preoperatively to help them understand the extreme difficulty in determining the correct IOL power. I make sure the patients understand the potential need for either an implant exchange or a piggyback lens after surgery. The final sentence of this paper should be read several times by any surgeon who is going to be performing cataract surgery on a patient who has had prior RK: "In some cases, an unexpectedly high refractive error still cannot be avoided."

R. Tipperman, M.D.

Choice of Lens and Dioptric Power in Pediatric Pseudophakia

Dahan E, Drusedau MUH (St John Eye Hosp, Johannesburg, South Africa)

J Cataract Refract Surg 23:618–623, 1997 1–5

Objective.—Intraocular lens (IOL) implantation in a young child's eyes should not cause corneal decompensation or myopia, and should not discolor or biodegrade over the years. Guidelines for lens choice and dioptric power based on the child's age, considering expected changes in axial length and refractive power, were created from information obtained

TABLE 1.—Patient Demographics

Group (Age Range)	Number of Eyes	Age at Implantation	Mean ± SD Follow-up (Years)	Last Age (Years)
Group A (1–18 mos)	68	9.36 ± 6.12 mos	6.93 ± 3.42	7.69 ± 3.30
Group B (19–36 mos)	36	2.37 ± 0.49 yrs	3.46 ± 1.62	5.84 ± 1.65
Group C (37 mos–8 yrs)	52	5.05 ± 1.43 yrs	3.83 ± 2.30	8.75 ± 2.35

(Courtesy of Dahan E, Drusedau MUH: Choice of lens and dioptric power in pediatric pseudophakia. *J Cataract Refract Surg* 23:618–623, 1997.)

TABLE 3.—First and Last Axial Length Refractions (Spherical Equivalent)

	Mean ± SD	
Group (Age Range)	First Refraction (D)	Last Refraction (D)
Group A (1–18 mos)	+5.54 ± 2.36	−0.83 ± 4.29
Group B (19–36 mos)	+3.63 ± 2.18	+0.90 ± 3.19
Group C (37 mos–8 yrs)	+2.20 ± 2.08	−0.40 ± 3.09

(Courtesy of Dahan E, Drusedau MUH: Choice of lens and dioptric power in pediatric pseudophakia. *J Cataract Refract Surg* 23:618–623, 1997.)

TABLE 4.—Last Visual Acuity and Range

Group (Age Range)	Last Visual Acuity (Mean)	Range
Group A (1–18 mos)	20/40	20/1200–20/20
Group B (19–36 mos)	20/30	20/100–20/20
Group C (37 mos–8 yrs)	20/25	20/400–20/20

(Courtesy of Dahan E, Drusedau MUH: Choice of lens and dioptric power in pediatric pseudophakia. *J Cataract Refract Surg* 23:618–623, 1997.)

TABLE 5.—Visual Acuity and Mean (±SD) Axial Length Growth

Group (Visual Acuity)	Number of Eyes	Mean Axial Length Growth (mm)
Group 1 (20/1200–20/100)	11	4.79 ± 1.50
Group 2 (20/80–20/60)	22	3.14 ± 1.83
Group 3 (20/40–20/20)	23	1.54 ± 1.68

(Courtesy of Dahan E, Drusedau MUH: Choice of lens and dioptric power in pediatric pseudophakia. *J Cataract Refract Surg* 23:618–623, 1997.)

- ***For children younger than 2 years...***

  Do biometry and undercorrect by 20%

  OR

  Use axial length only:

Axial Length (mm)	IOL Power (D)
17	28.00
18	27.00
19	26.00
20	24.00
21	22.00

- ***For children between 2 and 8 years...***

  Do biometry and undercorrect by 10%

FIGURE 1.—Guidelines for determining intraocular lens (IOL) power in pediatric eyes. (Courtesy of Dahan E, Drusedau MUH: Choice of lens and dioptric power in pediatric pseudophakia. *J Cataract Refract Surg* 23:618–623, 1997).

after a retrospective analysis of refractive development in pseudophakic eyes of children.

Methods.—Between June 1983 and April 1994, posterior chamber IOL implantation was performed in 156 pseudophakic eyes of 99 children, aged 1 month to 8 years, with unilateral congenital cataract (n = 42) or bilateral congenital and/or developmental cataract (n = 57). Children with unilateral cataract had extraction and implantation from the age of 1 month on. Children with bilateral cataract had cataract extraction but did not receive an IOL until they were older than 1 year. Children with developmental cataract had extraction and IOL implantation when visual acuity in the weaker eye was 20/80 or less. Patients were divided into 3 age groups on the premise that the eyes in the youngest group would grow the fastest (Table 1). Between 1983 and 1988, a 3-piece IOL or a 1-piece, adult-sized PMMA IOL with encircling haptics was used. After 1988, a custom, pediatric, 1-piece, PMMA IOL was used. Earlier IOL power calculations aimed at emmetropia, resulted in undercorrection. Patients, however, grew into emmetropia. After 1986 patients were intentionally undercorrected to compensate for myopic shifts. Axial lengths and refraction were measured before surgery and at the final visit. Amblyopia was treated aggressively.

Results.—The largest changes in axial lengths, refraction, and myopic shift occurred in the youngest group (group A) (Tables 3 and 4). Most severe amblyopia cases were in group A. Three IOL exchanges were necessary: 2 in group A because of large myopic shifts with extreme anisometropia in patients 3 months old at surgery, and 1 in group C because of severe amblyopia and progressive myopia in a 5-year-old patient. Axial length growth was greatest in patients with deep amblyopia and least in patients in group 3, who had good final visual acuity (Table 5). Many complications of IOL implantation in children result from the use of adult-sized lenses. Pediatric lenses used after 1988 were easy to insert and center. Most eye growth in children appears to occur during the first 2 years.

Conclusions.—The guidelines developed as a result of this analysis aim for an undercorrection of 20% in infants and 10% in toddlers (Fig 1). Induced initial hypermetropia is treated with glasses. Amblyopia is treated aggressively.

Longitudinal Changes in Axial Length in Pseudophakic Children

Sorkin JA, Lambert SR (Emory Univ, Atlanta, Ga)

J Cataract Refract Surg 23:624S-628S, 1997 1–6

Background.—Children who undergo cataract extraction generally have optical correction by means of intraocular lenses (IOLs). Because it is expected that myopic shift will occur with growth, some physicians implant IOLS that undercorrect current refractive error. To investigate the axial elongation occurring in children after implantation of IOL, a cohort of children who had cataract surgery with primary IOL implantation were studied for an average of 3 years.

Study Design.—A chart review was performed of all children who had cataract surgery with primary IOL implantation between 1990 and 1994 performed by a single physician. All patients had extracapsular cataract extraction with poly (methyl methacrylate) posterior chamber IOL implantation in the capsular bag at the time of surgery. Axial lengths were assessed, with the patient awake, before surgery in both eyes, if possible, using corneal applanation. Postoperative axial lengths were measured with the same A-scan unit, with the gain reduced to minimize IOL echoes. The SRK I or II formula was used to select the IOL power needed for emmetropia for patients at least 6 years of age. For younger children, an IOL with a power 1.00–2.00 D less than calculated was implanted. The primary variables were age at surgery, type of cataract, change in axial length, and change in spherical equivalent in the affected eye.

Findings.—During the study period, 28 eyes in 24 patients had cataract extraction with primary IOL implantation by the same physician. These patients comprise the study group. Eleven eyes were excluded because of incomplete follow-up, postoperative retinal detachment, IOL subluxation, or lack of axial length data. The patients were aged 3.5–9.6 years at the time of operation. Nine patients were boys and 6 were girls. Of the 17 cataracts in the study group, 9 were traumatic, 3 developmental, 3 congenital, and 2 were induced by steroids. Preoperative visual acuity was usually worse than 20/400. Visual acuity improved postoperatively and continued to improve during an average follow-up period of 3.1 years. At last follow-up, 94% of eyes had a visual acuity of at least 20/40. The overall average axial length change was 0.64 mm and the average myopic shift was −1.01 D. The average axial length change was significantly greater in the eyes with traumatic cataracts than in the eyes with developmental or congenital cataracts. There was a significant correlation between the age of the child at surgery and the preoperative axial length.

Conclusions.—Seventeen eyes of 15 children underwent cataract surgery with primary IOL implantation and were studied for an average of 3 years. The average mean axial length change during this period was 0.64 mm and the average myopic shift was −1.01 D. The average change in spherical equivalent mirrored the change in axial length. Patients with cataract surgery secondary to trauma had a greater average change in axial elongation and spherical equivalent. Although there was a trend for younger age to be associated with increased change in axial length, this association did not reach significance.

► Intraocular lens implantation is becoming increasingly routine for pediatric patients. Because of the rapid growth of the eye in extremely young patients, the best lens power to use for a given patient remains undetermined. These articles (Abstracts 1–5 and 1–6) help address some of the issues involved in implant power selection in extremely young patients. Surgeons need to be aware that the younger the child is, the greater a myopic shift will be seen and, therefore, the greater the emphasis should be placed on undercorrection initially with implant power so that the patients' final vision can be adjusted with spectacle correction. As the eye becomes progressively more myopic, there will be a tendency for the eye to move toward moderate myopia or emmetropia. Obviously, in addition to observing the patient for normal postoperative changes, great attention needs to be paid to the treatment of any underlying amblyopia.

R. Tipperman, M.D.

Anterior Chamber Irrigation With Unpreserved Lidocaine 1% for Anesthesia During Cataract Surgery

Koch PS (Koch Eye Associates, Warwick, RI)

J Cataract Refract Surg 23:551–554, 1997 1–7

Background.—Local anesthetic for cataract surgery is provided by many means. Injection anesthesia has been associated with brain stem anesthesia, ocular penetration, retrobulbar hemorrhage, retinal vascular occlusion, optic nerve trauma, and other complications. Fichman proposed topical application of anesthetic eye drops to help avoid these complications, but patients have reported discomfort from the microscope light and pressure changes during surgery, and pain from iris manipulation or injection of a miotic. Fichman suggested injecting unpreserved tetracaine directly into the anterior chamber to achieve additional anesthesia. Gills proposed irrigating the anterior chamber with unpreserved 1% lidocaine to achieve better anesthesia.

Methods.—In a prospective study, the ability of unpreserved 1% lidocaine irrigated into the anterior chamber to provide adequate anesthesia for cataract surgery was evaluated in 1,000 of 1,012 consecutive eyes in which temporal corneal incision cataract surgery was performed. The lidocaine was the only anesthetic used. After the initial corneal stab incision was made, 0.25–0.50 cc of unpreserved 1% lidocaine was irrigated into the anterior chamber.

Results.—Of the 1,000 patients, 996 were comfortable and pain free during the procedure after a single dose of anesthetic. One patient required supplemental retrobulbar anesthesia because of discomfort from the microscope. Another patient was also uncomfortable but did require additional anesthesia. Two patients were given additional anesthesia because of discomfort late in the procedure.

Discussion.—These results are encouraging. In most cases, unpreserved 1% lidocaine irrigated into the anterior chamber provided sufficient anesthesia for temporal corneal incision surgery. This technique was clearly unsatisfactory in 2 of the 1,000 patients. There were no signs of intraocular toxicity, but long-term monitoring with endothelial cell counts and morphologic analysis is needed to rule out this possibility.

Unpreserved Lidocaine to Control Discomfort During Cataract Surgery Using Topical Anesthesia

Gills JP, Cherchio M, Raanan MG (St Luke's Cataract and Laser Inst, Tarpon Springs, Fla; Ctr for Clinical Research, Chicago)

J Cataract Refract Surg 23:545–550, 1997 1–8

Background.—Topical anesthesia became possible in cataract surgery after small sutureless incisions through clear cornea or at the limbus were developed. Topical anesthesia can be difficult to use in some patients. After it was noted that there were no adverse effects after inadvertent injection of lidocaine into the anterior chamber, it was hypothesized that routine intraocular injection of lidocaine might be safe and effective.

Methods.—In a randomized, controlled, double-blind study, a determination was made of the ability of unpreserved 1% lidocaine to provide additional anesthesia during sutureless small-incision cataract surgery and intraocular lens implantation with topical anesthesia. Patients were randomized to receive 0.1 cc of unpreserved lidocaine 1% or 0.1 cc of saline. Pain and discomfort during phacoemulsification and intraocular lens insertion were rated on a predefined, uniform scale. A secondary study using an increased dose of 0.5 cc of unpreserved 1% lidocaine was also conducted.

Results.—Pain and discomfort scores of 2 or more were reported by 9% of patients given lidocaine and 26% of patients given saline; increased pressure or pain during phacoemulsification was reported by 10% of patients given saline. Patients given lidocaine had discomfort primarily during insertion of the intraocular lens, perhaps because of wound manipulation. Of patients given lidocaine, none reported pain and 2% felt increased pressure during phacoemulsification. Intraocular sensation was reported by 3% of patients given lidocaine when the dose was increased to 0.5% cc. There were no cases of significant cell loss and no adverse effects.

Discussion.—These results show that intraocular unpreserved 1% lidocaine used with topical anesthesia is safe and effective in controlling the intraocular discomfort and pain felt by some patients during cataract surgery and intraocular lens implantation. An increase in the lidocaine dose from 0.1 cc to 0.5 cc significantly reduced intraocular sensation during surgery.

▶ These excellent peer review articles (Abstracts 1–7 and 1–8) describe successful topical anesthesia methodology using anterior chamber injections of unpreserved 1% lidocaine for cataract surgery. For those readers not performing cataract surgery under topical anesthesia, the concept and technique may seem "daunting." Let me assure you that topical anesthesia works extremely well and, in the vast majority of cases, the surgery and patient response are no different from those of a standard peribulbar or retrobulbar bloc. Patient acceptance of the procedure is extremely high, and it is my opinion that the vast majority of patients are much more comfortable with this approach than with our standard injection techniques.

Although a few patients will find topical anesthesia difficult because of discomfort or excessive eye movement, these cases are really far and few between. I would reassure the reader that operating on these patients is not much different from operating on a patient with an "incomplete bloc."

Many surgeons make the transition to topical anesthesia around the time they also make the transition to working temporally. I believe that this can create some difficulties because of the "learning curve" associated with both procedures. As a surgeon who combines topical anesthesia with a temporal approach, I believe quite strongly that of the 2, the transition to topical anesthesia is much simpler. As noted above, for most patients, performing cataract surgery under topical anesthesia is no different from performing surgery with a bloc. Moving temporally, however, does have a number of obstacles to be overcome regarding the learning curve. It may be prudent for the surgeon in transition to master each of these techniques independently and then combine the 2. For more advice on performing topical cataract surgery, please see next article (Abstract 1–9).

R. Tipperman, M.D.

Indicators of Patient Suitability for Topical Anesthesia

Fraser SG, Siriwadena D, Jamieson H, et al (Whipps Cross Hosp, Leytonstone, London)

J Cataract Refract Surg 23:781–783, 1997 1–9

Background.—There are advantages to using topical anesthesia over injectable local anesthesia for small incision, self-sealing cataract surgery. However, not all patients are suitable for this technique. Many patients who have general anesthesia have a high anesthetic risk. It can be difficult to decide which anesthetic technique to use. It was hypothesized that patients who tolerated contact diagnostic techniques well also would perform well with topical anesthesia.

Methods.—In a prospective study, 50 patients who were thought to be suitable for phacoemulsification were enrolled. Three observers used a scoring system to assess how well each patient tolerated measurement of intraocular pressure and axial length. These scores were correlated to scores of how each patient tolerated phacoemulsification under topical anesthesia.

Results.—All patients underwent phacoemulsification and posterior chamber intraocular lens implantation. There was a high correlation between tonometry and A-scan scores and surgery scores. There was a significant discrepancy between tonometry and A-scan score and surgery scores in only 1 patient. This patient was one of the youngest in this investigation.

Discussion.—How well a patient tolerates tonometry and A-scan can be a good indicator of how the patient will tolerate phacoemulsification under topical anesthesia. The choice of anesthetic technique also should involve the age of the patient, as well as communication and cooperation abilities.

▶ Topical anesthesia works extremely well, but even the most ardent proponent of topical anesthesia agrees that appropriate patient selection is critical. Although topical anesthesia with intravenous supplementation can be used on virtually any patient, there are some cases where the operating surgeon is left wondering if the difficulties with patient head movement, lid squeezing, and overall movement are worth the effort.

Obviously, it would be nice to identify these patients ahead of time so that patients who would not be good candidates for topical anesthesia could have standard peribulbar or retrobulbar anesthesia. Typically, in my own practice, I just try to assess the patient's degree of "eye shyness." If on examining the eye and touching the adnexa they seem to squeeze and pull back a great amount, then I do consider whether or not they will be able to tolerate topical anesthesia. If, however, the patient is quite comfortable and relaxed during the examination, I find that topical anesthesia will be sufficient.

This article attempts to quantify this subjective approach. By grading the patient's ability to cooperate with tonometry and axial length measurements, they have been able to quantify the patient's ability to cooperate for cataract surgery with topical anesthesia.

To me, it is not a surprise that this relationship was not as accurate for younger patients. In general, younger patients are often poorer candidates for topical anesthesia. They seem to have much greater sensation during surgery, especially with chamber deepening. I found it helpful when performing cataract surgery using topical anesthesia in young patients to lower my infusion bottle height so that the chambers do not deepen quite as much, and there is not as much stretch on the zonules and ciliary apparatus. This seems to significantly increase the patient's comfort. The anxiety level and "sympathetic drive" of younger patients is often great, and many times, they are made more comfortable during surgery if supplemental intravenous sedation is used.

Topical anesthesia, especially with a temporal approach, can also be made much easier for the surgeon with a well-designed lid speculum. Because there is no facial bloc, the patient can easily blink. This is a problem with the standard wire specula, that were used in the past in that the patient could squeeze through the speculum, which made surgery much more difficult. In addition, because the conjunctiva and the lids are not anesthetized, if the assistant irrigates too vigorously, it will cause a blink response. These problems can be avoided by using a speculum specifically designed for a temporal approach and topical anesthesia. The speculum typically opens with a "rachet" mechanism, which will not allow the patient to squeeze or blink the eye. In addition, the assistant needs to be educated regarding appropriate corneal wetting techniques during topical anesthesia. Rather than squirting the eye with a vigorous stream of balanced salt solution, which will engage the lids and conjunctiva and cause a blink reflex, just a single drop or 2 should be placed directly on the cornea.

R. Tipperman, M.D.

Comparative Study of Silicone Versus Acrylic Foldable Lens Implantation in Primary Glaucoma Triple Procedure

Lemon LC, Shin DH, Song MS, et al (Wayne State Univ, Detroit)
Ophthalmology 104:1708–1713, 1997 1–10

Objective.—Whether small incision foldable intraocular lens (IOL) implantation in cataract surgery affects glaucoma control of visual outcome is not known. Results of an ongoing randomized prospective study comparing silicone and acrylic foldable IOLs in primary glaucoma triple procedure (PGTP) with selective use of mitomycin C (MMC) were reported.

Methods.—Primary glaucoma triple procedure was performed on 79 patients with primary open-angle glaucoma (POAG), with 36 receiving an IOLAB model L141U silicone lens and 43 receiving an Alcon Acrysof model MA60BM acrylic lens. Subconjunctival MMC was also selectively used in patients with a risk for PGTP failure. After surgery, patients were examined at 1, 2, 3, 4–6, and 9–12 months, and periodically thereafter.

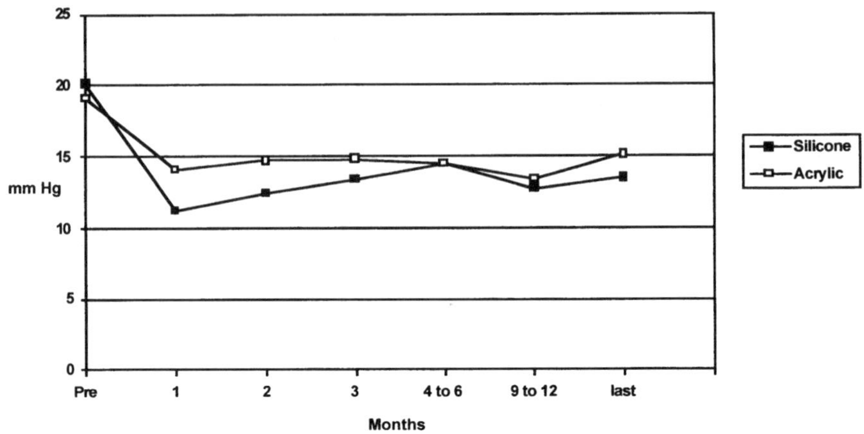

FIGURE 1.—Mean intraocular pressure vs. time (months). (From Lemon LC, Shin DH, Song MS, et al: Comparative study of silicone versus acrylic foldable lens implantation in primary glaucoma triple procedure. *Ophthalmology* 104:1708–1713, 1997. Published courtesy of *Ophthalmology*.)

Technique.—A primary trabeculectomy was performed followed by capsulorrhexis, phacoemulsion, and removal of the lens. The IOL was inserted, unfolded, and rotated. After a peripheral iridectomy, removal of viscoelastic material, and scleral flap closure, a balanced salt solution was injected through the paracentesis track, and the conjunctival flap was closed. All patients received identical postoperative medication. When necessary, digital or focal decompression and postoperative suture release was used to lower intraocular pressure (IOP) to target levels.

Results.—Postoperative IOPs were significantly lower than preoperative IOPs for both groups at all time points but not significantly different from each other at 2 months and beyond (Fig 1). Mean 1-month postoperative IOP was significantly lower in the silicone group than in the acrylic group. Significantly more patients with acrylic IOLs than with silicone IOLs had an IOP greater than 25 mm Hg (39.5% vs. 16.7%), and an IOP spike greater than 5 mm Hg above preoperative IOP in the first 2 weeks (37.2% vs. 16.7%) and first month (39.5% vs. 16.7%). Significantly more patients with acrylic IOLs than with silicone IOLs required suture release in the first month (48.8% vs. 25.0%) and the first 2 months (60.5% vs. 36.1%). Preoperative and postoperative medications, visual acuity, and complications were similar between groups.

Conclusions.—The acrylic IOL group had significantly higher mean IOPs 1 month postoperatively, and a significantly higher incidence of postoperative IOP spikes at 2 weeks and 1 month. The reason for this increased IOP with acrylic IOLs is unknown. The postoperative spike is easily managed if the cataract surgery is combined with trabeculectomy.

► This article attempts to demonstrate that patients who have acrylic lenses implanted at the time of combined cataract and glaucoma surgery have a greater incidence of elevated IOP at 1 month postoperatively and require more suture releases than patients with silicone lenses.

There are many possible reasons for these findings. I use acrylic lenses in a fair number of patients and have also used them for combined cataract and glaucoma surgery. My own personal experience has not mirrored that of this present article. Although the surgical techniques for both silicone and acrylic lenses used by the authors of this study were the same, I believe that may actually be the source of the differences noted by the authors.

The acrylic lens tends to be a much stiffer lens than the silicone lens once it is implanted. It is much easier for viscoelastic to be trapped behind the optic of the acrylic lens in the capsular bag than when using a silicone lens. If an aggressive attempt is not made to remove the viscoelastic from the capsular bag at the conclusion of cataract surgery in a patient with an acrylic lens, very often there will be a postoperative IOP spike related to the retained viscoelastic. In a patient with glaucoma or undergoing a glaucoma triple procedure, this could obviously be a confounding variable which the authors do not seem to have accounted for.

I chose this article because I think it may be used by both surgeons and lens manufacturers as a reason to recommend only silicone lenses in patients undergoing glaucoma triples.

R. Tipperman, M.D.

Management of Zonular Dialysis in Phacoemulsification and IOL Implantation Using the Capsular Tension Ring

Gimbel HV, Sun R, Heston JP (Univ of Calgary, Alta; Loma Linda Univ, Calif; Univ of California, San Francisco)

Ophthalmic Surg Lasers 28:273–281, 1997 1–11

Introduction.—Various types of rings have been developed to maintain the circular contour of the capsular bag after cataract removal in patients with extensive zonular dialysis. Fourteen cases in which loose or broken zonules were managed with polymethylmethacrylate capsular tension rings were selected for a retrospective review, with 5 cases presented in detail.

Patients and Methods.—All cataract surgeries were performed by a single surgeon using a standard phacoemulsification and posterior chamber intraocular lens (IOL) implantation technique. Patients were followed postoperatively for 2–11 months. Capsular tension rings were designed in 2 sizes: 12.5 mm compressible to 10.0 mm (Fig 1) and 14.5 mm compressible to 12.0 mm. The size of the capsule—estimated based on the size of the corneal white-to-white diameter—determined ring selection. Rings can be easily inserted into the capsular bag using Kelman-McPherson style forceps or lens positioning hooks. Large rings sometimes overlap on themselves, but this should not present any problem.

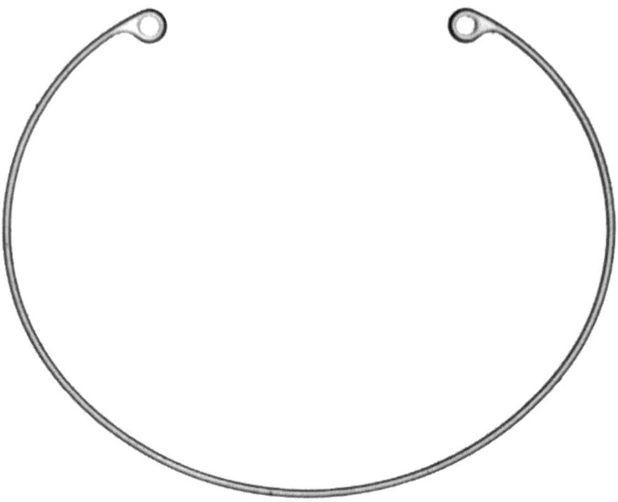

FIGURE 1.—Polymethylmethacrylate capsular tension ring type 14 (dimensions, 12.5 × 10.0 mm). (Courtesy of Gimbel HV, Sun R, Heston JP: Management of zonular dialysis in phacoemulsification and IOL implantation using the capsular tension ring. *Ophthalmic Surg Lasers* 28:273–281, 1997.)

Results.—The 14 patients had an average age of 66 years. One had 2+ loose zonules, 5 had 3+ loose zonules, 4 had a small zonular dialysis, and 4 had more extensive subluxation of the lens. Loose or broken zonules were discovered only at surgery in 8 cases (Table 2). The capsular tension rings were helpful in avoiding capsular collapse and vitreous presentation during surgery. By maintaining the circular contour of the capsular bag, capsular tension rings allow the IOL to be easily placed in the bag. The IOL had remained centered during short-term follow-up.

Discussion.—Use of a capsular tension ring in patients with zonular dialysis may have 5 potential benefits. The ring appears to enhance safety and efficacy during phacoemulsification and posterior chamber IOL implantation and may help to avoid vitreous herniation. By maintaining the circular contour of the capsular bag, IOL decentration may be reduced. Epithelial cell proliferation on the posterior capsule by compression may be inhibited, thus reducing the incidence of secondary cataract. When

TABLE 2.—Intraoperative Signs of Loose or Broken Zonules

1. Movement of lens during capsulorhexis.
2. Unusual movement of lens during hydrodissection, hydrodelineation, and nuclear rotation.
3. Unusual movement of lens during phacoemulsification or irrigation/aspiration.
4. Iris lifting or bulging from vitreous.
5. Vitreous herniation and around the lens and visible in the pupil.
6. Decentration of the crystalline lens.

(Courtesy of Gimbel HV, Sun R, Heston JP: Management of zonular dialysis in phacoemulsification and IOL implantation using the capsular tension ring. *Ophthalmic Surg Lasers* 28:273–281, 1997.)

loose or broken zonules are noted preoperatively, the ring should be placed in the capsular bag before phacoemulsification.

► Performing cataract surgery in patients with broken zonules is technically very challenging. The overall approach to the surgery is to try to avoid placing undue strain on the region of the zonular dialysis. Techniques that surgeons can use include low vacuum, low flow, reducing the infusion bottle height, and mechanical or "dry" stripping of cortex. Despite all these techniques, there can still be extension of the zonular dialysis, which can lead to vitreous prolapse and/or inadequate capsular support for in-the-bag posterior chamber IOL implantation.

In recent years, "capsular tension rings" have been used in Europe to treat these situations. Unfortunately, these have not been available in the United States. The "rumors" I have heard about these rings make it sound as if they would be extremely beneficial in managing patients with zonular dialysis. This article by Dr. Gimble, a world renowned and respected cataract surgeon, shows the great benefits that the capsular tension ring will have, once it is approved. In this article, several of the patients had zonular dialyses that were not recognized until the time of surgery. Nonetheless, once the ring was implanted, the patients were able to have phacoemulsification completed and a posterior chamber lens placed in the bag.

Several things I found interesting in this article that I had not realized before were that the capsular ring comes in several different sizes and that it can be placed quite early at the time of surgery, immediately after the capsulorhexis, before any lens material has been removed.

I certainly look forward to the availability of this device. I can think of several past cases in which I wish I had had it to use.

R. Tipperman, M.D.

Postoperative Contamination After Using Vancomycin and Gentamicin During Phacoemulsification

Ferro JF, de-Pablos M, Logroño MJ, et al (Hosp of Txagorritxu, Vitoria, Spain; Health District of Alava, Basque Country, Spain)
Arch Ophthalmol 115:165–170, 1997 1–12

Introduction.—Antibiotics are often added to the irrigating solution during cataract surgery in an attempt to prevent postoperative endophthalmitis, despite a lack of data on the efficacy and safety of this practice. A randomized clinical trial was designed to determine whether the addition of vancomycin and gentamicin to the irrigating solutions reduces the incidence of positive intraoperative cultures in patients who have undergone phacoemulsification with lens implantation.

Methods.—The 2-part trial was placebo-controlled and conducted in a double-blind manner. In a preliminary study, intracameral antibiotic concentrations were measured immediately after surgery in 10 eyes and 2 hours after surgery in an additional 10 eyes. The primary study was carried out after validity of the assay was confirmed. Participants in the primary study were 117 consecutive patients (120 eyes) with cataracts. In the treatment group (60 eyes), vancomycin (20 μg/mL) and gentamicin (8 μg/mL) were added to the irrigating fluid. The placebo group received only irrigating fluid. Patients in both groups underwent anterior chamber aspiration, with culturing performed 2 hours later.

Results.—Analyses performed for the preliminary study showed the half-life of both antibiotics to be less than 2 hours. The primary study yielded 120 samples adequate for analysis. Positive culture results were obtained in 7 patients (12.0%) in the placebo group and 3 patients (5.0%) in the treatment group. The total number of isolates was 10 in the placebo group and 5 in the antibiotic treatment group. *Staphylococcus* coagulase-negative organisms were the most commonly isolated, and all *Staphylococcus* species organisms were sensitive to gentamicin. During the 12-month follow-up period, postoperative endophthalmitis did not develop in any eyes.

Discussion.—In this group of patients who underwent phacoemulsification for cataracts, the addition of antibiotics to the irrigating solution did not significantly reduce the proportion of cultures positive for organisms. After 2 hours of contact between microorganisms and the antibiotic solution, not every susceptible bacteria was killed. Because the odds of a positive culture result were 2.51 times greater for the placebo group, a larger sample size could have demonstrated statistically significant results in favor of antibiotic prophylaxis.

► Almost every article which talks about endophthalmitis has a statement describing how "endophthalmitis is one of the most feared problems after intraocular surgery." Obviously, to any anterior segment surgeon, the "devastating" consequences of endophthalmitis are well known. Numerous studies have evaluated different preoperative, intraoperative, and postoperative regimens to determine whether any of them will be effective in reducing the incidence of endophthalmitis. These studies have had great difficulty in showing a statistically significant difference with treatment. Part of the difficulty is the (fortunately) low incidence of endophthalmitis.

Recently, several studies have documented the beneficial effect of instilling sterile povidone-iodine into the cul de sac prior to surgery. Many high volume anterior segment surgeons have also recommended using intraocular vancomycin and gentamicin in the infusion fluid to help decrease the incidence of endophthalmitis. Dr. James Gills published in one of the ophthalmology magazines reported performing over 25,000 cases using this regimen without a single incidence of endophthalmitis.

It is interesting that this article could not show a statistically significant result when comparing the incidence of positive postoperative cultures with a placebo treated group versus a group treated with gentamicin and vancomycin at the time of surgery. They did document, however, a 2.51 "odds ratio" increase in the risk of developing a positive postoperative culture in the placebo group.

Currently, I am using antibiotics (vancomycin only) in my infusion fluids because of my "belief" that it does decrease the incidence of postoperative endophthalmitis. I base this on the recent American Society of Cataract and Refractive Surgery review led by Samuel Masket, M.D. which demonstrated that the intraoperative use of antibiotics was the only parameter that surgeons could control that seem to decrease the risk of a patient developing endophthalmitis. Pre- and postoperative topical antibiotics did not have an effect in reducing the incidence of endophthalmitis.

The great fear of using antibiotics in the infusion fluid, especially gentamicin, is the risk of macular toxicity. As a result, surgeons should never utilize this technique in secondary lens implantation when the posterior capsule is open. In addition, if the posterior capsule is compromised at the time of surgery, then the surgeon should probably switch to an infusion fluid which does not contain antibiotics. Readers should carefully review the next article (Abstract 1–13).

R. Tipperman, M.D.

Gentamicin Retinal Toxicity After Cataract Surgery in an Eye That Underwent Vitrectomy

Rosenbaum JD, Krumholz DM, Metz DM (Mt Sinai School of Medicine, New York; State Univ of New York; Brookdale Hosp Med Ctr, Brooklyn, NY)
Ophthalmic Surg Lasers 28:236–238, 1997 1–13

Introduction.—To reduce the risk of postoperative infectious endophthalmitis, antibiotics such as gentamicin are often added to the infusion solution during cataract surgery. Retinal toxicity should not be a problem in normal eyes when gentamicin is used as an anterior chamber irrigant. In the case reported here, however, gentamicin-related macular toxicity developed after phacoemulsification with antibiotic-fortified infusion solution.

Case Report.—A man, 23, underwent cryopexy for retinal dialysis caused by blunt trauma. The treatment was successful, but 18 months later a retinal detachment that did not involve the macula developed in the same eye. Pars plana vitrectomy, endolaser treatment, and an air-fluid exchange yielded good results. Several months later, however, a dense cataract started to form and a large amount of inflammatory debris formed in the anterior chamber. Four months after vitrectomy the patient underwent phacoemulsification with placement of a posterior chamber intraocular lens. The irrigating solution used for the procedure contained gentamicin (0.008 mg/mL) and vancomycin (0.01 mg/mL). One month later, the first retinal examination revealed a large area of atrophic retinal pigment epithelium and retinal sclerosis with vaso-occlusive changes in the macula. Fluorescein angiography demonstrated an oval zone of complete retinal vascular obliteration, consistent with gentamicin toxicity of the retina. The patient's eye has remained stable, with 20/200 vision.

Discussion.—Because this patient's eye had undergone blunt trauma and a vitrectomy, gentamicin used in the irrigating solution for phacoemulsification appears to have seeped from the anterior chamber into the vitreous cavity. Gentamicin was thus able to settle over the macula during the procedure, resulting in macular toxicity. Antibiotic prophylaxis should be avoided in the infusion fluid of patients who have undergone vitrectomy.

▶ This case report describes an unfortunate patient who developed a macular infarct secondary to gentamicin toxicity which reduced the final visual acuity to the 20/200 level. This type of result needs to be kept in mind by any ophthalmologist who is considering the use of antibiotics in the infusion fluid. It obviously produces just as "devastating" a result as endophthalmitis.

Given this case report, avoidance of antibiotics in the infusion fluid would be prudent for any patient who has undergone a vitrectomy. It is probably worth sharing this case report and other case reports which document the "devastating" effects of gentamicin toxicity with whichever pharmacist is going to be responsible for mixing the antibiotic additives to the infusion fluid. The nursing staff, as well, who will be responsible for adding antibiotics to the infusion fluid should also understand the potential problems should there be a miscalculation in the dosing of gentamicin.

This is also one of the reasons why I only add vancomycin to my infusion—in hopes of avoiding the macular toxicity associated with gentamicin.

R. Tipperman, M.D.

Cataract Extraction as a Means of Treating Postfiltration Hypotony Maculopathy

Sibayan SAB, Igarashi S, Kasahara N, et al (Harvard Med School, Boston)
Ophthalmic Surg Lasers 28:241–243, 1997 1–14

Background.—The adjunctive use of antimetabolites in glaucoma filtration surgery has led to an increase in ocular hypotony, associated in some cases with maculopathy and significant visual loss. Patients with postfiltration hypotony maculopathy can be treated by measures to incite inflammation at the bleb site. Cataract extraction is one means of promoting such inflammation, which promotes scarring and retards aqueous flow. Cataract extraction in this setting can also lead to a postoperative increase in intraocular pressure (IOP). In the 2 cases reported here, pre-existing cataracts were extracted to deliberately increase IOP in patients with postfiltration hypotony maculopathy.

Case Reports.—A woman, 59 (case 1), and a man, 56 (case 2), were referred for management of glaucoma. Both had undergone argon laser trabeculoplasty and were receiving maximum tolerated medical therapy. Visual acuity was 20/20 in both patients; IOP was 17 mm Hg in case 1 and 21 mm Hg in case 2. Both patients underwent trabeculectomy and received either mitomycin-C or 5-fluorouracil. Visual acuity decreased to 20/60 after surgery (at 5 months in case 1 and at 10 months in case 2); IOP measured at the same time was 2 mm Hg in case 1 and 5 mm Hg in case 2. Both patients eventually underwent phacoemulsification with posterior chamber intraocular lens implantation. The operation was successful in improving IOP and visual acuity. The first patient had no evidence of maculopathy or metamorphopsia 30 months after phacoemulsification, and both conditions improved significantly in the second patient (examined 28 months after phacoemulsification). Filtration blebs were less diffuse in both cases.

Discussion.—Inducement of inflammation at the filtration area is recommended as a means of treating hypotony. Although scleral incisions can incite a greater degree of inflammation than clear-corneal incisions, the latter are preferred to prevent excessive scarring of the conjunctiva and filter failure. In patients with pre-existing cataracts and postfiltration hypotony maculopathy, cataract extraction can increase IOP and resolve the maculopathy. Inflammation can also be increased by decreasing the dose of steroids after surgery.

► I have had several patients referred to me whose case reports fit quite closely with the clinical history of patients in this article. They have typically had aggressive glaucoma filtering surgery with mitomycin-C and ended up with diffuse blebs and extremely low pressures. In my experience, extremely mature cataracts developed in these patients. Although cataract surgery is no different for these patients than for a "routine cataract patient," 1 problem I have noticed regarding these patients, which the authors do not report, is difficulty in obtaining an accurate axial length measurement. Because of the profound hypotony, there is often a small degree of globe collapse, which makes it difficult to obtain an accurate axial length measurement.

Interestingly, once hypotonus eyes obtain "normalized" IOP, their axial lengths do not necessarily return to "normal." The operating surgeon is, therefore, left with difficulty in choosing the correct implant. If the axial lengths of both eyes are measured, the measurement in the nonhypotonus eye is often found to be significantly larger. In general, I have compared implant power calculations for both the hypotonus and nonhypotonus eye and tended to pick and implant closer to that which would be determined by the hypotonus eye. I do, however, have a lengthy discussion with these patients regarding the difficulty in implant power calculations so that they will understand should an implant error occur.

As noted earlier, the surgery itself is no different from routine surgery. However, I tend to taper and discontinue steroids much more quickly in hopes of increasing postoperative inflammation so that the IOP in these eyes will rise. I have found, as the authors have, that cataract surgery tends to work quite well in treating the postfiltration hypotony.

R. Tipperman, M.D.

A Comparison of Retrobulbar Versus Sub-Tenon's Corticosteroid Therapy for Cystoid Macular Edema Refractory to Topical Medications

Thach AB, Dugel PU, Flindall RJ, et al (Walter Reed Army Med Ctr, Washington, DC; Retinal Consultants of Arizona, Phoenix)
Ophthalmology 104:2003–2008, 1997 1–15

Introduction.—Cystoid macular edema (CME) continues to be a potential complication after extracapsular cataract extraction. A number of treatments have been used for clinically significant CME with visual loss, including oral, topical, and periocular steroids. Two approaches to the treatment of CME refractory to topical medications were retrospectively compared: retrobulbar and posterior sub-Tenon's injection of corticosteroids.

Methods.—A total of 48 patients (49 eyes) who had decreased visual acuity with clinical and fluorescein angiographic evidence of CME at least 4 weeks after cataract surgery were studied. The patients showed no improvement with topical corticosteroids or nonsteroidal anti-inflammatory agents. Eighteen eyes were treated with a single retrobulbar injection of triamcinolone acetonamide, 40 mg in 1 mL. Thirty-one eyes were treated with 3 biweekly posterior sub-Tenon's injections of triamcinolone in the same concentration. The patients were followed up monthly for best-corrected visual acuity, intraocular pressure, and clinical evidence of CME. The study definition of treatment success was clinical improvement of CME with improved visual acuity.

Results.—The 2 groups had similar demographic characteristics, and neither had complications of corticosteroid injection. Median time since surgery was 3 months in the retrobulbar group and 4 months in the sub-Tenon's group. Median follow-up was 10 and 12 months, respectively. Before treatment, average visual acuity was 20/97 in the retrobulbar group and 20/92 in the sub-Tenon's group. Vision improved to 20/58 in the retrobulbar group and 20/50 in the sub-Tenon's group. There was no significant difference in either best or final visual acuity, although vision improved significantly within both groups. In neither group was intraocular pressure significantly higher after treatment than before. The success rate of corticosteroid injection was 89% in the retrobulbar group and 94% in the sub-Tenon's group.

Conclusions.—In patients with postoperative CME causing loss of visual acuity, both retrobulbar and posterior sub-Tenon's corticosteroid injections are effective treatments. No adverse effects are noted with either technique; both provide a high rate of clinical and visual improvement. To clarify the roles of corticosteroids, topical medications, and systemic anti-inflammatory drugs in CME, a multicenter, randomized, controlled trial is needed.

► Cystoid macular edema remains a vexing problem for most cataract surgeons. Although its incidence in routine cases, and even in complicated cases, is low, because of the sheer magnitude of numbers of patients undergoing cataract surgery, CME remains an important clinical problem.

Most ophthalmologists have their own "regimen" for patients with CME. This typically begins with topical anti-inflammatories and/or nonsteroidal anti-inflammatories. However, if a patient does not improve, at some point periocular injection of steroid is considered.

I was pleased to see in this article how successful the injections were in improving patients' overall vision. Obviously, patients do not find these injections the most pleasant of experiences. Because there seems to be no clinically different significance between a single retrobulbar injection or 3 biweekly posterior sub-Tenon's injections, it makes sense to probably treat patients with a single retrobulbar injection. Parenthetically, I would state that I do know several patients who did not improve with a single retrobulbar injection but did improve with multiple injections.

Hopefully, an effective topical agent for CME will be developed. Until that time, however, depo-steroid injections will remain a valuable treatment for CME.

R. Tipperman, M.D.

Posterior Capsule Opacification After Cataract Surgery in Patients With Uveitis

Dana MR, Chatzistefanou K, Schaumberg DA, et al (Massachusetts Eye and Ear Infirmary, Boston; Harvard Med School, Boston; Univ of Athens, Greece; et al)

Ophthalmology 104:1387–1394, 1997 1–16

Background.—Posterior capsule opacification (PCO) is the most common long-term cause of reduced visual acuity after modern cataract surgery. Younger patients are at higher risk for PCO, possibly because of the more vigorous postoperative inflammatory reponse in these patients. Patients with uveitis may be at increased risk of PCO after cataract surgery. The incidence of PCO in uveitic eyes undergoing phacoemulsification and standard extracapsular cataract extraction (P/ECCE) was compared to the incidence in a group of eyes without uveitis.

Study Design.—A chart review was performed on P/ECCE records from 1982 to 1995 from the Immunology and Uveitis Service of the Massachusetts Eye and Ear Infirmary. The presence, type, and duration of uveitis, the treatment regimen and the type and grade of cataracts were obtained from these charts. Intraocular inflammation was controlled by regional corticosteroids injections and topical corticosteroids. If disease recurred, oral nonsteroidal anti-inflammatory drugs (NSAIDs) were added. If disease persisted, oral corticosteroids were added to the regimen. Peripheral cryopexy was performed for recurrent pars planitis. Systemic immunosuppressive therapy was instituted if inflammation could not be controlled by previous methods. A standard preoperative regimen of topical mydriatic, cycloplegic, and NSAID was instituted for all patients before surgery. A 1-piece polymethylmethacrylate posterior chamber intraocular lens was implanted into the capsular bag whenever possible. A pars plana vitrectomy was performed if inflammatory debris was present. The primary end point of this study was the requirement for a neodymium:yttrium-aluminum-garnet posterior capsulotomy. Indications for this procedure included microscopic evidence of PCO and subjective visual complaint.

Findings.—The study group consisted of 108 eyes of 78 patients with uveitis and 122 eyes of 106 patients without uveitis treated by P/ECCE. The patients with uveitis were significantly younger than the patients without uveitis. Crude PCO incidence rates were 54% over an average of a 4.3-year follow-up for patients with uveitis and 40% over an average 3.9 years for patients without uveitis. The rates of PCO differed significantly between patients with and without uveitis. However, after adjustment for the significantly younger age of patients with uveitis, this statistically significant difference disappeared.

Conclusions.—This study of a large group of patients undergoing cataract surgery demonstrates that the apparently higher incidence of PCO detected among patients with uveitis after cataract surgery is predominantly attributable to the younger age of these patients at the time of surgery.

► I found the results of this article quite interesting. I typically have always felt, as I believe the authors of this study did, that patients with uveitis were more prone to have PCO after cataract surgery. The results of this excellent article really show this to be a "myth." It appears that when appropriate statistical evaluation is done, the increased incidence of PCO is really not related to the patient's uveitis but actually to the young age and cataract formation in patients with uveitis.

When I counsel young patients regarding cataract surgery, I discuss with them the increased incidence of PCO and the need for a neodymium:YAG capsulotomy following cataract surgery, given their young age. In patients with uveitis, I discuss this as well, although I typically tell the patients that the increased incidence of PCO is probably related to their uveitis. This article will therefore change the way I counsel patients and discuss with them the etiology of PCO.

It should be noted that in patients with severe ocular inflammatory conditions such as cytomegalovirus who are treated with silicone oil, PCO will develop very rapidly regardless of their age.

R. Tipperman, M.D.

Pseudophakic Retinal Detachment in High Axial Myopia

Jacobi FK, Hessemer V (Univ of Giessen, Germany)

J Cataract Refract Surg 23:1095–1102, 1997 1–17

Background.—Patients with axial myopia who undergo extracapsular cataract surgery (ECCS) are at risk of retinal detachment. Intraocular lens (IOL) implantation during ECCS, however, provides structural support, and may cause fewer cases of retinal detachment. These authors evaluated the incidence of retinal detachment in eyes with high axial myopia that were operated on with ECCS and IOL implantation.

Methods.—A total of 253 surgical procedures were evaluated in 190 patients with high axial myopia. Mean patient age was 66 ± 11.8 years, and each had a minimum axial length of 27.0 mm. All patients completed a questionnaire regarding whether they had experienced retinal detachment or had undergone laser treatment for opacification of the posterior capsule. Follow-up ranged from 7 months to 8 years 7 months (mean 3.8 ± 2 years).

Findings.—The mean axial length was 29.2 mm (range 27.01 to 37.50 mm), and mean postoperative refraction was −3.54 ± 2 D (range −0.32 to −13.30 D). Neodymium:yttrium-aluminum-garnet (Nd:YAG) laser capsulotomy was performed in 74 of 253 procedures (29.2%). Over the follow-up period, pseudophakic retinal detachment occurred in only 2 of 353 procedures (0.8%). In 1 case retinal detachment occurred 3 years 7 months after Nd:YAG laser capsulotomy, and in the second case retinal detachment occurred in the superior retina 8 days after surgery, along with a superonasal quadrant tear and temporal peripheral degeneration. A third patient had retinal detachment 3 years after IOL explantation because of lens subluxation. One patient experienced expulsive choroidal hemorrhage during IOL implantation in the anterior chamber. In 4 cases (1.6%), vitrectomy was required because of posterior capsule rupture. Patients in whom retinal detachment developed were younger (mean age 46.5 ± 13.2 years) and more often underwent Nd:YAG laser posterior capsulotomy.

Conclusions.—In these patients with high axial myopia, ECCS was associated with little risk of retinal detachment. Retinal detachment was more common in patients with complications such as IOL explantation and vitreous loss. Also, younger patients were more likely to have retinal detachment, as were those undergoing Nd:YAG laser capsulotomy. Thus, if special diligence is used during the surgical procedure to ensure that no complications develop, ECCS with IOL implantation is a safe procedure for these high-risk patients.

► Patients with high axial myopia often are counseled against having cataract surgery or are at least told of the extremely high risks of surgery because of their axial myopia. The results of this study show that if surgery is uncomplicated, the risk of retinal detachment in high axial myopia is probably no greater than that for any other patient.

Because patients with high axial myopia tend to have cataracts at a much earlier age and tend to be significantly compromised by the cataracts, these are often some of the patients who can be helped the most by cataract/lens implant surgery. In addition, the ability to correct their refractive error with appropriate intraocular lens power selection offers a great potential of visual rehabilitation in these patients. Obviously, for any individual patient, the potential risks and benefits of the surgery need to be reviewed and discussed. However, on the basis of the results of this study, if the surgery is uncomplicated, patients probably are not a higher risk for retinal detachment because of their high axial myopia.

R. Tipperman, M.D.

Corneal Autograft Patches for Covering Exposed Transscleral Sutures

Lifshitz T, Wender A, Lapid-Gortzak R (Ben Gurion Univ of the Negev, Beer Sheva, Israel)

Ophthalmic Surg Lasers 28:426–427, 1997 1–18

Background.—The protrusion of suture ends is a problem in transscleral suturing of a posterior chamber intraocular lens. The most common methods for preventing this problem are scleral flaps, buried sutures, and conjunctival flaps. These methods have their own shortcomings. Scleral flaps provide less suture support, weaken the sclera, and are complicated by suture erosion. Buried sutures require double passage with the needle, which increases the risk of infection. Conjunctival flaps are not always thick enough to prevent the suture ends from protruding. In addition, all these methods leave an open tract into the eye, which increases the risk of endophthalmitis. The authors prefer the use of corneal autograft patches for covering exposed suture ends.

> *Technique.*—The use of autograft patches includes a combined perforating keratoplasty and transscleral fixation of a posterior chamber intraocular lens. Two freehand, partial-thickness buttons prepared from the excised recipient cornea are sutured with 10-0 nylon over the exposed suture ends.

Results.—Corneal autograft patches were used in 4 patients. The follow-up period was 14–27 months. The sutures were well-covered by the patches. After the recipient patches cleared, visualization of the covered sutures was possible. There was no local reaction to suture exposure, infection, erosion, dellen, graft migration, or thinning. There were no complications related to the corneal autograft patches.

Discussion.—Corneal autograft patches were used successfullly in these 4 patients undergoing a combined penetrating keratoplasty and transscleral fixation of a posterior chamber intraocular lens. None of the common complications occurred. This technique is not commonly used, but is a safe easy method of covering exposed suture ends. It is recommended by the authors to solve the problem of protruding suture ends during transscleral suturing of a posterior chamber intraocular lens.

► I included this article for review because I think it is a nice technique and not one you hear about that often for transscleral sutures. Many times, sutured posterior chamber lenses are used at the time of penetrating keratoplasty. I think it is clever to use the patient's own corneal tissue as a protective cover for the exposed sutures.

Normally when placing transscleral sutures for posterior chamber lens fixation, I try to rotate the suture into the globe so the knot is buried and all that is exposed is the suture itself. However, I have had to treat patients with exposed sutures. Sometimes, the suture can be carefully trimmed. Other times, the suture tails can be shrunk with light cautery. However, there are times when a "patch graft" is the best approach.

R. Tipperman, M.D.

Effect of Cataract on Corneal Topography Results
Singh D (Joshi Colony, Amritsar, India)
J Cataract Refract Surg 22:1506–1508, 1996 1–19

Introduction.—The case presented here demonstrates that certain ocular conditions can cause K-readings taken with a videokeratoscope to be inaccurate. Discrepancies between K-readings taken with a keratometer and those taken with a TMS-1 videokeratoscope were attributed to the presence of an advanced cataract and a dilated pupil.

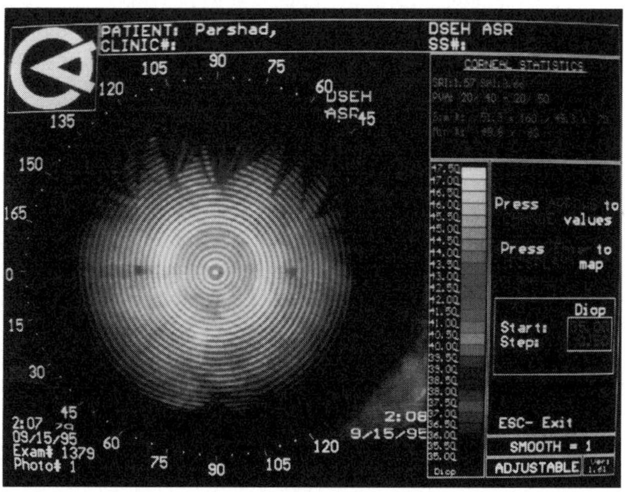

FIGURE 1.—Videokeratoscopy of the eye with advanced cataract and a widely dilated pupil shows that the reflection from the cataract mixes with the reflection from the cornea. The corneal reflection rings beyond the pupil edge are difficult to see. (Courtesy of Singh D: Effect of cataract on corneal topography results. *J Cataract Refract Surg* 22:1506–1508, 1996.)

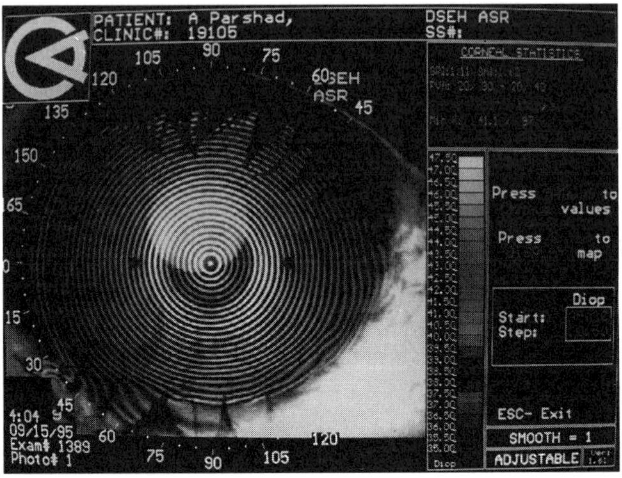

FIGURE 2.—Videokeratoscopy after the dilated pupil has been contracted shows a bright, round area above the center caused by a reflection from the cataract. All rings up to the periphery of the cornea are fairly well defined. (Courtesy of Singh D: Effect of cataract on corneal topography results. *J Cataract Refract Surg* 22:1506–1508, 1996.)

Case Report.—Man, 65, had advanced cataract. Routine keratometry performed with a manual Appaswamy keratoscope and a Humphrey autokeratometer yielded a difference of 0.60 D between the 2 readings. Very high K-readings were obtained with TMS-1 videokeratoscopy. Repeated keratometry and videokeratoscopy readings showed a large discrepancy (42.50 and 54.00 D, respectively). Videokeratoscopy images differed considerably for a dilated pupil (Fig 1) compared with a contracted pupil (Fig 2). With contraction, the videokeratoscopy readings were close to those obtained by keratometry. Corneal topography maps of the same eye under dilation and contraction showed many differences. Topography readings were high in the pupillary area when the pupil was dilated, whereas contraction yielded low topography readings except in the central area.

Discussion.—The findings in this patient with advanced cataract suggest that keratometry may be more accurate than computerized videokeratoscopy for routine cataract surgery, especially in eyes with a dilated pupil.

▶ Although this is just a case report, I thought it was worth including because the use of corneal topography is becoming "routine" even in standard cataract surgery. Obviously, corneal topography has played an important role in refractive surgery in the last several years.

As anterior segment surgeons begin to increasingly view cataract surgery as a "refractive" procedure, it is only natural that corneal topography would be used in evaluating patients preoperatively. If the surgeon was unfortunate enough to have missed this case report, he might not realize the significant effect that a moderate cortical or mature cataract could have on keratometer readings obtained on an automated corneal topography. This underscores the need for still performing manual keratometry readings in these patients.

R. Tipperman, M.D.

2 Refractive Surgery

Managing Corneal Haze After Excimer Laser PRK

by Christopher J. Rapuano, M.D.

Excimer laser photorefractive keratectomy (PRK) has become a common treatment for low to moderate degrees of myopia, both in the United States and around the world. While other techniques, such as laser in situ keratomileusis (LASIK), are gaining in popularity, they are often more technically difficult and consequently are performed primarily by high volume refractive surgeons. One of the main risks of PRK is postoperative corneal haze/scar. The terminology of *haze* and *scar* is ambiguous. Generally, mild corneal opacity, which does not affect best corrected Snellen visual acuity, is termed *haze*. Corneal opacity which decreases best corrected visual acuity is usually called *scar*. One of the main challenges of the PRK surgeon is managing PRK haze/scar.

The first question to address is the etiology of corneal haze after PRK. Numerous animal and human studies have been performed on corneas after PRK. In general there is cellular infiltration, fibroblast proliferation and new connective tissue/collagen formation. These changes typically result in a decrease in corneal clarity during the initial healing phase after PRK. Occasionally this nontransparency of the cornea is clinically significant.

The second issue is the quantification of corneal haze after PRK. The most common method to quantify haze is clinical slit lamp appearance. A common grading system is listed in Table 1. Numerous other methods have been used in attempt to classify haze in a more objective manner. Computerized analysis of standardized slit lamp photographs[1] and Scheimpflug anterior segment photography[2] can both produce more objective analyses of haze, but require additional equipment and a well-trained technician for effective use. A scatterometer, used to measure back scatter of light, may be a more physiologic method to evaluate patients' visual symptoms from corneal opacities, but is not widely available.[3] Recently, confocal microscopy has been used to objectively quantify abnormalities in the cornea at the cellular level after PRK.[4] Confocal microscopy technology is steadily improving and may become the standard of care in evaluation of PRK haze. As an added benefit, confocal microscopy may be

TABLE 1.—Clinical Grading of Post-PRK Corneal Haze

0 haze	clear, no haze
0.5+ haze	barely detectable
1+ haze	mild, not affecting refraction
1.5+ haze	mildly affecting refraction
2+ haze	moderate haze, refraction possible but difficult, best corrected vision decreased
3+ haze	opacity prevents refraction, anterior chamber easily visualized
4+ haze	view of anterior chamber difficult
5+ haze	unable to view anterior chamber

useful for early diagnosis of certain corneal ulcers, such as from fungus or acanthamoeba.

As PRK haze is determined by the individual's healing process, the clinical course varies from patient to patient. Typically, mild corneal haze is noted in almost all (if not all) patients between 2 and 6 weeks after PRK. The haze peaks by 2–4 months (occasionally 6 months) and then dissipates between 4 and 12 months, with continued disappearance over years. In rare cases, the onset of haze can occur after 6 months and even more rarely after several years.[5, 6] Therefore, it is extremely important to tell all PRK patients to seek follow-up care if they notice decreased vision even years after PRK. The actual incidence of PRK haze is difficult to determine because there are so many variables, such as method of determining haze, severity of haze, time after PRK, type of excimer laser, and amount of myopia treated. In general, visually significant haze at 1 year is thought to be in the 1% to 2% range for low myopia (−1 to −4 D), 2% to 5% for moderate myopia (−4 to −7 D) and even greater for higher myopia.

Clinical management of PRK haze is divided into prevention, medical therapy, and surgical treatments. The PRK procedure involves creating a large epithelial defect, typically about 6-mm in diameter. Prolonged healing of the epithelial defect is known to predispose the patient to increased corneal haze, at least in the short-term, and probably in the long-term, too. Anything that promotes more rapid resolution of the epithelial defect would tend to decrease PRK haze.

Mechanical scraping ideally creates a circular epithelial defect 6-mm in diameter, but in reality a larger epithelial defect often occurs. A laser-scrape epithelial removal technique creates a perfectly circular 6-mm diameter epithelial defect by using the phototherapeutic mode of the laser to remove approximately 40 microns of epithelium. The remaining 10 microns or so of epithelium is removed by mechanical scraping. Another technique to limit the epithelial removal to a 6-mm diameter circle was recently studied by Abad et al.[7] They placed 20% alcohol in a 6-mm optical zone marker on the cornea to soften the epithelium. After 20 seconds the alcohol was removed from the optical zone marker and a 6-mm diameter circular epithelium defect was easily created by gentle epithelial scraping. Epithelial scrubbers, such as the Amoils and Pallikaris brand brushes, have been used to mechanically remove a precise 6-mm circle of epithelium.[8] Potential disadvantages of these single-use instruments include their cost and potential damage to the stromal surface from the rough brush surface.

Post-operatively, many surgeons use a bandage soft contact lens to aid in reepithelialization. While certainly helpful to reduce painful symptoms in most patients, a tight contact lens can actually impede epithelialization and can sometimes cause significant corneal edema and a tight lens syndrome.

An often overlooked therapy which can improve reepithelialization is lubrication. Preservative-free tear supplements, with or without the use of a bandage contact lens, can greatly improve both patient comfort and epithelial healing. Punctal occlusion, either with removable silicone plugs or even temporary collagen plugs, can be used to maintain a moist surface after PRK. In addition, surgeons need to keep in mind that postoperative medications can be epithelial-toxic, and should be kept to a minimum. There is anecdotal evidence that ultraviolet light exposure in the early postoperative period may be associated with increased risk of haze. It is probably best for patients to minimize such exposure for several months after PRK.

Topical corticosteroid use after PRK is rather controversial. Even so, many PRK surgeons employ steroids for several months postoperatively in attempts to prevent corneal haze and refractive regression. In the United States most clinicians are using a tapering dose of fluorometholone for a period of time after PRK. The duration of steroid use ranges from several weeks (especially in lower myopes) to several months.

Despite the physician's best attempts to prevent corneal haze, it does occur in certain patients. The next step is to determine whether the haze should be treated. In general, haze associated with decreased best spectacle corrected visual acuity should be treated. Specifically, if the haze is mild, not affecting vision, and the refraction is satisfactory, no treatment is required at this time. However, the haze, vision, and refraction should be followed closely. If the haze is moderate and affecting vision and the refraction is more *myopic* than intended, then increase the topical steroids. If the haze is moderate and affecting vision, but the refraction is more *hyperopic* than intended, then be very cautious about increasing the topical steroid regimen because permanent overcorrection can result.

When topical steroids are increased, the frequency or the potency can be increased depending on the severity of the haze and myopia. Treatment can range from a mild increase in fluorometholone frequency to changing to prednisolone acetate four times or more a day. When steroids are increased, frequent follow-up is required to determine the response and monitor for side effects, such as elevated intraocular pressure. If there is no perceptible response in 2–4 weeks of prednisolone acetate at least 4 times a day, then a response is unlikely to occur with steroids—they should be promptly tapered. If there is a positive response to the increased steroid regimen, then they need to be tapered rather slowly depending on the haze and refraction. Needless prolonged steroids can have serious ocular side effects.

When clinically significant corneal haze persists despite medical intervention, then surgical treatment may be required. The surgeon should wait *at least* 6 months before contemplating surgical treatment of haze. Ideally, the wait should be even longer because haze tends to improve with time, although it can take many months. Additionally, the refraction needs to be stable for several months on low-dose or no steroids before retreatment.

A repeat PRK can be performed for treatment of myopia and haze. When significant haze is present, the surgeon needs to be very cautious about believing the manifest refraction because there is a tendency for the patient to be overminused. An objective measurement of corneal curvature (such as keratometry readings) comparing pre- and postoperative measurements should be obtained to validate the refraction.

If just haze (and no undercorrection) is being treated, a mechanical scraping of the epithelium can be attempted, but the results are quite variable. A phototherapeutic keratectomy, that is, a *plano cut* can be performed, but overcorrection can result. The best technique is to use as large an ablation zone as possible and to ablate as little tissue as necessary to remove the bulk of the haze. These two steps will minimize induced hyperopia. One hundred per cent of the haze does not need to be removed, especially if it requires an excessively deep ablation; the deeper the ablation, the greater the risk of corneal flattening.

In retreatments, whether for residual myopia, corneal haze, or both, the epithelium tends to be rather adherent to the stroma, and mechanical débridement is much more difficult than in primary treatments. The laser-scrape technique (described earlier) may be used, but the basal epithelial cells can still be quite tenacious. Many surgeons prefer a transepithelial approach to retreatments. In this case a phototherapeutic, plano ablation is set for the entire depth of the epithelium, approximately 50 microns, and then the refractive ablation proceeds immediately afterward. There is no mechanical removal of epithelium at all. Since a small amount of central epithelium tends to remain once the peripheral epithelium is completely ablated, an additional 0.50–0.75 D "fudge factor" is added to the refractive ablation. An aggressive topical steroid regimen should be used following all retreatments to minimize the risk of haze and refractive regression. The surgeon and patient need to be aware that retreated eyes are at higher risk or overcorrection when compared to primary treatments.

While PRK has been used around the world in hundreds of thousands of patients for many years, and is a mature procedure when compared to such newcomers as LASIK, it is still undergoing improvements in hardware, software, procedure techniques, and postoperative regimens. Some of the most promising developments will likely occur in the arena of adjunctive medical therapy. Gillies et al[9] used topical interferon α 2b in humans and found slightly prolonged epithelial healing, but they noted decreased haze and a trend to improve best spectacle corrected visual acuity after PRK for greater than 5 D of myopia. My colleagues and I at Wills Eye Hospital[10, 11] topical anti-TGF β 1,2,3 in rabbits and found decreased post-PRK haze when compared to placebo. While these postoperative medical therapies are not yet ready for wide clinical use, they highlight the fact that advances in PRK are still proceeding.

PRK is not a perfect procedure, but the perfect refractive surgery has not yet been developed. LASIK, the intrastromal ring and phakic intraocular lenses, some the newest refractive surgery procedures with the brightest futures, have both advantages and disadvantages when compared to PRK. As we do a better job in preventing and managing PRK haze, these newer procedures will have a higher standard of care to meet in the future.

References

1. Maldonado MJ, Arnau V, Naves A, et al: Direct objective quantification of corneal haze after excimer laser photorefractive keratectomy form high myopia. *Ophthalmology* 103:1970–1978, 1996.
2. Binder PS, Bosem M, Weinreb RN: Scheimpflug anterior segment photography assessment of wound healing after myopic excimer laser photorefractive keratectomy. *J Cataract Refract Surg* 22:205–212, 1996.
3. Braunstein RE, Jain S, McCally RL, et al: Objective measurement of corneal light scattering after excimer laser keratectomy. *Ophthalmology* 103:439–443, 1996.
4. Moller-Petersen T, Vogel M, Li HF, et al: Quantification of stromal thinning, epithelial thickness, and corneal haze after photorefractive keratectomy using in vivo confocal microscopy. *Ophthalmology* 104:360–368, 1997.
5. Meyer JC, Stulting RD, Thompson KP, et al: Late onset of corneal scar after excimer laser photorefractive keratectomy. *Am J Ophthalmol* 121:529–539, 1996.
6. Lipshitz I, Lowenstein A, Varssano D, et al: Late onset corneal haze after photorefractive keratectomy for moderate and high myopia. *Ophthalmology* 104:369–374, 1997.
7. Abad J-C, An B, Power WJ, et al: A prospective evaluation of alcohol-assisted versus mechanical epithelial removal before photorefractive keratectomy. *Ophthalmology* 104:1566–1575, 1997.
8. Pallikaris IG, Karoutis AD, Lydataki SE, et al: Rotating brush for fast removal of corneal epithelium. *J Refract Corneal Surg* 10:439–442, 1994.
9. Gillies MC, Garrett SK, Shina SM, et al: Topical interferon alpha 2b for corneal haze after excimer laser photorefractive keratectomy: The Melbourne Excimer Laser Group. *J Cataract Refract Surg* 22:891–900, 1996.
10. Myers JS, Gomes JAP, Siepser SB, et al: Effect of transforming growth factor beta 1 on stromal haze following excimer laser photorefractive keratectomy in rabbits. *J Refract Surg* 13:356–361, 1997.
11. Thom SB, Myers JS, Rapuano CJ, et al: Effect of topical anti-transforming growth factor-beta on corneal stromal haze after photorefractive keratectomy in rabbits. *J Cataract Refract Surg* 23:1324–1330, 1997.

Refractive Outcome of Radial Keratotomy: Does the Result of the First Eye Predict Outcome in the Second Eye?

Batra VN, Maloney RK (Univ of California, Los Angeles)

Am J Ophthalmol 123:165–173, 1997 2–1

Background.—Currently available nomograms predict the mean outcome of refractive surgical procedures. However, they provide no information on variability of outcomes. Although nomograms for radial keratotomy can provide a mean predicted refractive change, the results obtained for an individual eye may vary substantially from that prediction (Fig 1). Most patients undergoing refractive surgery are operated on first in 1 eye and then later, in the other. It has been suggested that the results

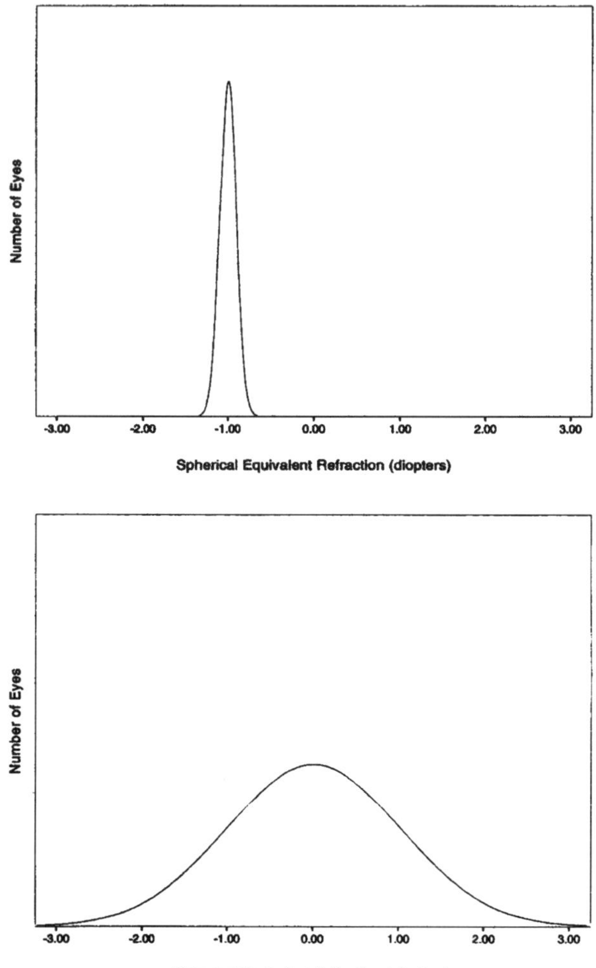

FIGURE 1.—Distribution of postoperative refraction for 2 hypothetical surgical procedures. **Left**, results of a hypothetical procedure with a mean postoperative refraction of −1.0 diopter and an SD of 0.1 D. Fifty percent of treated eyes are within 1 D of emmetropia. **Right**, results of a hypothetical procedure with a mean postoperative refraction of emmetropia and an SD of 1.0 D. Sixty-six percent of treated eyes are within 1.0 D of emmetropia. Despite the greater percentage of eyes within 1.0 D of emmetropia in the procedure at right, the procedure shown at left is clearly superior because it has less variability. The percentage of eyes within 1 D of emmetropia is a poor measure of variability for refractive surgical procedures. (Courtesy of Batra VN, Maloney RK: Refractive outcome of radial keratotomy: Does the result of the first eye predict outcome in the second eye? *Am J Ophthalmol* 123:165–173, 1997.)

from the first eye may be useful in refining surgery on the second eye. This study examined the ability of the results of radial keratotomy in the first eye to predict the results in the second eye.

Methods.—The retrospective study included 129 eyes of 81 patients undergoing 8–incision radial keratotomy. Each operation was done using a Russian or centripetal incision technique, planned by a modified Case-beer nomogram. The results were analyzed by regression analysis and used to create a nomogram that assessed variability in the outcome of the first eye. The findings were included in a statistical technique for incorporating the results in the first eye into surgical planning for the second eye. Bilateral surgery was performed and adequate follow-up was obtained in 39 patients.

Results.—After operation on the first eye, the distribution of the residuals was normal, with no correlation between the residual and attempted corrections. In the patients who had bilateral surgery, the variability of the second eye was 0.79, according to the standard deviation of the residuals. Including the residual from the first eye into the regression prediction did not significantly improve the ability to predict the refractive change in the second eye.

Conclusion.—The findings suggest that the difference between the expected and achieved refractive correction is a superior measure of variability in the results of radial keratotomy. The refractive results in the first eye operated on do not appear to predict the results in the second eye. Thus, refractive accuracy in the second eye is not reduced by performing radial keratotomy on both eyes at the same operation.

► To answer the question posed in the title of this paper, the authors use a statistical concept not generally used in ophthalmology, namely, that variability of outcome is best measured by using the standard deviation of the difference between expected and actual results. For example, if every patient after radial keratotomy is 1.5 D undercorrected, the variability of the surgery would be minimal (excellent), but the nomogram would need to be modified by 1.5 diopters. Standard evaluation of outcomes, such as mean deviation from intended and percentage within 1D of intended would be rather poor in this case.

On the other hand, if there were a normal distribution of outcomes, centering around plano but with many patients undercorrected by 1.5 D and overcorrected by 1.5 D, the mean deviation from intended and the percentage within 1.0 D would be fairly good, but the variability of actual results would be large (poor). (See Fig 1.) Although this statistical model seems like an excellent idea, the paper was otherwise quite confusing.

Using this concept, the authors examined the radial keratotomy results of the first eye vs. the second eye and found no improvement in the second eye results when using data from the first eye. They also found that radial keratotomy for low myopia was no less variable than for moderate myopia. The authors conclude that first eye results should not be used when planning second eye surgery; however, they also acknowledge that surgeons should use their own judgement. For example, if a first eye is grossly overcorrected, it would be prudent to adjust the technique accordingly for the fellow eye.

C.J. Rapuano, M.D.

Clear Lensectomy and Implantation of a Low-Power Posterior Chamber Intraocular Lens for Correction of High Myopia: A Four-Year Follow-up

Colin J, Robinet A (Centre Hospitalier Universitaire de Brest, France)
Ophthalmology 104:73–78, 1997 2–2

Introduction.—Five years ago, a prospective study was conducted of retinal prophylaxis, clear lensectomy, and posterior chamber lens implantation. The 1-year results have been reported previously. The 4-year results are now presented.

Methods.—This study included 52 eyes in 30 patients with preoperative myopia greater than 12 D. Argon laser photocoagulation was performed before clear lens extraction in patients with lattice degeneration, retinal tear, or hole.

Results.—A 4-year evaluation was done in 28 patients and 49 eyes; 2 patients were lost to follow-up. A 30-year-old woman patient had retinal detachment 18 months postoperatively. Neodymium: yttrium-aluminum-garnet (Nd:YAG) capsulotomy for posterior capsular opacification was performed in 18 eyes during the 4-year follow-up period. Refractive changes of greater than 1.0 D did not occur in any patient. Postoperative acuity was better in patients who had Nd:YAG capsulotomy.

Discussion.—The risk of visual loss after intraocular surgery is greater than the risk after refractive corneal surgery, which can be significant. The current series used modern cataract surgical techniques for clear lensectomy and prophylactic retinal treatment. These 4-year results confirm the accurate refractive results seen at 1 year and confirm stability of refraction at 4 years. With this surgical procedure, there is concern for inevitable vitreous-retinal degeneration and later retinal detachment. At 4 years, the rate of retinal detachment was 1.9%. In an earlier report by Barraquer, this rate was 3.7% at 2 years and 5.4% at 4 years.

► In this forum 3 years ago, I commented on the authors 1-year follow-up of clear lensectomy and posterior chamber intraocular lens implants for high myopia and stated that longer term follow-up was needed. Here the authors have provided excellent follow-up of 49 of the original 52 eyes at 4 years.

Only 1 eye (1.9%) had a retinal detachment. It occurred 18 months postoperatively, requiring 3 vitreoretinal surgeries and ended up with 20/200 best-corrected vision secondary to macular edema. Carmen Barraquer previously reported a 5.4% incidence of retinal detachment at 4 years. With prophylactic retinal treatment and newer cataract surgery techniques, the 1.9% incidence may be closer to current reality. Whatever the real number, the question remains for the surgeon and patient, does the risk (generally to both eyes) outweigh the benefits? Although 4-year data are excellent, even longer term numbers are important to obtain for an operation on relatively young patients (mean age in this study was 36 years).

C.J. Rapuano, M.D.

The Intrastromal Corneal Ring Segments: Phase II Results for the Correction of Myopia

Schanzlin DJ, Asbell PA, Burris TE, et al (St Louis Univ; Mount Sinai School of Medicine, New York; Northwest Corneal Services, Portland, Ore; et al)

Ophthalmology 104:1067–1078, 1997 2–3

Objective.—Intrastromal corneal ring segments (ICRS) is a new technique being evaluated for correcting myopia, The ICR has an "arc shortening" effect on the cornea. A modification of the original 360 degree ICR was used in phase II clinical trials in 1995 (Fig 1). Results for the first 102 patients are presented.

Methods.—ICRS from 0.25 to 0.45 mm were inserted into 1 eye of each of 150 patients requiring myopic correction from −1.00 to −6.00 D. Of these, 102 have been monitored for 3 months.

> *Technique.*—The procedure was performed using topical anesthesia in 99 patients and with intravenous-conscious sedation and parabullar (local) anesthesia in 3. A single diamond knife set to 68% of this pachometry reading to ensure that a radial incision would be made no deeper than two thirds of the way through the cornea. Corneal tissue was separated, the Vacuum Centering Guide (KeraVision, Inc., Fremont, CA) was placed over the center, and the globe was stabilized as the vacuum was slowly increased. The stromal lamellae were blunt dissected with specially designed dissectors. Intrastromal segments were inserted, and the incision was closed with 2 interrupted 10-0 nylon sutures. The duration of the procedure averaged 15.1 minutes and ranged from 10 to 25 minutes.

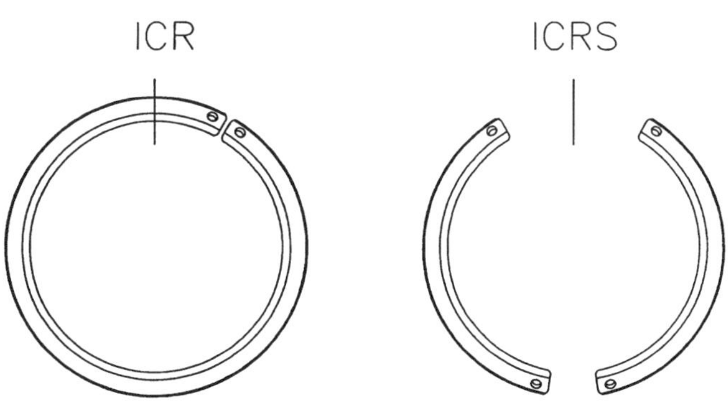

FIGURE 1.—The 360 degree intrastromal corneal ring (*ICR*) (KeraVision, Fremont, Calif.) (*left*) and the intrastromal corneal ring (*ICRS*) segments (*right*) are both composed of the same optically transparent polymethylmethacrylate. The 1.8–2 mm long radial incision, through which the device is inserted, is pictured at the 12 o'clock position. (Published courtesy of *Ophthalmology*, from Schanzlin DJ, Asbell PA, Burris TE, et al: The intrastromal corneal ring segments: Phase II results for the correction of myopia. *Ophthalmology* 104:1067–1078, 1997.)

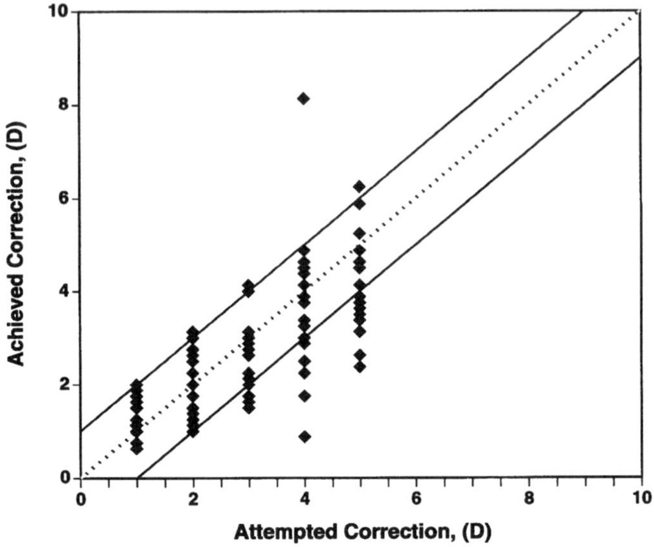

FIGURE 4.—Attempted vs. achieved correction at month 3. Cycloplegic refraction spherical equivalent (n = 99). (Published courtesy of *Ophthalmology*, from Schanzlin DJ, Asbell PA, Burris TE, et al: The intrastromal corneal ring segments: Phase II results for the correction of myopia. *Ophthalmology* 104:1067–1078, 1997.)

Results.—At 3 months, 5 of 99 patients had lost 2 lines or more of best spectacle-corrected visual acuity (BSCVA). There were 75 of 99 (77%) patients who attained a refraction within ±1.00 D of their intended correction and 94 (95%) who were within ±2.00 D (Fig 4). After surgery, patients had contrast sensitivity without glare similar to what they had before surgery. Corneal sensation losses were at least 20 mm for 8 (8%) patients. Twenty patients had astigmatism at least 1.00 D in cylinder at 3 months. Intrastromal corneal ring segments were removed in 2 patients. Complications have been managed easily and have been related to the new technique learning curve. The refractive effect was found to be reversible in those patients with explanted ICRS.

Conclusion.—Preliminary results with ICRS are good with no significant contrast differences after surgery. Additional investigation is justified to evaluate the corrective effect.

► The authors report the surgical results for 99 patients 3 months after ICRS placement (see Fig 1). They found 77% are within 1 D of attempted correction, and 95% are within 2 D of attempted correction at the 3 month follow-up visit (see Fig 4). Five percent lost 2 or more lines of BSCVA. Twenty percent had induced astigmatism greater than or equal to 1 D. Two surgical complications occurred requiring explant of the ICRS within 5 days of surgery (1 inadvertent placement of a ring into the anterior chamber and 1 infectious keratitis). The initial procedure took between 10 and 25 minutes, averaging 15 minutes.

This study offers mediocre results at best. The saving grace is that this is an early study, and improvements in techniques and nomograms are sure to improve accuracy and safety. In addition, the postoperative cornea appears to retain its natural aspheric shape. Perhaps most importantly, it is potentially reversible, and if it is reversible, it should be *modifiable*, for example, allowing the possibility to exchange implant size to improve refractive results.

C.J. Rapuano, M.D.

Laser Intrastromal Keratomileusis for High Myopia and Myopic Astigmatism

Condon PI, Mulhern M, Fulcher T, et al (Waterford Regional Hosp, Ireland; Mater Private Hosp, Dublin)

Br J Ophthalmol 81:199–206, 1997 2–4

Background.—The correction of high myopia by photorefractive keratectomy results in more corneal haze and regression, compared with correction of lower degrees of myopia. Pallikaris, et al. introduced the concept of hinging the corneal cap to minimize displacement and irregular astigmatism. It is generally believed that corneal haze and regression can be minimized by preserving Bowman's membrane. This new technique is discussed in several reports, but the use of laser intrastromal keratomileusis (LASIK) to correct compound myopic astigmatism is described in only one.

Methods.—There were 52 patients with myopia greater than 8.0 D: 32 patients were classified as *myopic LASIK* and 16 as *astigmatic myopic LASIK*. Three patients had retreatment, and 1 patient canceled. Patients were subdivided into 3 groups: group 1 with -8 to -15 D, group 2 with greater than -15 D to -20 D, and group 3 with greater than -20 D. In the myopic LASIK group, 8 patients were treated with the Summit laser, and the rest were treated with the Meditec laser. The Meditec laser was used in all patients in the astigmatic myopic LASIK group and in all cases of retreatment. Ablation was performed at a single optical zone: 5.0 mm with the Summit laser and 5.5 mm with the Meditec laser.

Results.—In 7 of the primary cases, the best-corrected visual acuity was reduced by 1 Snellen line; 3 patients were in the myopic LASIK group, and 4 were in the astigmatic myopic LASIK group. A reduction in best-corrected visual acuity by 1 Snellen line also was seen in 1 patient who had retreatment. Eight patients had significant ablation decentration; the Summit laser was used in 7 patients, and the Meditec laser was used in 1. There were 17 cases of corneal complications, including epithelial cell nests and active epithelial ingrowth (Table 5). Interface haze was graded 0–2 and was seen in 9 patients; 1 patient with grade 2 haze had severe difficulty with night driving. Three patients had particulate debris. At 6 months, specular microscopy showed no significant reduction in endothelial cell count. Two patients had severe glare, and 1 patient had monocular dip-

TABLE 5.—Complications of LASIK

Undercorrection greater than −1.5 D	35 cases
Retreatment required*	6 cases
Corneal haze	9 cases
Decentred ablation	8 cases
Epithelial ingrowth	3 cases
Interface debris	3 cases
Cap stress lines	2 cases

*One retreatment is scheduled, and 1 patient could not be retreated because the residual cornea was too thin.

(Courtesy of Condon PI, Mulhern M, Fulcher T, et al: Laser intrastromal keratomileusis for high myopia and myopic astigmatism. *Br J Ophthalmol* 81:199–206, 1997. Copyright BMJ Publishing Group.)

lopia. No patient had halo phenomena. Five eyes had astigmatism induced by treatment, but were not associated with decentration.

Discussion.—LASIK is becoming the preferred treatment for correcting myopia greater than 8.0 D. For higher degrees of myopia, photorefractive keratectomy is associated with regression and subepithelial haze. It has been shown that preservation of Bowman's membrane can reduce regression and haze, and for this reason a flap is created and the stromal bed is ablated rather than the cap. Regression after LASIK was not a serious problem in these patients. Vector analysis showed that surgically induced astigmatism was 0.93 D in the astigmatic myopic LASIK group; the range was 0–5.0 D. The most common complications with LASIK was undercorrection and decentration. The rate of overcorrection was 20% for the total sample. Centration was compared in myopic photorefractive keratectomy and myopic LASIK groups. The magnitude of displacement was almost twice as high in LASIK group. Advantages of LASIK included little or no postoperative pain or haze, a simple postoperative regimen, no pad, and a short course of antibiotics without topical steroids. Disadvantages included the need for a fully functioning operatory suite and the purchase of an expensive microkeratome. The procedure is technically difficult and should only be done by experienced ophthalmic surgeons.

▶ Over the past 6 months, many papers on early LASIK results for the treatment of high myopia have appeared in the peer review literature. This paper is one of the best by virtue of the number of eyes (51) and follow-up (8–24 months, mean 16 months). In addition, one third had astigmatism correction with the laser. It is not perfect however because 2 different excimer lasers were used (Summit and Meditec) with relatively small ablation zones of 5.0 and 5.5 mm.

The pros of LASIK are "safety," minimal pain, rapid visual recovering, minimal corneal haze, and little post-operative medication and need for follow-up.

The cons include 15% loss of 1 line of best-corrected visual acuity, 70% undercorrected by greater than 1.5 D, 20% overcorrection, 16% significant decentered ablations, 18% corneal haze, and 6% epithelial ingrowth (see

Table 5). In addition, the surgeon needs access to an expensive microkeratome, and the intraocular pressure is raised to greater than 65 mm Hg during the creation of the flap, with potential side effects.

I agree with the authors' comments that a safer, more user-friendly microkeratome would be extremely helpful, and more accurate nomograms are needed. They conclude, "There is still a long way to go with this technique."

C.J. Rapuano, M.D.

Excimer Laser Photorefractive Keratectomy for Hyperopia

Dausch D, Smecka Z, Klein R, et al (Marienhospital; Aniberg, Germany; Klinika Ocni A Esteticke Chirurgue, Zlin, Czech Republic; Hôpital de l'Orangerie, Strasbourg, France; et al)

J Cataract Refract Surg 23:169–176, 1997 2–5

Background.—Recent studies of myopic eyes after photorefractive keratectomy (PRK) suggest that the problems associated with this procedure may be alleviated by the use of a larger ablation zone, resulting in less variation in refractive outcomes. The outcomes associated with the use of an enlarged treatment zone for hyperopic PRK were evaluated.

Methods.—Sixty-eight hyperopic eyes in 62 patients underwent PRK using an MEL 60 excimer laser. The average attempted correction was +4.85 D. The patients were followed up for up to 12 months.

Findings.—Eighty-one percent of the eyes were within 1 D and 59% were within 0.5 D of the intended correction 1 year after PRK. In 92% of the eyes, the best corrected visual acuity was unchanged or improved. Six percent of the eyes lost 1 line of visual acuity; 1%, 2 lines; and 1%, 3 lines.

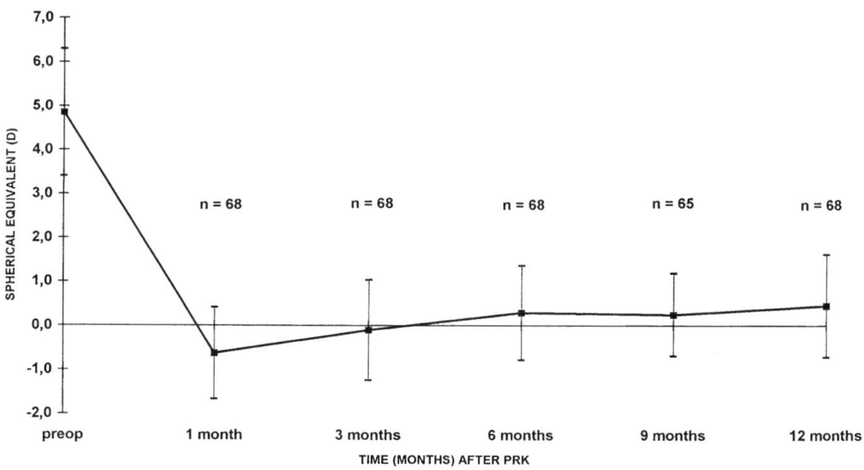

FIGURE 2.—Mean spherical equivalent (*D*) and standard deviation over time. (Courtesy of Dausch D, Smecka Z, Klein R, et al: Excimer laser photorefractive keratectomy for hyperopia. *J Cataract Refract Surg* 23:169–176, 1997.)

Ninety-seven percent of the eyes had an uncorrected visual acuity of 20/40 or better, and 40%, 20/20 or better (Fig 2).

Conclusions.—The use of a 9-mm treatment zone in PRK is an efficient, relatively safe way to correct hyperopia of up to 8.25 D. The predictability of this procedure was good. Ophthalmologists must be very careful to improve the centration of the optical zone.

► Dieter Dausch, the lead author of this article, is one of the pioneers of hyperopic PRK, reporting the first hyperopic PRK study in 1993. Originally, a 7-mm ablation zone was used, but this study investigated a 9-mm ablation zone. Although only 68 eyes were treated, with 1 year of follow-up, the results are quite reasonable. Best spectacle corrected vision decreased slightly at 1 month and then returned to baseline by 3 months. Refractions were slightly over corrected at 1 month and slightly under-corrected at 3 months, at which point the refractions were stable (see Fig 2). The large epithelial defects healed by 6 days and haze and halos resolved by 6–12 months. Decentration occurred in 2 patients, associated with decreased best spectacle corrected vision. Hyperopic PRK appears promising but more work certainly needs to be performed.

C.J. Rapuano, M.D.

Influence of Patient Age on Refraction and Corneal Haze After Photorefractive Keratectomy

Hefetz L, Domnitz Y, Haviv D, et al (Tel Aviv Univ, Israel)

Br J Ophthalmol 81:637–638, 1997 2–6

Objective.—Photorefractive keratectomy (PRK) has been particularly successful in low and moderate myopes. Results of a retrospective study of the effect of age on outcome are presented.

Methods.—Spherical equivalent and anterior corneal haze were measured at 3, 6, and 12 months after PRK in 599 eyes categorized into the following 3 groups based on preoperative baseline refraction: group 1, −2.00 to −6.00 D; group 2, −6.25 to −10.00 D; and group 3, ≥−10.25 D. Each refraction group was divided into the following 3 age-groups: group 1, younger than 30 years: group 2, 30–39 years; and group 3, 40 years or older.

Results.—At 12 months, residual myopia readings in the 3 age-groups of the low myopic group were −0.24 D, −0.46 D, and −0.28 D. Residual myopia readings in the moderate myopia group were −0.70 D, −0.87 D, and −0.81 D. Residual myopia readings in the high myopic group were −1.51 D, −1.63 D, and −1.54 D. Similarly, degrees of haze in the refraction groups were 0.26, 0.29, and 0.34 for the low myopia group; 0.53, 0.57, and 0.54 for the moderate myopia group; and 0.66, 0.78, and 1.15 for the high myopic group.

Conclusion.—Residual myopia and degree of anterior corneal haze were unrelated to age. Residual myopia and corneal haze were highest in the high myopic group, regardless of age.

► The party line, as taught in excimer laser PRK courses and based on multiple PRK studies, is that PRK results are not dependent on a patient's age. However, a number of PRK surgeons feel that older patients not infrequently end up somewhat overcorrected.

This paper, which includes almost 600 eyes with 1 year of follow-up, found no differences in refractive results or post-operative haze, depending on the patient's age. However, an important piece of information is missing. The authors do not specify whether the refractions were cycloplegic or not. Although it may not have made a difference in the results, the best way to standardize refraction and its analysis, especially when examining different age-groups, is with cycloplegic refractions.

C.J. Rapuano, M.D.

Effect of Variations in Surgical Technique and Patient Management on Outcomes of Photorefractive Keratectomy

McCarty CA, for the Melbourne Excimer Laser Group (Univ of Melbourne, East Melbourne, Australia)

J Refract Surg 13:55–59, 1997 2–7

Objective.—The prevalence of complications after excimer laser photorefractive keratectomy (PRK) increases with higher amounts of myopia and eccentric ablations. This has been blamed on less experienced surgeons. No previous study has specifically examined the effects of variations in surgical and patient management on the clinical outcomes of PRK. The influence of these variations on the outcomes of PRK for myopia and myopic astigmatism was studied.

Methods.—A wide range of surgical and patient management variables were evaluated for their impact on the outcomes of PRK or photoastigmatic keratectomy in 645 eyes. All operations were done using a VISX Twenty/Twenty excimer laser. The 27 participating surgeons all used the same treatment protocol with allowances for some variation (Table 1). Spherical equivalent manifest refraction, spectacle-corrected visual acuity, and uncorrected visual acuity were the 1-year clinical outcomes assessed.

Results.—The study included 347 eyes of 221 low myopes, 240 eyes of 172 high myopes, and 58 eyes of 47 extreme myopes. The patients' mean age was 37 years. Seventy percent of the procedures included astigmatic corrections. The mean time to epithelial healing was 3 days, slightly faster when the epithelium was "replaced." Lesser amounts of preoperative myopia were associated with better results in terms of spherical equivalent refraction and uncorrected visual acuity. However, none of the management variables tested had a significant impact on outcomes in a univariate analysis. After controlling for preoperative spherical equivalent refraction,

TABLE 1.—Frequency of Variation in Surgical and Patient Management in Eyes Treated with Photorefractive Keratectomy

Variation	Frequency (percent)
Treatment based on cycloplegic refraction (versus manifest)	18 (3)
Use of pledget to apply anesthesia	4 (1)
Marking of visual axis	110 (17)
6.5-mm diameter zone marker (versus 7.0 mm)	47 (7)
Epithelium removal	
Paton spatula	410 (66)
Blade	216 (34)
Articificial tears after epithelium removal	51 (8)
Fixation	
Patient fixation	459 (73)
Forceps	160 (26)
Suction	6 (1)
Cellulose sponge	1 (0.2)
Replace epithelium after surgery	96 (15)
Bandage contact lens	70 (11)
Use of two semipressure patches (versus one)	43 (7)
NSAIDs	202 (31)

Abbreviation: NSAIDs, nonsteroidal anti-inflammatory drugs.

(Courtesy of McCarty CA, Aldred GF, Couper T, et al: Effect of variations in surgical technique and patient management on outcomes of photorefractive keratectomy. *J Refract Surg* 13:55–59, 1997.)

variations in surgical practice had no effect on the occurrence of adverse reactions or loss of spectacle-corrected visual acuity.

Conclusion.—The tested variations in patient and surgical management have no apparent impact on the clinical outcomes of PRK. As shown previously, the preoperative spherical equivalent refraction determines the predictability of PRK.

► The Melbourne Excimer Laser Group has, once again, effectively gathered and reported their excimer laser results. They retrospectively analyzed several variations of surgical technique and patient management during and after excimer laser PRK, including different methods of epithelial removal, patient fixation, bandage soft contact lens, and nonsteroidal anti-inflammatory drug use (see Table 1). They found no significant difference in refraction or uncorrected and best corrected visual outcomes for the variations studied.

This finding corroborates the experience of many PRK surgeons, namely, that clinical results are quite consistent from surgeon to surgeon and institution to institution. The authors also document mean uncorrected vision of 20/30 for low myopes (less than −5.25 D), 20/40 for high myopes (−5.37 to −11.37 D) and 20/100 for extreme myopes (−11.50 to −18.25 D), emphasizing the need for a better refractive surgery option for extreme myopes.

C.J. Rapuano, M.D.

Lack of Diurnal Variation in Vision, Refraction, or Keratometry After Excimer Laser Photorefractive Keratectomy

Goldberg MA, Dorr DA, Pepose JS (New York Eye and Ear Infirmary; Washington Univ, St Louis)

Am J Ophthalmol 123:407–408, 1997 2–8

Purpose.—In the correction of myopia, excimer laser photorefractive keratectomy (PRK) offers better preservation of the corneal structure than does radial keratotomy. Other potential sequelae of radial keratotomy include hyperopic drift and diurnal shifts in visual acuity, refraction, and keratometry. Eyes undergoing excimer laser PRK were studied for diurnal variations in visual acuity, refraction, and keratometry.

Methods and Findings.—The study included 29 eyes of 29 patients undergoing excimer laser PRK using a 5 mm optical zone. The degree of myopia ranged from −1.00 to −6.00 D spherical equivalent. Postoperatively, the eyes were examined for diurnal variations in visual acuity, spherical equivalent, keratometry, and intraocular pressure. The operated and fellow eyes had no significant differences in the magnitude of these diurnal variations.

Conclusion.—This small study finds no evidence of diurnal variation in visual acuity, spherical equivalent, or keratometry in eyes undergoing excimer laser PRK. The findings should be confirmed in larger samples.

► This relatively small study (29 eyes) also confirms the impression of PRK surgeons that there is minimal to no diurnal fluctuation in vision after excimer laser PRK. The authors found a trend toward post PRK diurnal variation in intraocular pressure and definite diurnal variation in the untreated fellow eye, but no difference in diurnal variation between treated and nontreated eyes. They did not discuss whether post-PRK eyes had a lower intraocular pressure than nontreated fellow eyes. This study is limited however, because of its small size, use of a 5-mm PRK ablation zone, and only evaluating patients treated for −1.00 to −6.00 D of myopia.

C.J. Rapuano, M.D.

The Effect of Excimer Laser Photorefractive Keratectomy on Intraocular Pressure Measurements Using the Goldmann Applanation Tonometer

Mardelli PG, Piebenga LW, Whitacre MM, et al (Washington Univ, St Louis; Univ of Missouri—Kansas City)

Ophthalmology 104:945–949, 1997 2–9

Background.—Laser photorefractive keratectomy (PRK) changes the thickness and curvature of the central cornea. Corneal curvature may affect the accuracy of Goldmann tonometer readings. The effect of PRK on Goldmann applanation tonometry readings was investigated in a group of healthy myopic patients.

Methods.—One hundred eleven patients were included in the study. Intraocular pressure (IOP) was measured using Goldmann applanation tonometry at baseline and 12 months after PRK. In addition, ultrasonic corneal thickness was measured and keratometry performed. Contralateral eyes were studied as controls.

Findings.—Mean tonometer readings were significantly lower in the treated eyes than in the untreated eyes. Treated eyes also had a significant decrease in mean central pachymetry. The mean spherical equivalent and central keratometry readings were significantly reduced in the treated eyes, by a mean of 3.3 and 2.2 diopters, respectively.

Conclusions.—Goldmann tonometer readings are mildly reduced in eyes treated with PRK. Reductions in IOP measurements are probably not great enough to change treatment decision making for at individual patient with glaucoma but may delay its recognition and treatment.

▶ This paper confirms Chatterjee et al.'s findings (*Ophthalmology*, March 1997) that intraocular pressure measurements decrease after excimer laser PRK. Chatterjee et al paper used non-contact tonometry while Mardelli and colleagues used the gold standard, Goldmann applanation tonometry. Mardelli and associates found a 0.5 mmHg decrease in intraocular pressure in the treated eye when compared to the untreated eye. They did not find a statistically significant relationship between depth of ablation and decrease in intraocular pressure measurement; however, with larger numbers and a wider range of treatment, a difference might be found.

C.J. Rapuano, M.D.

Influence of Ablation Plume Dynamics on the Formation of Central Islands in Excimer Laser Photorefractive Keratectomy

Noack J, Tönnies R, Hohla K, et al (Medizinisches Laserzentrum Lübeck GmbH, Lübeck, Germany; Chiron Technolas GmbH, Munich, Germany)

Ophthalmology 104:823–830, 1997 2–10

Objective.—As experience was gained with excimer photorefractive keratectomy, larger zone diameters came into use, particularly in patients with high myopia. This improved the predictability and stability of the refractive outcome. However, central islands—areas of reduced central ablation—have been reported in more than 70% of patients. Central islands occur only in patients treated with a series of concentric ablation patterns, not in those treated with scanning laser beams. Time-resolved laser flash photography was used to study the ablation plume during excimer laser photorefractive keratectomy, and its effects on the formation of central islands.

Methods.—A clinical ArF-laser with a radiant exposure of 120 mJ/cm^2 was used to ablate plane polymethyl-methacrylate (PMMA) targets, spherical PMMA targets, and the corneas of enucleated porcine eyes. The ablation zone ranged from 1 to 7 mm, with a 10-Hz ablation rate.

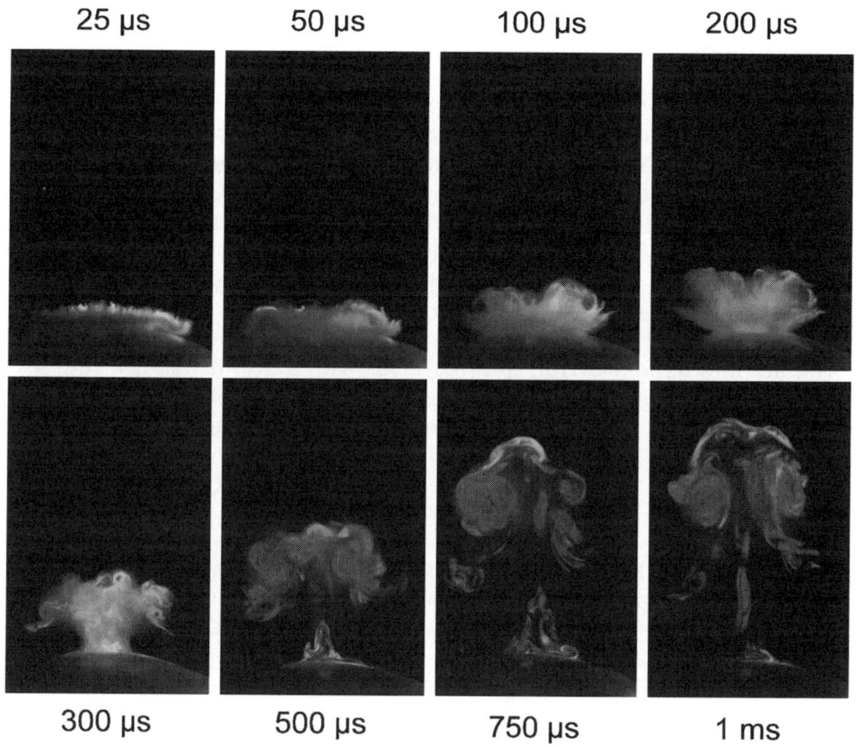

FIGURE 5.—Images of the ablation plume obtained at various times after ablating a 7-mm circular zone of the cornea sample. The length of the *bar* corresponds to the zone diameter. (Published courtesy of *Ophthalmology*, from Noack J, Tönnies R, Hohla K, et al: Influence of ablation plume dynamics on the formation of central islands in excimer laser photorefractive keratectomy. *Ophthalmology* 104:823–830, 1997.)

Time-resolved laser flash photography was performed to visualize the dynamics of the laser ablation products.

Results.—All zone diameters were associated with central islands, which were significantly higher for larger ablation zones. In the corneas, the laser ablation plume scattered much more light than in PMMA (Fig 5). With a 5-mm ablation zone on the cornea, very few particles were observed 25 msec or later after the excimer laser pulse. However, the 7-mm zone was associated with larger amounts of ablated material, with a denser particle cloud observed over the center of the zone, even after 100 msec.

Conclusion.—The findings suggest that deposition of particles in the center of the ablation zone may be a major cause of central islands after excimer laser photorefractive keratectomy. Re-ablation of the deposited material takes part of the energy of the subsequent laser pulse. Reduced ablation rates in the center of the zone, where the redeposition tends to occur, lead to the formation of a central island. Fewer particles accumulate over the center in smaller ablation zones. The best way to eliminate central islands may be through additional laser pulses to the central area of the ablation zone.

► This paper, together with the next paper (Abstract 2–11), investigated the issue of central island status post photorefractive keratectomy, using a broad beam excimer laser. Here, the authors used laser flash photography to visualize the ablation products as they were ejected off the surface of the ablated material (see Fig 5). They found that these particles accumulate centrally and that the larger the ablation zone, the more significant the accumulation. This debris would then block some of the laser light in subsequent pulses, leading to decreased ablation centrally, resulting in central islands.

The authors used a Chiron excimer laser with a 10–Hz ablation rate (like the Summit excimer laser ablation rate). It would be interesting to learn whether the effect was similar using a slower ablation rate, such as 5–6 Hz, as used by the VISX excimer laser.

C.J. Rapuano, M.D.

Corneal Ablation Profilometry and Steep Central Islands

Shimmick JK, Telfair WB, Munnerlyn CR, et al (VISX Incorporated, Santa Clara, Calif; Univ of Alabama at Birmingham; Columbia Univ, New York)

J Refract Surg 13:235–245, 1997 2–11

Purpose.—In excimer laser ablation, surface power within the treated zone is usually distributed with relative uniformity, with a smooth power transition to the peripheral cornea. However, a central area of undercorrection—or "steep central island" is sometimes seen within the ablated area. Optical profilometry was performed to determine the shape of the

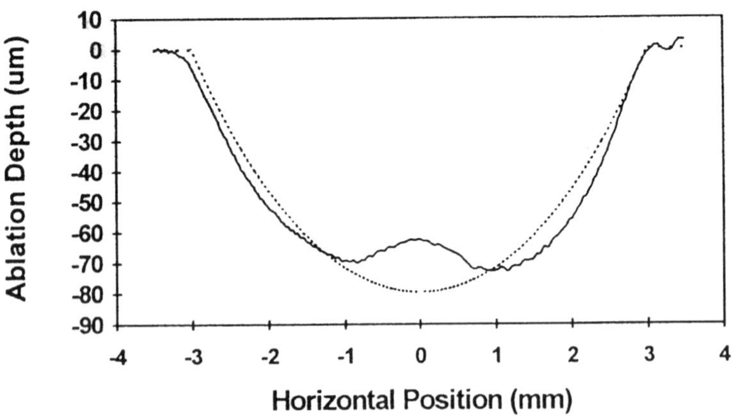

FIGURE 8.—Live rabbit eye 6 mm, −6.00 D ablation profiles (*dashed line*, intended ablation; *solid line*, measured ablation). (Courtesy of Shimmick JK, Telfair WB, Munnerlyn CR, et al: Corneal ablation profilometry and steep central islands. *J Refract Surg* 13:235–245, 1997.)

ablated anterior corneal surface immediately after photorefractive keratectomy.

Methods.—Studies were performed in enucleated porcine eyes as well as living rabbit eyes. Ablations were performed using a VISX Twenty Twenty B excimer laser system with Vision Key System. For this study, profile adjustment to correct for steep central islands was eliminated. This permitted study of the effects of spatially varying ablation rates with an ablation algorithm that assumed constant tissue ablation. Corneal ablation profiles were measured using a custom optical profilometer.

Results.—The shape of the corneal stromal ablation did not precisely match the laser beam profile. Corneal ablation rates varied with ablation diameter and were not uniform across a uniform beam (Fig 8). The cause of the variable ablation rates was unclear. However, modifying the ablation algorithm to correct for spatial variation permitted spherical ablations.

Conclusion.—The findings suggest that spatial variance of tissues ablated with a uniform laser beam irradiance is the cause of steep central islands after photorefractive keratectomy. Risk may be greater in patients undergoing greater dioptric corrections, larger ablation diameters, and transepithelial ablations that do not correct for spatial variance. The laser ablation algorithm can be modified to produce spherical ablations. This correction should help to avoid problems with corneal topographic abnormalities, hasten recovery of spectacle-corrected vision, and increase the safety and efficacy of excimer laser photorefractive keratectomy.

► This paper, like the previous one (Abstract 2–10), investigated central islands after broad-beam excimer laser photorefractive keratectomy. Here, the authors used a profilometer to evaluate the exact amount of tissue ablated off the target (either polymethyl-methacrylate or corneal tissue). They found that somewhat more tissue was ablated peripherally and somewhat less tissue was ablated centrally than expected, leading to "central island formation" (see Fig 8).

The authors discussed numerous theories for this difference from expected ablation, including persistent debris/fog over the ablation zone blocking subsequent ablations. They then undertook a software modification of the ablation, redistributing pulses to give more effect centrally and less peripherally, resulting in elimination of the central islands. The current VISX software has this "anticentral island" modification, and, clinically, it works quite well.

C.J. Rapuano, M.D.

Excimer Laser Reablation

Loewenstein A, Lipshitz I, Varssano D, et al (Ichilov Hosp, Tel-Aviv, Israel)
Ophthalmic Surg Lasers 28:282–287, 1997 2–12

Background.—Repeated laser keratectomy is often needed to rectify undercorrection, regression, and haze after photorefractive keratectomy (PRK) that is unresponsive to topical steroids. The results of repeat PRK in one group of patients observed for 12 months or longer were reported.

Methods.—The first 100 consecutive patients who had completed at least 12 months of follow-up after PRK were reviewed. In all patients, the diameter of the ablation zone was 5 mm. Postoperative treatment included dexamethasone 0.1% 4 times a day for the first month, with steroid reduction by 1 drop per day every month. In 32 eyes requiring repeat excimer laser keratectomy, the repeat procedure was comparable to the first one, except that the epithelium was removed by a phototherapeutic keratectomy procedure, using up to 200 pulses in a 6 mm zone. Immediately after, PRK was done, adjusted to remove all residual myopia.

Findings.—Of the 32 eyes undergoing repeat treatment, 22% initially had low myopia; 34.4%, moderate myopia; and 44%, high myopia. Mean time between the first PRK and the repeat laser keratectomy was 12 months. Mean SE was −4.77 before reoperation, declining to −0.57 D after retreatment. Sixty-two percent of the eyes had moderate or severe haze before retreatment. After treatment, none had severe haze, and 3% had moderate haze.

Conclusions.—The overall results of repeated PRK in the treatment of regression after PRK appear to be good. A small reduction in best vision occurred only in a small subgroup with regression and haze after the initial procedure.

► Since it takes a while to organize findings in a thousand PRK patients with at least 1 year of follow-up, the techniques originally used in this study are outdated, namely, a 5-mm ablation zone in all eyes. When the FDA finally approved PRK in the U.S., it was using a 6-mm ablation zone. Consequently, much of the specific numbers in this paper are not applicable. However, several general conclusions regarding PRK retreatment can be made: 1) even with a 5 mm ablation zone, there was only a 3.2% reoperation rate; 2) best corrected vision tended to improve with retreatment; and 3) retreatment for regression *without* haze faired better than regression *with* haze. Overall, the small percentage of PRK patients who need retreatment tend to improve but not generally to the level of the eyes that did not require retreatment.

C.J. Rapuano, M.D.

Combined PRK and PTK in Myopic Patients With Recurrent Corneal Erosion

Kremer I, Blumenthal M (Ein Tal Eye Ctr, Tel Aviv, Israel)
Br J Ophthalmol 81:551–554, 1997 2–13

Objective.—Recurrent corneal erosion (RCE), a disorder of the epithelial basement membrane, is often associated with a history of shallow corneal injury and sometimes with epithelial basement dystrophy (EBMD). Although there are a variety of therapies used to treat this condition, the efficacies have not been definitively evaluated. Results of pancorneal excimer laser photoablation, including the combination of photorefractive keratectomy (PRK) and phototherapeutic keratectomy (PTK), for myopic patients with recalcitrant recurrent erosion syndrome are presented.

Methods.—Sixteen patients (6 men), age 32–52 years, with unilateral EMBD and myopia ranging from −2.0 to −7.0 D and astigmatism ranging from −1.0 to −3.5 D were treated using the excimer laser. Patients were monitored for an average of 31 months. Using combined PRK and PTK, the whole epithelium was scraped up to the limbal zone with a Beaver blade. Then the Visx 20/20 B excimer laser was used to correct the myopia by ablating a 6 mm diameter area centered on the pupil. Thereafter, the computer program was switched to the PTK mode, and the 3.0 mm zone was treated to a depth of 6 μm (Fig 1).

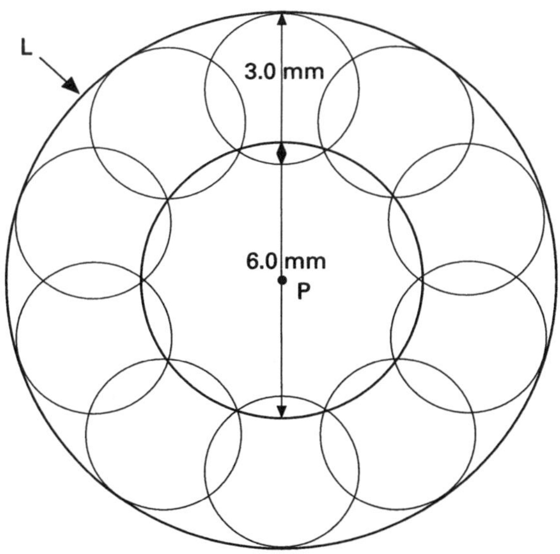

FIGURE 1.—PRK-PTK treatment scheme illustrating the central 6 mm diameter zone of PRK, surrounded by confluent 3 mm diameter circular zones of PTK, reaching the corneal limbus (*L*). (Reprinted with permission of the BMJ Publishing Group, from Kremer I, Blumenthal M: Combined PRK and PTK in myopic patients with recurrent corneal erosion. *Br J Ophthalmol* 81:551–554, 1997.)

Results.—Reepithelialization occurred between 7 and 9 days, symptoms were gone within 1 month, and no recurrence of corneal erosion was observed during the follow-up period. A myopic shift of −1.0 D, small compared with the hyperopic shift reported in other studies, was seen in 14 eyes. Although recalcitrant RCE initially appears to be a local abnormality, the authors suspect that it is really a diffuse disease of the corneal epithelium.

Conclusion.—Combined PRK and PTK successfully relieved RCE and corrected myopia in myopic patients.

► Drs. Kremer and Blumenthal report on combined PRK, centrally for myopia, and PTK, in the periphery for recalcitrant RCE, after complete mechanical de-epithelialization (Fig 1). Intellectually, it seems like a logical combination of 2 excellent techniques, but performing them together has theoretical problems. For example, creating a 12 mm epithelial defect, with a re-epithelialization time that is twice as long as normal after PRK, could predispose to increased haze with decreased best corrected vision and regression. In this study, best-corrected vision was the same or better in most eyes but did decrease 1 Snellen line in 2 eyes.

Additionally, the peripheral PTK treatment might tend to steepen the cornea, leading to greater undercorrection. In fact, although the refractive results were good, not one patient achieved 20/20 uncorrected visual acuity, probably because the mean undercorrection was about 0.5 D. Perhaps this technique could be modified by adding −0.25 to −0.50 D to the tempted correction to compensate for the peripheral PTK treatment.

C.J. Rapuano, M.D.

Epithelial Growth Within the Lamellar Interface After Laser In Situ Keratomileusis (LASIK)

Helena MC, Meisler D, Wilson SE (Cleveland Clinc Found, Ohio)

Cornea 16:300–305, 1997 2–14

Background.—Laser in situ keratomileusis (LASIK), a refractive technique, involves performing a lamellar keratotomy of about 130–160 μm deep using an automated microkeratome. The resulting flap is retracted and excimer laser applied to the stromal bed. After the ablation, the flap is repositioned without suturing. Little information is available on the complications of LASIK. The occurrence and follow-up of ectopic, interface, epithelial growth after LASIK were documented in 4 eyes in 3 patients.

Patients and Findings.—The patients were 2 men, aged 44 and 22 years, respectively, and 1 woman, aged 29 years. The affected eyes were examined by slit-lamp biomicroscopy. Corneal topography was obtained with the Tomey TMS-1 instrument. Interface opacities and surface irregularity developed in each eye with epithelium in the interface after LASIK. Early surgery was performed in 1 eye, and the other 3 were observed. All eyes lost at least 1 line of best spectacle-corrected visual acuity and had visual disturbance at the last follow-up visit.

Conclusions.—The presence of epithelium in the lamellar interface is a significant complication associated with LASIK. Interface epithelium may be associated with early postoperative inflammation in some eyes. When reoperation is necessary, both sides of the interface should be scraped with a metal blade. In some eyes, light excimer laser therapy can facilitate the removal of epithelium.

► While the LASIK honeymoon hasn't ended yet, these authors report an important, if infrequent, complication of LASIK, epithelial growth in the flap interface. While often considered "part of the learning curve" and "extremely rare in experienced hands," it is an important, potentially serious, complication. It is one of those complications where avoidance is key, since treatment is often problematic. With new techniques, come new problems. Surgeons need to be vigilant in reporting such new complications.

C.J. Rapuano, M.D.

Dilute Topical Proparacaine for Pain Relief After Photorefractive Keratectomy

Shahinian L Jr, Jain S, Jager RD, et al (Stanford Univ, Calif; Pacific Laser Eye Centre, Vancouver, BC)

Ophthalmology 104:1327–1332, 1997 2–15

Objective.—Because patients who have undergone photorefractive keratectomy (PRK) often have a lot of pain after surgery, a prospective, randomized, double-masked clinical investigation was conducted to determine if there is a nonanesthetic and nontoxic concentration of topical proparacaine that can be applied repeatedly to the cornea to reduce pain after PRK.

Methods.—Corneal sensation was measured in the eyes of 50 healthy volunteers before and after instillation of 1 drop of 0.01%, 0.025%, 0.05%, 0.1%, and 0.2% topical proparacaine. Corneal sensation was determined in 10 healthy volunteers before and 1 minute after instillation of 1 drop of 0.05% proparacaine every 15 minutes for 2 hours. The highest nonanesthetic dose (0.05%) was evaluated for toxicity compared with placebo after hourly instillation for 12 hours a day for 7 days. After surgery, eyes were fitted with a soft bandage contact lens and treated with topical diclofenac sodium 0.1% 4 times daily for 2 days and by 0.3% tobramycin and 0.1% dexamethasone 4 times daily for the first week. Patients were given topical 0.05% proparacaine or artificial tears to use as needed and asked to evaluate pain control.

Results.—Nonanesthetic concentration determination studies showed no significant difference in corneal sensitivity between placebo and 0.05% proparacaine. No adverse events were reported or found in the toxicity studies. In the analgesia study, the average change in pain score was significantly greater and the average oral narcotic use was significantly lower in the proparacaine group than they were in the placebo group.

Conclusion.—Dilute proparacaine (0.05%) provides analgesia without corneal anesthesia after PRK.

▶ "Less pain" and "faster visual recovery" are the 2 reasons many patients select laser in situ keratomileusis (LASIK) PRK. Shahinian, et al. offer a potential solution to one of these problems with PRK. They demonstrate significant pain reduction (analgesia) without loss of the protective corneal touch sensation (anesthesia) with the use of topical 0.05% proparacaine. It appeared nontoxic after 1 week of frequent use in normal volunteers and after PRK. When compared with artificial tears, it was associated with a slightly longer time to reepithelialization, 3.48 days, compared with 3.13 days, but the difference was not statistically significant. Prolonged epithelial defects after PRK have been associated with increased corneal haze. These authors did not address postoperative haze and refractive results in their patients.

If shown to be safe and effective in a larger number of patients with longer term follow-up, it may become standard care after PRK. If safe after PRK, it may be beneficial after traumatic abrasions, recurrent erosions, or corneal ulcerations.

C.J. Rapuano, M.D.

Lack of Virus Transmission by the Excimer Laser Plume

Hagen KB, Kettering JD, Aprecio RM, et al (Loma Linda Univ, Calif; Jules Stein Eye Inst, Los Angeles; Univ of California, Los Angeles)

Am J Ophthalmol 124:206–211, 1997 2–16

Objective.—Papilloma virus, HIV-1, and *Escherichia coli* bacteria have been found in carbon dioxide laser plume. Because the excimer laser pulse removes approximately one third of a micrometer of corneal tissue, it is possible that intact viral particles from a ruptured cell could escape into the plume. Virus transmission through airborne excimer laser debris during refractive and therapeutic corneal procedures was investigated in an in vitro experiment.

Methods.—Tissue culture plates infected with pseudorabies virus (ATCC VR-L35), a porcine herpesvirus, were lasered with the Excimer UV 200 laser (Summit Technologies, Waltham, Mass.) at fluences of 180 mJ/cm^2 and 150 mJ/cm^2. There was a 35 mm distance (plate height, 15 mm; space between plates, 5 mm) between infected and uninfected cells. The negative control was treated the same way except that it was not lasered. The positive control consisted of a mist of supernatant from infected PK-15–cell monolayers sprayed in 10 uninfected cell monolayers.

Results.—None of the uninfected cell culture plates was infected. Uninfected PK-15 cells were not contaminated. All 20 of the positive control plates showed growth within 24 hours.

Conclusion.—There was no in vitro transference of viable pseudorabies virus by the excimer laser plume at fluence levels of 180 mJ/cm^2 and 150 mJ/cm^2. Because pseudorabies virus shares characteristics with HIV and herpes simplex, it is a good and safe model for testing viral survival and transmission using the excimer laser. Viral transmission to the surgeon is unlikely under the conditions used.

Do Intact Viral Particles Survive Excimer Laser Ablation?

Taravella MJ, Weinberg A, Blackburn P, et al (Univ of Colorado, Denver)
Arch Ophthalmol 115:1028–1030, 1997 2–17

Objective.—It is possible that viruses such as HIV, herpes simplex, and adenovirus could survive excimer laser ablation and escape into room air. Whether the ablation plume could potentially pose a health risk to personnel performing or assisting in excimer laser ablation was investigated.

Methods.—A confluence monolayer of human embryonic lung fibroblasts was inoculated with varicella-zoster virus (VZV) and ablated in 4 separate experiments with an excimer laser set. The plume was collected by suction, sampled using an in-line bubble chamber, and subjected to polymerase chain reaction (PCR) analysis. Culture isolation of VZV from the bubble chamber and inlet tubing was performed. Positive (inoculated) and negative (uninoculated) controls were included in each experiment.

Results.—Polymerase chain reaction results from the bubble chamber were positive for ablations 1, 3, and 4, and negative for the controls. Polymerase chain reaction results from the inlet tubing also were positive for ablations 1 and 3. Inlet tubing was not sampled for ablation 4. None of the viral cultures showed growth.

Conclusion.—No VZV appeared to be transferred in the excimer laser plume. Because VZV is a large virus, there exists the possibility that smaller viruses could survive the ablation process. Additional investigations are being conducted. Wearing a surgical mask is recommended. Evacuation of the laser plume is suggested.

► These 2 studies (Abstracts 2–16 and 2–17) attempted to answer the same basic question: Can a live virus be spread from patients to others during excimer laser surgery? Happily, they both concluded from their limited studies that the answer appears to be no. Hagen, et al. used a very simple but clever system of placing a hole through a culture plate through which to ablate live virus and collect potentially infectious virus from the laser plume. Taravella et al. used a much more complicated collection system but performed PCR analysis in addition to viral cultures. Not surprisingly, using PCR, they found evidence of viral particles in the laser plume, but there was no growth on the culture plates, suggesting that the laser ablation fragments the virus to a point where it is no longer infectious. Even so, Taravella et al. advised surgeons to wear surgical masks capable of filtering out small particles when performing PRK.

C.J. Rapuano, M.D.

3 Glaucoma

Introduction

by George L. Spaeth, M.D.

It could be looked at either of two ways. Either 1997 was the year that everything finally fell apart or the year that things first started coming together. Those with e-mail have watched an impassioned debate about the very most fundamental aspect regarding glaucoma, specifically, *What is glaucoma?*

So, what is glaucoma? Is it an optic neuropathy with characteristic disc and field changes? Is glaucoma always related to some abnormality of intraocular pressure? Is glaucoma always related to some effect of intraocular pressure, whether or not the intraocular pressure is normal or abnormal? Is glaucoma independent of intraocular pressure? Are changes in intraocular pressure related to glaucoma in a way that is causal or casual? Does a person have glaucoma when he has genes that will certainly cause the manifestations of glaucoma but have not yet expressed themselves in a way that can be detected? Does a person have glaucoma when the intraocular pressure is 60 mm HG, but the disc and the visual field are normal, and the patient has no pain? Is glaucoma a set of findings, or is it a disease which requires symptoms for it to be present? Or is it some or all of these things? Until there is some commonality of agreement regarding the answers to these questions, there can be no meaningful discussion about how to diagnose, monitor, or treat glaucoma.

At the American Glaucoma Society meeting held toward the very end of 1997, Dunbar Hoskins, in the Shaffer Lecture, made a plea for trying to keep things simple. He reminded us that around the world millions of individuals lose vision from an entity (or related group of entities) that has been shown to be helped in many of those individuals by lowering intraocular pressure. This review emphasizes his point. For while it is important for us to do better in the future, patients will not be well served if we forget what we know while trying to learn what we don't know. So, what is it that we know?

We know that the eye can be damaged by the pressure inside the eye, and that the potential for the eye to be damaged by that pressure varies markedly from individual to individual and from time to time in the same individual. Depending on the level of pressure and the sensitivity of the tissues, many different tissues of the eye can become damaged: the lens, the iris, the cornea, the retina, the ciliary body, and the optic nerve. The damage to the eye shows itself in different patterns, some of which have become sufficiently well defined that are called "characteristic changes in the optic nerve and the visual field." Experimental models of all sorts cast valuable light on the pathogenesis of glaucoma and provide clues regarding appropriate treatment, but such models can be misleading as well as helpful. What *is* definite is that some individuals get better when their intraocular pressure is lowered. They get better in two senses: in the first place, some patients show a definite improvement; that is, the cornea clears up, the optic nerve shows less damage, or the visual field improves. More typically, what is meant by "getting better" is a change in the rate at which patients had been getting worse. For example, if a patient has been consistently losing vision for a period of 10 years, and then, in response to an intervention, stops getting worse, there is a reasonable likelihood that the change in the patient's course was related to the intervention. This kind of beneficial effect has been noted anecdotally for many years. Recently it has been shown to occur in appropriately designed studies. It can no longer be doubted that lowering intraocular pressure can benefit some patients who show the signs and symptoms of glaucoma.

It is also important to remember that to date no form of treatment other than lowering intraocular pressure has been demonstrated to have any definite beneficial effect in patients with glaucoma. There have been studies that have suggested that the visual fields might be benefited by certain types of other therapy, such as the use of systemic calcium channel blockers, but the results are controversial, and there are other interpretations. For example, patients receiving calcium channel blockers may have an improvement in their visual field in response to improved cerebral function, unrelated to any change in the eye.

In the simplest terms, there are three reasons why patients with "glaucoma" get worse: (1) they do not really have glaucoma, (2) their intraocular pressure continues to be at a level that causes continuing damage, or (3) prior damage set into motion a process that will cause continuing damage.

Patients who do not have glaucoma, that is to say, who do not have a condition that has the potential for being benefited by lowering intraocular pressure, will not be benefited by lowering intraocular pressure. Patients with conditions such as shock-induced optic neuropathy, traumatic evulsion of the optic nerve, and pituitary adenomas will not be benefited by lowering intraocular pressure. One of the first things that any physician must consider when caring for a patient with glaucoma who seems to be getting worse despite treatment, is "Does this patient really have glaucoma?" Many conditions can mimic glaucoma, that is, can mimic the changes that occur in patients that appear to be caused by pressure within the eye. It is not always possible to determine whether or not the patient has a pressure-dependent condition. To some degree, the very diagnosis of glaucoma is a retrospective one, that is, one that can be made with certainty only when the patient has been shown to improve when the intraocular pressure has been lowered.

It is controversial whether patients with "low-tension glaucoma" are benefited from lowering pressure. One of the reasons for this controversy is certainly that the diagnosis "low-tension glaucoma" is a duffle bag full of many different conditions, some of which are probably true "glaucoma" and some of which are probably not. If the patient does not have a pressure-sensitive condition, then lowering the intraocular pressure is not likely to be of benefit. It is, then, not correct to say, "Patients with low-tension glaucoma are not benefited by lowering intraocular pressure." Rather, it is correct to say, "It is difficult to differentiate those patients with glaucoma occurring in association with normal intraocular pressure from those who have similar findings but in which the intraocular pressure is not currently causing the damage."

By definition, if a patient has a condition in which damage is occurring because the intraocular pressure is too high and the damage is continuing to occur, then the intraocular pressure is too high. One of the serious misunderstandings in the field of glaucoma is that physicians really have a good idea about what a patient's intraocular pressure is. Physicians measure intraocular pressure in an artificial setting, and then generalize from that about what is happening for the rest of the patient's life. In the first place, the measurement of intraocular pressure is only an approximation; pressure varies depending upon compliance of the scleral coats, thickness of the cornea, method of measurement, etc. Again, at the American Glaucoma Society meeting, Joel Schuman reported on the marked inaccuracy of applanation tonometry in infants. If the patient seems to have what we currently think of as "glaucoma" and the patient is getting worse from glaucoma, then the first thing that the ophthalmologist should think about is that the intraocular pressure is too high. But before putting the patient at risk by increasing medications or performing surgery, it has to be determined that the patient is in fact getting worse, *and* that the worsening is being caused by glaucoma. Visual fields vary markedly from time to time and frequently appear to be getting worse when in fact the "change" is mere variability of testing. Is it certain that the visual field has indeed gotten worse? Is it certain that the cause for the worsening is the glaucoma? May it be caused by cataract, fatigue, central nervous system deterioration, or an angioma?

The first consideration, then, is to make sure that the patient actually has a condition in which the ocular tissues are being damaged (or were damaged in the past) by intraocular pressure higher than those tissues can tolerate. The second consideration requires focusing in on the essentials: Has the optic disc gotten worse? Is the visual field really worse? Are the patient's symptoms worse? Changes in the optic disc cannot be noted unless the disc is properly examined. Changes in the visual field can be misleading because the information obtained seems to be "objective" when in fact it is by no means as hard as it appears to be on the printout. Physicians have been trained to pay primary attention to "objective" findings and to give less credence to subjective complaints. We will return to this matter later, but for purposes of the discussion here, this tendency is unfortunate from the point of view of the patient. Especially towards the end stages of glaucoma the objective demonstration of deterioration is difficult; on the other hand, even slight changes in the patient's condition are noted by the alert patient. Thus, the patient who says, "I'm getting worse" must be believed. The worsening may not be caused by glaucoma, but if in fact the patient has glaucoma and the patient says he or she is getting worse, appropriate steps should be taken to confirm or deny the condition objectively and appropriately.

The third issue, the idea that damage may progress inexorably, is an issue about which there is a great deal of heat but not much light. It has been generally assumed that when the optic nerve has become damaged it becomes even more easily damaged. This can be supported theoretically and seems to be supported by some clinical experience, which notes that people who have gotten worse tend to continue to get worse. However, it could be argued with equal logic that the reason why patients with damage are likely to have continuing damage is not because the existing damage predisposes them to the continuing damage, but rather because they were predisposed to getting damage even before the damage occurred. Many of the formulas used to arrive at a "target pressure" advise adding a modifying factor that relates to the amount of damage that is already present. Supposedly the pressure needs to be lower for those in whom marked damage is already present. But, to repeat, the validity of this concept has not been demonstrated. Is lowering intraocular pressure of any benefit in a patient whose optic nerve has become so deformed that the laminar tunnels are now almost totally collapsed on each other? When a patient has far-advanced glaucomatous visual loss, and is getting worse, is the patient more likely to be helped or harmed by having his or her pressure lowered? I believe it is important for us to remember that that question cannot at this time be answered with certainty. My own decisions are determined by the *rate* at which the patient is getting worse and by the patient's own wishes. If the patient's visual loss is continuing at a rate that will cause the patient to be substantively worse before he or she dies, then I usually advise patients to seriously consider surgery. They are told there is a chance they could lose central vision at the time of the surgery (somewhere between 2% and 10%), but that if they do not have surgery, it seems likely they are going to lose vision before they die. Thus, though the surgery promises them nothing and subjects them to significant risks, it may be an option they should consider.

It has been demonstrated by Shiose's study[1] that patients can develop glaucomatous cupping and visual field loss and still have complete return of function. It has not been demonstrated whether that reversible change predisposes the patient to being more susceptible to damage in the future. Unfortunately, at this point the inexorable damage that may occur to patients who already have damage is an issue that it is important to consider but about which there is in fact more heat than light.

There is almost no information in the literature on what makes patients with glaucoma get worse. There is almost no information in the literature on the rate or the way in which patients with glaucoma get worse. There is a vast amount on how *optic discs* get worse or *visual fields* get worse. There is virtually nothing on how *patients* get worse.

To date, almost all studies on the course of glaucoma have centered on what happens to the intraocular pressure, what happens to the optic disc, or what happens to the visual field. These are the three classic measurements of the glaucomatous condition. But, unless patients have been "educated" by physicians or others, patients do not really care what happens to their intraocular pressure, their optic disc, or their visual field. And they are right in not particularly caring. Patients are concerned with whether they are feeling well, whether they are going to continue to feel well, whether they are seeing well, and whether they are going to see well. What justification is there for making a patient who is asymptomatic become symptomatic? How can we really think we are doing our jobs properly when the patient who has no visual complaints is given visual complaints by our treatment or is made sick by the medicine we advise or the surgery we perform?

The objective measurements we make in our patients with glaucoma are only of value insofar as they are *accurate* indicators of the patient's present or future *functional* ability. Our responsibility as physicians is to do what we can to help our patients celebrate life fully. If a patient with "glaucoma" develops optic nerve damage and visual field loss but does not develop any limitation in his or her function, the patient has done well. Our goal is not to prevent any visual field loss. Our goal is only to prevent visual field loss that is so severe that it causes the patient to have some symptomatology. Optic disc damage and visual field damage, then, are only of significance insofar as they are valid indicators of current or future problems. A serious shortcoming in the way glaucoma patients have been approached has been the lack of a system of staging that went from beginning to end. Most of our considerations have merely measured the middle period of glaucoma, that period of time when damage is worsening. I suggest we use a more comprehensive staging system, which encompasses the patient from start to finish (Table 1).

Stage 1 describes the period during which the patient manifests indicators that suggest he or she has a likelihood to develop glaucoma damage. Such indicators include a gene known to be associated with glaucoma, elevated intraocular pressure, an abnormality of the visual field suggestive of glaucoma damage, or other risk factors or signs that are suggestive but not definitive.

Stage 2 is the stage of damage. Here the patient has unquestionable optic disc damage or unquestionable visual field loss, the damage believed to be caused, at least in part, by intraocular pressure higher than the ocular tissues can tolerate. However, in stage 2 the patient is still asymptomatic. That is, at this point the patient is damaged but totally unaware of having been damaged. Serial disc photographs, serial visual fields, estimates of change in nerve fiber layer thickness—all of these are methods of measur-

TABLE 1.—Stages of Glaucoma

- I. Glaucoma Suspect
  - A. Positive Family History of
    - 1. angle-closure attack
    - 2. visual loss caused by chronic glaucoma
  - B. Bearer of Gene for Glaucoma
  - C. Elevation of Intraocular Pressure in Response to Topical Steroids
  - D. Intraocular Pressure 20–30 mm Hg
  - E. Occludable Anterior Chamber Angle
    - 1. C10r or narrower angle
    - 2. D10r or narrower angle
    - 3. C15s or narrower angle
    - 4. D10s or narrower angle
    - 5. Schaffer 0 or 1
  - F. Disc Appearance
    - 1. Cup asymmetry 0.1–0.2 C/D
    - 2. Rim width at inferior or superior pole 0.2–0.3 C/D
    - 3. Cup 0.5 C/D or larger
    - 4. Vertical cup 0.1 C/D larger than horizontal cup
  - G. Exfoliation Syndrome or Pigment Dispersion Syndrome
- II. Asymptomatic Damage
  - A. Questionable Damage
    - 1. Intraocular pressure 31–40 mm Hg
    - 2. Disc appearance
      - a. asymmetry 0.2–0.3 C/D
      - b. rim width 0.1–0.2 C/D
      - c. questionable notch
      - d. questionable saucer
      - e. temporal/inferior rim ratio less than ½
      - f. temporal/superior rim ratio less than ⅔
    - 3. Visual field loss
      - a. nasal hemifield loss, 2 contiguous spots, 5–10 dB
      - b. nasal hemifield loss, 1 spot, 10–15 dB
      - c. paracentral hemifield loss, 2 contiguous spots, 5–10 dB
      - d. paracentral hemifield loss, 1 spot, 10–15 dB
      - e. generalized loss, mean defect 5 dB
    - 4. Optically closed angle with questionable peripheral anterior synechiae
  - B. Definite Damage
    - 1. Intraocular pressure 41–50 mm Hg
    - 2. Disc appearance
      - a. asymmetry 0.3 or greater
      - b. rim lost in no more than 1 quadrant
      - c. definite notch
      - d. definite acquired pit of optic nerve
      - e. disc hemorrhage crossing rim edge
    - 3. Visual field loss
      - a. nasal hemifield loss, 3 contiguous spots, 5–15 dB
      - b. nasal hemifield loss, 2 contiguous spots, 10–20 dB
      - c. arcuate loss, 3 contiguous spots, 10–20 dB
      - d. arcuate loss, 4 contiguous spots, 10–15 dB
      - e. generalized loss, mean defect 5–10 dB
    - 4. Peripheral anterior synechiae less than 50% of angle
  - C. Marked Damage
    - 1. Intraocular pressure above 51 mm Hg
    - 2. Disc appearance
      - a. rim lost in more than 1 quadrant
      - b. superior and inferior notch
    - 3. Visual field loss
      - a. nasal hemifield loss, 4 contiguous spots, 5–15 dB
      - b. nasal hemifield loss, 3 contiguous spots, 15–20 dB
      - c. arcuate loss, 4 contiguous spots, 10–20 dB
      - d. arcuate loss, 3 contiguous spots, 20–30 dB
    - 4. Peripheral anterior synechias more than 50% of angle

(*Continued*)

TABLE 1 (cont.)

III. Symptomatic Damage
- A. Questionable Symptoms
  1. No limitation of function, but sense that vision is not "right"
  2. Intermittent minimal discomfort
- B. Early Functional Loss
  1. Unable to do activities requiring good vision: loses place on page, sees poorly in dark, etc.
  2. Mild, definite pain or discomfort
- C. Moderate Functional Loss
  1. Major change in lifestyle required because of loss of vision: can no longer drive, difficulty reading, etc.
  2. Pain severe enough to interfere with daily activities
- D. Severe Loss
  1. Incapacitated by visual loss or pain

ing the amount of damage and determining whether the damage is worsening, and all of these are concerned primarily with measuring changes occuring within stage 2.

Stage 3 is the stage of symptoms. In stage 3 the damage has worsened to the point that the patient notices that something is wrong. There are presently surveys that question patients about their symptomatology. However, there are no objective scales to monitor change in this stage.

The end of stage 3 is that point at which the patient has become incapacitated by the glaucoma.

Hoskins was right. It is not helpful to think of glaucoma in a way that is so complex that we and our patients are paralyzed by the complexity. It is not advisable to ignore the complexity, but there must be a clarity of definition and purpose. Glaucomatous disease is that condition in which a person has lost visual function or feels pain because of damage to the ocular tissues caused at least partially by intraocular pressure higher than those tissues can tolerate. Before contracting glaucomatous disease, a patient may exhibit the findings of glaucoma, and before that the patient may have the precursory signs of glaucomatous disease. But these should not be confused with or substituted for the disease itself. The goal of therapy is to try to prevent patients from having disease and to achieve that goal with methods that do not cause additional problems.

Reference

1. Shiose Y, Ohmi Y, Kawase Y, et al: Glaucoma and the optic disc: I. Studies on the cup and pallor in the optic disc. *Jpn J Clin Ophthalmol* 32:51, 1978.

Misdiagnosis of Acute Angle Closure Glaucoma

Siriwardena D, Arora AK, Fraser SG, et al (Whipps Cross Hosp, London)
Age Ageing 25:421–423, 1996 3–1

Background.—Approximately 0.1% to 0.2% of the general population develops acute angle closure glaucoma, which is characterized by a sudden onset of severe ocular pain, nausea, vomiting, and significant reduction in vision in the affected eye. The diagnosis can be missed in patients who do not have these classic symptoms, and a delay in diagnosis can permanently affect the patient's vision.

Methods.—Thirty-eight patients with primary acute angle closure glaucoma were identified from the records of a hospital eye unit. The initial diagnosis by the referring physician was obtained, as well as the time between the patients first symptoms and the first treatment given. Of the 38 patients, 25 were women. The mean patient age was 72.9 years.

Results.—The correct diagnosis was made by the referring physician in only 39.5% of patients. Treatment was delayed by a mean of 5.8 days in patients who had a misdiagnosis. General practitioners were the most likely to misdiagnose, and emergency ward physicians were most likely to diagnose acute angle closure glaucoma correctly.

Discussion.—Patients with acute angle glaucoma do not always have typical symptoms. Physicians should have a high degree of suspicion regarding this diagnosis because delayed treatment can severely compromise vision. Expensive equipment or a high level of training is not needed to diagnose acute angle glaucoma. Patients with a red eye and a reduction in vision should immediately be referred to an ophthalmologist.

▶ Ophthalmologists assume that the diagnosis of angle closure glaucoma is fairly straightforward. This article, however, points out the high percentage of patients with angle closure glaucoma in whom the diagnosis is made incorrectly by referring practitioners, with a resultant mean delay of treatment of slightly less than a week! This is a tragic situation. Primary angle-closure glaucoma is a remarkably treatable condition, as long as the diagnosis is made promptly and correctly. In a setting in which an ever-increasing number of patients are receiving their diagnosis from "gatekeepers" or other nonspecialists, it is certain that the number of patients who are improperly diagnosed is going to increase. What is the solution? It is as follows:

1. Ophthalmologists need to educate their professional colleagues regarding the signs and symptoms of angle closure glaucoma.
2. Ophthalmologists need to educate their colleagues regarding the nature of the eye predisposed to the development of an angle closure attack.
3. The public needs to be made aware of the significance of misdiagnosis of angle closure glaucoma and encouraged to take those steps necessary to assure that patients are referred to those able to make an appropriate diagnosis and to initiate appropriate treatment.

G.L. Spaeth, M.D.

Reduction in Intraocular Pressure After Excimer Laser Photorefractive Keratectomy: Correlation With Pretreatment Myopia

Chatterjee A, Shah S, Bessant DA, et al (Optimax Laser Eye Clinic, Manchester, England; Inst of Ophthalmology, London)

Ophthalmology 104:355–359, 1997 3–2

Introduction.—Previous studies have described reduced intraocular pressure (IOP), as measured by applanation tonometry, in eyes undergoing excimer laser photorefractive keratectomy (PRK). However, the accuracy of these measurements can be questioned because of the reduction in central corneal thickness and flattening associated with excimer laser PRK. Reductions in IOP after excimer laser PRK were assessed and correlated with the degree of myopia treated.

Methods.—The study included data on 1,320 patients who had undergone non-simultaneous bilateral excimer laser PRK. The IOP values measured in both eyes at the initial consultation were compared with those recorded at the time of operation in the second eye. The IOP values of the yet-untreated second eyes served as controls for the initially treated eyes. All IOP values were the average of 3 measurements performed on a Nidek NT-1000 automated noncontact tonometer.

Results.—In the untreated eye, measured IOP values were 13.1 mm Hg preoperatively and 12.8 mm Hg postoperatively. In the treated eye, the measurements were 13.0 mm Hg preoperatively and 9.6 mm Hg postop-

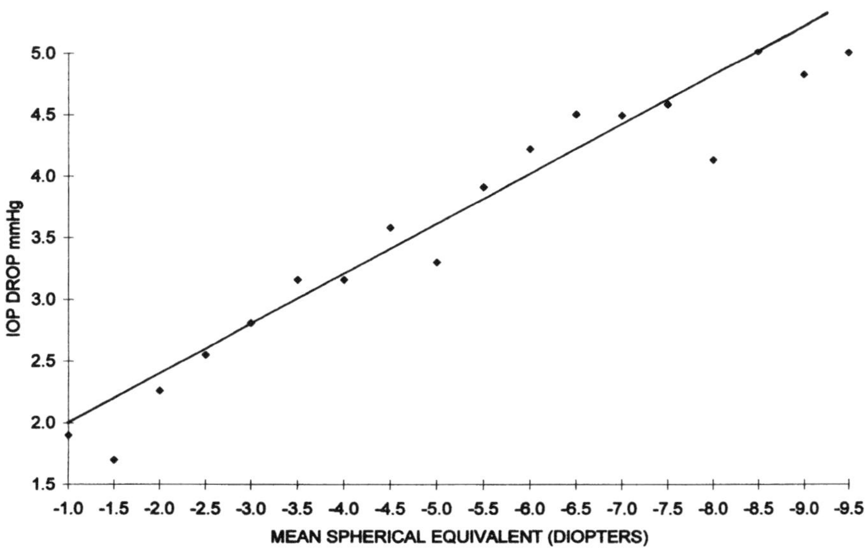

FIGURE 2.—Mean intraocular pressure (*IOP*) drop in treated eye, allowing for diurnal variation (using untreated eye as control). (Published courtesy *of Ophthalmology*, from Chatterjee A, Shah S, Bessant DA, et al: Reduction in intraocular pressure after excimer laser photorefractive keratectomy. *Ophthalmology* 104:355–359, 1997.)

eratively. The mean difference from before to after surgery was 0.3 mm Hg in the untreated eye vs. 3.5 mm Hg in the treated eye. After adjustment for diurnal variation using the fellow eye as a control, the difference was significant at 3.1 mm Hg (Fig 2).

Conclusion.—In eyes undergoing excimer laser PRK, there is a linear relationship between the observed reduction in IOP and the degree of myopia corrected. Determination of the true IOP value in an eye that has undergone PRK requires correction, based on the equation: IOP drop (mm Hg) = 1.6 − [0.4 × treatment MSE (diopters)] where MSE is the mean spherical equivalent. Failure to recognize this phenomenon could lead to failure to recognize dangerous glaucoma.

▶ The authors have performed a great service, using their large excimer laser PRK patient population to confirm what has been noted and discussed recently in refractive circles, which is that IOP measurements seem artificially lowered after PRK. A similar phenomenon is seen in patients with keratoconus, in whom IOP measurements appear falsely low. The main criticism of this study is that *noncontact* tonometry was performed. It is believed by many to not be as accurate as Goldmann applanation tonometry. However, the large patient population makes up for that shortcoming.

The authors demonstrate a highly statistically significant decrease in IOP after PRK, which is directly correlated with the amount of myopia treated when compared with the untreated fellow eye (see Fig 2). This drop is about 4 mm Hg. for a −6.00-D treatment. Although not huge, it should certainly be kept in mind when considering whether a patient's IOP is too high for the optic nerve. As such studies are reproduced and the numbers verified with Goldmann applanation tonometry, perhaps a certain value should be added to a PRK patient's IOP measurement each time the pressure is taken to remind those involved with the patient's care that the measurement may be artificially low.

C.J. Rapuano, M.D.

▶ Several authors have noted that intraocular pressure is lower after certain types of refractive surgery. Indeed, some authors have even suggested refractive surgery as a treatment for glaucoma, arguing that the surgery lowers intraocular pressure. This important contribution shows that excimer laser photorefractive keratectomy does not actually lower intraocular pressure, but lowers the reading on the applanation tonometer. Because the cornea of patients who have had such surgery is thinner, the intraocular pressure is measured as lower than it actually is.

G.L. Spaeth, M.D.

Repeatable Diffuse Visual Field Loss in Open-Angle Glaucoma

Chauhan BC, LeBlanc RP, Shaw AM, et al (Dalhousie Univ, Halifax, NS)

Ophthalmology 104:532–538, 1997 3–3

Introduction.—In glaucoma, diffuse loss may be pressure mediated and localized loss may be caused by nonpressure-related factors. Studies to date on diffuse visual field loss in glaucoma have used only single fields, which could subject the studies to sampling biases. The frequency with which repeatable purely diffuse loss occurred was evaluated in 113 patients with glaucoma.

Methods.—Patients with glaucoma were tested at 6-month intervals using program 30–2 of the Humphrey Field Analyzer. Cumulative defect curves were created for all visual fields at a median of 7 per patient. Visual fields were rated by 2 observers as being: "normal" or showing "diffuse," "localized," or "diffuse and localized" loss. Repeatable diffuse loss was defined as occurring when at least two thirds of the number of fields in the follow-up were determined to be "diffuse."

Results.—Cumulative defect curves indicated that 14 patients (12.4%) had repeatable diffuse loss. Six patients were excluded because of early lens changes despite good visual acuity, and 3 patients were excluded because of a suggestion of localized loss. Repeatable diffuse loss was caused solely by open-angle glaucoma in the remaining 5 patients (4.4%).

Conclusion.—Diffuse visual field loss may be exaggerated by other factors than glaucoma but can occur repeatedly in a small number of patients as the only sign of visual field damage.

► "Glaucoma" suggests a homogeneity that is not present. Of course, there are many different mechanisms for causing intraocular pressure to become elevated. But there are also many different mechanisms that account for the optic nerve damage that occurs in patients, even when they have the same mechanism responsible for elevating their intraocular pressure.

The article by Chauhan and associates is a nice addition to the literature, documenting the fact that some types of glaucoma are associated with widespread damage over the entire visual field. This clearly represents a different pathogenesis than the other types of glaucoma, in which visual field damage is sharply circumscribed, becoming deeper and deeper in 1 small area before spreading. This type of field defect is specifically considered and quantitated in some visual field software and testing programs.

The more diffuse types of visual field loss are generally not considered to be so "real" and are often attributed to other factors, such as a decrease in the clarity of the media or fatigue. As knowledge of the subtypes of glaucoma becomes more complete, we will learn more about the various subtypes of visual field damage that occur in these different clinical entities.

G.L. Spaeth, M.D.

Variability in Patients With Glaucomatous Visual Field Damage is Reduced Using Size V Stimuli

Wall M, Kutzko KE, Chauhan BC (Univ of Iowa, Iowa City; Dahousie Univ, Halifax, NS)

Invest Ophthalmol Vis Sci 38:426–435, 1997 3–4

Introduction.—The automation of perimetry has provided many benefits. However, variability of conventional automated perimetry continues to be too high in areas of visual field damage. An analysis of frequency-of-seeing curves was performed in patients with glaucoma and normal controls using Goldmann stimulus sizes I, III, and V.

Methods.—Ten patients with glaucoma and 5 age-matched controls underwent testing with the Humphrey Field Analyzer program 24-2 or 30-2. The method of constant stimuli was used to measure frequency-of-seeing curves by controlling the perimeter with a custom computerized program. Using 2 widely separated visual field locations on the program 24-2 or 30-2 grid, stimuli were presented in 2-dB intervals to at least 10 dB on either side of the estimated program 24-2 or 30-2 threshold for Goldmann sizes I, III, and V. In patients with glaucoma, 1 test location was used in an area of normal visual field sensitivity and 1 was in an area of 10 to 20 dB loss. Controls were tested at the (3°, 3°) and (−21°, −9°) test locations. There were 15 repetitions at each intensity.

Results.—Variance was lowest at the abnormal test location in patients with glaucoma using a size V stimulus. There were significant differences between results from the V to III and V to I stimuli. This trend in estimated standard deviations was also observed in tests of the area of normal sensitivity in patients with glaucoma and for the controls' peripheral test locations, but not the central location. The smaller decrease in variability between estimated standard deviations of the size I and III stimuli was not significant at any test location.

Conclusion.—Findings are in agreement with earlier reports regarding high test result variability in patients with glaucoma and moderate visual field loss. The size V stimuli decreased variability in tests of moderately damaged and normal sensitivity test locations in patients with glaucoma.

▶ Most ophthalmologists performing automated perimetry use the size III stimulus. The size III stimulus is used even in patients who have advanced glaucoma. There are, however, valid reasons for using a larger stimulus size, such as stimulus V. When there is no response to stimulus size III, so that the test is recorded as a zero, and the test is repeated and again there is no response, so that the field chart again shows a zero, the ophthalmologist may conclude that there has been no change in the visual field. After all, both results are zero.

But this is not the case. A zero does not mean an absolute loss of vision. A zero with test III stimulus simply means that the patient was unable to see the brightest size III test size stimulus. However, that patient may well have been able to see the brightest size V test stimulus. If at the time of the initial test a size V stimulus had been used and the patient had been able to see that stimulus, then at a retest the size V stimulus objects had been used again, but at the time of the retest the patient was unable to see that stimulus, then one could conclude that the patient had become worse.

Using a larger stimulus, then, increases the ability to detect change when the amount of visual field loss is advanced. The authors have indicated in this paper that in patients with significant glaucoma damage, a larger test object also decreases the variability of the test results.

Specificity and sensitivity tend to move in opposite directions. Smaller test objects tend to be able to pick up smaller defects, that is, smaller test objects may be more sensitive than larger test objects in finding visual field defects. But smaller test objects tend to be less specific than larger test objects. A defect found by a larger test object is more likely to be a real defect.

G.L. Spaeth, M.D.

Clinical Presentation and Initial Treatment Patterns With Exfoliation Glaucoma Versus Primary Open-Angle Glaucoma

Konstas AGP, Stewart WC, Stroman GA, et al (Aristotelian Univ of Thessaloniki, Greece; Pharmaceutical Research Corp, Charleston, SC)

Ophthalmic Surg Lasers 28:111–117, 1997 3–5

Introduction.—Patients with exfoliation glaucoma (PXE) are thought to be more difficult to manage medically than patients with primary open-angle glaucoma (POAG). Patients with PXE and POAG were prospectively evaluated to compare initial findings and response to treatment.

Methods.—Evaluations of optic disc, visual field, and intraocular pressure (IOP) were compared in 22 and 24 consecutive newly diagnosed patients with PXE and POAG, respectively. Treatment response was also compared.

Results.—Optic disc and peripapillary parameters were similar between patients with PXE and POAG at initial evaluation. The mean defect was significantly worse in patients with PXE, compared with patients with POAG. Loss variances were similar between groups. The mean initial IOP for patients with PXE was significantly higher than for patients with POAG. Significantly more treatment steps were required to control IOP in patients with PXE, compared with patients with POAG. Thirteen of 24 patients with PXE and 3 of 22 patients with POAG needed either laser or conventional surgical techniques to decrease IOP; the difference was significant.

Conclusion.—On initial examination, patients with PXE had higher IOP and greater visual field loss than patients with POAG. Intraocular pressure was more difficult to manage in patients with PXE than in patients with POAG.

► The exfoliation syndrome is probably more common than is generally recognized. The amount of variability of expression of the exfoliation syndrome is also probably more common than is generally recognized. Overall, about 50% of patients with exfoliation syndrome ultimately receive a diagnosis of glaucoma.[1]

But those patients in whom glaucoma develops in association with the exfoliation syndrome tend to have a glaucoma that is unstable and in which progressive damage often occurs more rapidly than in open-angle glaucomas without the exfoliation syndrome. The article by Konstas and associates should make us more aware of how potentially damaging glaucoma in association with the exfoliation syndrome can be. As such, once glaucoma develops in patients with the exfoliation syndrome, these patients probably need to be followed more closely than would be true for most of the other types of open-angle glaucoma.

G.L. Spaeth, M.D.

Reference

1. Johnson DH: The exfoliation syndrome: A continuing challenge, in Albert DM, Jakobiec FA (eds): *Principles and Practice of Ophthalmology*, vol 3. Philadelphia, WB Saunders, 1993, pp 1400–1412.

Topical Beta-blockade With Intrinsic Sympathomimetic Activity Offers No Advantage for the Respiratory and Cardiovascular Function of Elderly People

Diggory P, Cassels-Brown A, Fernandez C (St James's Univ Hosp, Leeds, England; Mayday Hosp, London)

Age Ageing 25:424–428, 1996 3–6

Background.—Chronic open-angle glaucoma becomes more common with age and occurs in 5% of individuals older than 65 years. It is asymptomatic until visual field is lost. Chronic open-angle glaucoma is responsible for 15% of registrations for blindness in this older population. The aim of therapy is to lower intraocular pressure. Application of topical β-antagonists is the most common treatment but may result in unrecognized impairment of respiratory and cardiovascular funtion in elderly patients. The β-antagonists carteolol and betaxolol may cause less impairment because of their intrinsic sympathomimetic or cardioselective properties.

Methods.—In a randomized, double-blind study, the effects of carteolol and betaxolol were compared with those of timolol. The study included 60 patients older than 60 years with glaucoma and no history of bronchospasm. Patients underwent spirometry and pulse and blood pressure were measured at baseline and at 4 weeks.

Results.—Mean spirometric values did not change significantly in patients given timolol or carteolol. After patients changed to betaxolol from timolol, mean peak flow improved by 9.1% and forced expiratory volume in 1 second (FEV_1) improved by 9.4%. Differences in the changes in peak flow and FEV_1 between betaxolol and timolol and between betaxolol and carteolol were significant. Clinical improvement in FEV_1 was seen in 21% of patients given betaxolol. When carteolol was substituted for timolol, pulse and blood pressure did not change, but mean resting pulse increased by 10 beats per minute in patients given betaxolol.

Discussion.—In older patients, the intrinsic sympathomimetic activity of carteolol has no advantage over timolol in spirometry, pulse or blood pressure in patients with glaucoma. Carteolol was well tolerated by these patients and is an excellent ocular hypotensive agent. When these patients changed from timolol to betaxolol, spirometry improved, and respiratory symptoms and resting pulse rate improved slightly. Routine monitoring of pulse, blood pressure, and spirometry is recommended for elderly patients treated with β-antagonists. If bradycardia, hypotension, or a decrease of more than 15% in peak flow and FEV_1 occurs, alternatives to topical β-antagonists should be sought.

► Systemic symptoms are common in patients with glaucoma who are receiving topical or systemic medications to treat the glaucomatous condition. Family practitioners and internists frequently do not obtain full histories regarding the use of ophthalmic medications. Ophthalmologists frequently do not obtain full histories regarding systemic side effects. The consequence is that patients not infrequently have systemic side effects caused by ophthalmic medications, but the cause for the side effect is not attributed to the ophthalmic medication. This paper by Diggory and colleagues establishes the significantly lesser likelihood of respiratory side effects in patients who are receiving betaxolol compared with timolol or carteolol.

Ophthalmologists should not conclude, however, that betaxolol is always the β-blocker of choice or that betaxolol is free of pulmonary, much less other, systemic side effects. Timolol can lower intraocular pressure more markedly than betaxolol and, thus, may offer an advantage over betaxolol. However, when timolol, carteolol, or other topical β-blockers are used to treat patients with glaucoma, both the patient and the physician must be aware of the propensity of these medications to cause pulmonary side effects. In many cases, the side effect is minimal, and the patient manages to cope with it fairly well. In many other cases, the side effect is attributed by the patient to aging, "chronic bronchitis," or some source other than the topical β-blocker. Especially in the elderly, who are predisposed to respiratory problems, betaxolol offers the advantage of a decreased likelihood of pulmonary side effects.

G.L. Spaeth, M.D.

A Review of the Outcome of Trabeculectomy in Open-Angle Glaucoma

Vesti E, Raitta C (Helsinki Univ)

Ophthalmic Surg Lasers 28:128–132, 1997 3–7

Introduction.—Glaucoma surgery is the most effective means of decreasing intraocular pressure (IOP), but it is rarely used as a primary treatment. Trabeculectomy outcome at 1-year follow-up was evaluated in 87 consecutive eyes of 87 patients with open-angle glaucoma.

Methods.—Outcome of trabeculectomy was associated with a biomicroscopic appearance of the filtering bleb. Visual acuity, myopic shift in refraction, and lens opacity measurements were used as determinants for cataract progression. The effects of viscoelastics on complications and short-term outcome were evaluated in a randomized series of 107 eyes. Fifty-six percent and 44% of eyes, respectively, had exfoliative glaucoma and primary open-angle glaucoma (POAG). Success was defined as an IOP of less than 22 mm Hg with, or preferably without, additional glaucoma medication.

Results.—When the success rate was defined as an IOP of less than 22 mm Hg without glaucoma medication, 77% of eyes with POAG and 72% of eyes with exfoliative glaucoma were considered to have been treated successfully with trabeculectomy. Preoperative treatment with miotics and possibly with laser trabeculoplasty, anterior fistulation, and postoperative hypotony was associated with unfavorable flap-sized blebs and bleb failure. In the randomized, prospective trial of 107 eyes, there was no significant change in incidence of complications or short-term outcome when sodium hyaluronate was used.

Conclusion.—Treatment was unsuccessful in about 30% of eyes when success was defined as an IOP of below 22 mm Hg without glaucoma medication. The use of sodium hyaluronate had no significant effect on the incidence of complications or short term outcome in 107 eyes.

▶ Vesti and Raitta have noted that the preoperative use of miotics and the postoperative occurrence of a very low IOP predispose to poor results of glaucoma filtering surgery. This article, especially when considered with the previous one, stresses the importance of caring for glaucoma patients in a way that results in the least damage to the tissues, either by medications used before surgery or medications used at the time of surgery itself.

G.L. Spaeth, M.D.

Combined Cataract and Glaucoma Procedures Using Temporal Cataract Surgery

Gayton JL, Van Der Karr MA, Sanders V (EyeSight Associates, Warner Robins, Ga; Ctr for Clinical Research, Chicago)

J Cataract Refract Surg 22:1485–1491, 1996 3–8

Background.—When cataract and glaucoma surgery are performed at the same time, the additional morbidity and cost associated with 2 surgeries are eliminated. However, it has been reported that combined surgeries can induce 2.00 diopters or more of against-the-rule astigmatism.

Methods.—A comparison was made of 50 consecutive eyes that received a superior cataract incision with a superonasal trabeculectomy, and of 65 eyes that received a temporal cataract incision with a superonasal trabeculectomy. The mean patient age was about 75 years.

Results.—At 3 months, significantly more patients who had had a temporal incision had controlled intraocular pressure without medication. Significantly more patients who had had a superior incision had uncontrolled intraocular pressure at each postoperative visit. At every postoperative visit, the mean surgically induced cylinder was higher in patients who had had a superior incision. Patients who had had a superior incision had early with-the-rule mean induced cylinder that decayed to against-the-rule. At more than 3 months, this group had a mean induced cylinder with keratometry of −1.01 D. Patients who had had a temporal incision initially had a negligible induced cylinder of −0.13 D that drifted somewhat with the rule to a final mean induced cylinder of +0.49 D. At the last follow up visit, 31% of patients who had had a superior incision and 57% of patients who had had a temporal incision had an uncorrected visual acuity of 20/40 or better; 72% of patients who had had a superior incision and 94% of patients who had had a temporal incision had a best corrected visual acuity of 20/40 or better.

Discussion.—Separating cataract and glaucoma surgical procedures to a temporal cataract incision frees the surgeon to use the more astigmatically neutral techniques of temporal, sutureless cataract surgery. The advantages of performing both procedures are maintained. Patients who had had a temporal incision had less surgically induced cylinder.

► The goal of surgery in a patient with a cataract is clear: obtain the best possible visual acuity with the least morbidity and cost. This goal is, of course, not a new one; nor is it an absolute one. Improvements continue to be made in the technique of cataract surgery, but the goal today is the same as it was 2 years, 5 years, 50 or 500 years ago.

In contrast, the goal of glaucoma surgery is far more complex, because the disease is far more complex. The goal is not simply to lower intraocular pressure, because pressure below approximately 8 mm Hg is associated with increasing complications, poorer vision, and less patient satisfaction. Nor is the goal merely to lower intraocular pressure to an "acceptable" level. In the first place, who knows *a priori* what is an acceptable level? Presumably, if the patient's glaucoma has been getting worse with a pressure of 25 mm Hg, an acceptable level would be below 25 mm Hg. But is it 20 mm Hg, or 15 mm Hg, or 10 mm Hg?

In the second place, by an "acceptable," level does one mean the intraocular pressure during the first 2 weeks postoperatively, at the end of 1 month, or at the end of 5 years? A badly damaged optic nerve may become more badly damaged in the first two postoperative weeks, at which time a pressure is characteristically quite high in a glaucoma patient having cataract surgery unassociated with a filtration procedure. However, 1 year after surgery, the intraocular pressure will probably be lower than it was preoperatively. Such findings have been used to support the performance of a cataract extraction without a filtering procedure in a patient with glaucoma. But an intraocular pressure that is "acceptable" at 1 year in the patient just mentioned, was completely unacceptable 2 weeks after the surgery!

In the third place, lowering intraocular pressure is achieved at a cost, and a pressure level "acceptable" from the point of view of pressure may be associated with such unpleasant symptoms for the patient that the surgery surely could not be called successful. For example, a patient may have an intraocular pressure of 10 mm Hg, which the surgeon thought was going to be perfect, but also have a filtering bleb which produces photophobia and tearing and is predisposed to recurrent infections. One could hardly call such a surgical procedure "totally successful."

In the most generic sense, then, a successful glaucoma surgical procedure would be one that was as inexpensive as possible and resulted in as rapid improvement in a patient's visual function as possible (or at least was associated with no further deterioration) immediately after the surgery and for the duration of the patient's life. Unfortunately, there is no procedure that comes anywhere close to fulfilling this generic goal.

When one combines glaucoma surgery with cataract surgery, one introduces into the glaucoma part of the procedure a completely unwanted aspect, specifically, an increased degree of ocular inflammation, which appears to be (at this point) an unavoidable aspect of cataract surgery. Consequently, studies that have evaluated intraocular pressure 3 months after surgery (a fairly common time period in reports of combined cataract-glaucoma surgery) have only dealt with 1 aspect of the need to control intraocular pressure after cataract extraction in a patient with glaucoma.

The authors of the study abstracted here have shown that they can achieve less astigmatism by placing the incision for the cataract surgery temporally and performing the filtration aspect of the surgery superonasally. Their study did not involve a prospective random design, and the results suggest—but by no means confirm—their hypothesis that using separate incisions will result in less astigmatism. Additionally, the authors report better control of intraocular pressure at 2–4 weeks postoperatively in those patients having 2 incisions in comparison with those having one incision. This is helpful information, but, unfortunately, the authors do not provide information regarding the results during the first few days postoperatively, which is a critically important time in patients with glaucoma.

Selecting the procedure that is most appropriate for a patient who has both glaucoma and a cataract demands individualization of the procedure. There is no generic "best" operation for a patient with glaucoma, and there is no generic "best" operation for a patient who has a cataract in addition to glaucoma. In some individuals, cataract extraction alone is most appropriate; in others, glaucoma surgery alone is most appropriate; and combinations of the 2 surgeries are most appropriate for other individuals.

What Gayton, Van Der Karr, and Sanders have done is to provide helpful information that suggests that performing a guarded filtration procedure superonasally and a cataract extraction temporally may be a highly appropriate approach to surgery in some patients with glaucoma who need a cataract extraction. This is an important contribution. However, it would be unfortunate if those reading their report concluded that the authors had established what is now "the best way" to remove a cataract in a patient with glaucoma.

G.L. Spaeth, M.D.

Clinicopathologic Features and Surgical Management of Dissecting Glaucoma Filtering Blebs

Ulrich, GG, Proia AD, Shields MB (Duke Univ, Durham, NC)

Ophthalmic Surg Lasers 28:151–155, 1997 3–9

Introduction.—Glaucoma filtering blebs are associated with many postoperative complications. A filtering bleb extending over the cornea is a late complication that is uncommon but potentially serious. Three cases of glaucoma filtering bleb migrating over the cornea that required surgical treatment are described.

> *Case Report.*—Man, 73, had a history of open-angle glaucoma and underwent posterior lip sclerectomy of the left eye in 1972. After 4 years, a large, white filtering bleb extending over the superior cornea had developed. The bleb continued to migrate toward the visual axis and reduced his vision to 20/80. Bleb revision was done in 1977. The bleb healed with no leakage or recurrence of the excessive bleb and retention of good intraocular pressure control. The patient's visual acuity improved to only 20/60. The patient later had cataract extraction by an inferior incision.

Discussion.—Three different revision techniques were used in these patients, and the revised blebs have continued to function. After a 15- to 17-year follow-up in 2 of these 3 cases, the dissecting filtering blebs have not recurred. Various terms are used to describe a glaucoma filtering bleb that crosses the limbus and extends over the cornea, including extension, migration, dissection, overhanging, and overlying. The lack of agreement of terms reflects the incomplete understanding of the mechanism of this complication. It is unclear if it is a true dissection between layers of the cornea, or a massaging by lid action of a large conjunctival bleb over the surface of the cornea. The authors suggest that aqueous humor dissects between the corneal epithelium and stroma, resulting in abnormal hydration of the superficial lamellae. A large, high-flow surgical fistula may be associated with the development of a dissecting glaucoma filtering bleb.

The 3 cases in the current report had full-thickness scleral fistulae, which also was true in most cases previously reported.

► This paper reminds us of a highly useful method of managing a rare condition, specifically the bleb that spreads down over the cornea over a period of many years. The method the authors suggest would be totally inappropriate for most of the bleb problems that are bothering patients today. The most common problems now are a consequence of the use of mitomycin C. Conjunctiva and Tenon's capsule treated with mitomycin C have a proclivity to become totally ischemic and virtually necrotic. Where that occurs, the tissue covering the pocket of aqueous humor in the subconjunctival space is a thin layer. It may be so thin that aqueous leaks through it spontaneously, or holes develop in the layer. If this thin layer were incised, it would leave bare sclera underneath it and an eye in serious trouble.

A second type of bleb associated with mitomycin C is that in which the tissue covering the sclerostomy consists of loculated cysts, as is true for the filtering bleb that follows standard guarded filtration procedures and full-thickness filtration procedures. However, the surface layer of this loculated collection of small cysts becomes so thin that the aqueous leaks through it excessively, or holes in the layer develop, threatening the well-being of the eye. Were this superficial layer to be cut and excised, it would leave the underlying cysts, which would provide some protection of the globe and could reepithelialize. However, where the tissue had been significantly damaged by the antimetabolite, excessive filtration would be likely to recur.

The type of bleb problem described in this article is quite different. The bleb that forms after a full-thickness filtration procedure is usually multiloculated. This is also the case for the blebs that follow guarded filtration procedures, except these blebs tend to be a bit thicker. After many years, these multiloculated blebs can spread down over the cornea, and as pointed out by the authors, this spreading is subepithelial. There is no actual attachment of the underlying tissue to the corneal stroma. This type of bleb must be distinguished from the thin-layered antimetabolite bleb. The loculated bleb is far more opaque; the sclera cannot be seen; there may be small blood vessels in the interstices of the cysts; and there is real substance to the bleb. If the bleb is compressed with an instrument, it is noted to have resistance, much like boggy tissue whereas the antimetabolite-damaged thin conjunctival layer can be flattened out, there being nothing between the surface and the sclera except aqueous.

The amputation of the excessive tissue spreading down the cornea is well described. The method, however, also can be used in the same type of bleb that has become too florid and elevated, and is causing dellen or other symptoms. In such cases one can simply cut off the surface layers of the bleb, thinning the bleb markedly, with prompt relief of the patient's symptoms. In most cases, there is no change in intraocular pressure. Although there may be a short duration of seepage of aqueous humor through the cut edge, in most cases this does not occur at all, and it is rarely a problem.

Again, however, such a method would be totally inappropriate in blebs that are not thick and multiloculated.

G.L. Spaeth, M.D.

Identification of a Gene That Causes Primary Open Angle Glaucoma
Stone EM, Fingert JH, Alward WLM, et al (Univ of Iowa, Iowa City; Univ of California, San Francisco; Alcon Labs Inc, Fort Worth, Tex; et al)
Science 275:668–670, 1997 3–10

Background.—Glaucoma is a common cause of blindness. The most common form of glaucoma is primary open angle glaucoma (POAG), which affects 1% to 2% of the population older than 40 years. The molecular basis of POAG is not well understood. Juvenile POAG refers to a subset of POAG with an earlier age of onset. A genetic locus (GLC1A) associated with juvenile POAG was identified on chromosome 1q21-q31 by genetic linkage analysis. This interval was narrowed, using observed recombination in large kindreds, to a 3-centimorgan region of chromosome 1q between D1S3665 and D1S3664. Two potential POAG genes in this region, APT1LG1 and TIGR (trabecular meshwork-induced glucocorticoid response protein), were screened for mutations in juvenile POAG kindreds.

Methods and Results.—The TIGR gene assay was used to screen affected members of 4 different chromosome 1q-linked large glaucoma families and 4 smaller families. A tyrosine to histidine mutation in codon 430 (Tyr430His)was detected in all 22 affected members of 1 family. A glycine to valine mutation in codon 357 was detected in 2 families. A nonsense mutation at codon 361 was detected in 2 families. The prevalence of these TIGR mutations was estimated by screening patients with glaucoma with a family history, unselected POAG probands, the general population and unrelated volunteers older than 40 years with normal intraocular pressures and no history of glaucoma. Eight additional individuals with the Gln361STOP mutation and 1 with the Tyr430His mutation were identified. No amino acid-altering mutations were detected in those known to be free of glaucoma. The Gln361STOP mutation was detected in 1 person from the general population. This mutation was also detected in 3 of 103 unrelated patients with POAG seen in a glaucoma clinic. These findings indicate that mutations in the GLC1A gene are involved in a significant fraction of all cases of glaucoma. Missense or nonsense mutations were detected in 13 of 330 unrelated patients with glaucoma and 1 of 471 controls. This difference was highly significant.

Conclusions.—Genetic linkage analysis and screening for shared haplotypes was used to narrow the previously identified glaucoma disease gene interval on chromosome 1q. A gene that lies within this region and is known to be expressed in the ciliary body and trabecular meshwork, TIGR, was analyzed. Mutations in this gene were detected in 13 unrelated patients with glaucoma. This provides evidence that TIGR mutations may be responsible for the cases of glaucoma linked to chromosome 1q. Identification of this gene is important, because although treatment for glaucoma is available, it is difficult to detect before the onset of optic nerve damage. Specific glaucoma-causing mutations would be useful for identifying patients at high risk and directing them toward screening and treatment to prevent loss of vision.

Exclusion of One Pedigree Affected by Adult Onset Primary Open Angle Glaucoma From Linkage to the Juvenile Glaucoma Locus on Chromosome 1q21-q31

Avramopoulos D, Kitsos G, Economou-Petersen E, et al (Inst of Child Health, Athens, Greece; Univ Eye Clinic of Ioannina, Greece; Univ of Athens, Greece; et al)

J Med Genet 33:1043–1044, 1996 3–11

Background.—Glaucoma is a common cause of blindness. The most common form of glaucoma is primary open angle glaucoma (POAG), which affects 1% to 2% of the population older than 40 years. The molecular basis of POAG is not well understood. Juvenile POAG refers to a subset of POAG with an earlier age of onset. A genetic locus (GLC1A) associated with juvenile POAG was identified on chromosome 1q21-q31 by genetic linkage analysis. Blood samples were collected from 50 members of a large POAG kindred identified in Epirus, Greece, and investigated with microsatellite markers to examine linkage.

Methods.—This kindred had clinical findings that were consistent with POAG. The age at diagnosis was at least 30 years and POAG appeared to be transmitted in an autosomal dominant fashion.

Findings.—Lod score analysis demonstrated no linkage between adult onset POAG in this kindred and the entire 1q21-q31 chromosomal region previously associated with juvenile POAG.

Conclusions.—These linkage data indicate that the POAG gene mutated in this kindred does not lie in the previously identified region on chromosome 1q associated with juvenile POAG. This suggests that juvenile and adult onset POAG may be distinct genetic entities.

► The articles from Stone and colleagues (Abstract 3–10) and Avramopoulos and colleagues (Abstract 3–11) are among the continuing contributions to the understanding of the genetic basis of glaucoma. Some glaucomas appear to have a primary genetic basis, whereas others are solely the result of environmental influences. The overwhelming majority of glaucomas are a consequence of genetic factors interacting with environmental forces. One type of glaucoma that appears to be strongly related to a genetic abnormality is the noninflammatory, open-angle glaucoma that occurs in individuals between the ages of around 10 and 40 years. This type of glaucoma has been related to an abnormality located on chromosome 1q21-q31. Further study of pedigrees of individuals with juvenile POAG have allowed the position of the responsible abnormality to be narrowed to the region between markers D1S3665 and D1S3664. The 2 articles mentioned here deal with noninflammatory, open-angle glaucoma that occurs in older individuals, the type of glaucoma that recently has been called primary open-angle glaucoma. Avramopoulos and colleagues noted that, in their pedigree, no abnormality was found in the locus that has been held responsible for at least one type of juvenile POAG. They conclude that juvenile POAG and POAG are probably genetically distinct conditions. In contrast, the paper by Stone and colleagues found an abnormality in the same area in around 3% of an unselected population of adult patients with POAG.

The glaucomas are conditions in which it appears that the sequence of damage is initially pressure that is higher than the tissue can tolerate, then functional loss secondary to the tissue damage. Usually this damage occurs to the optic nerve and is manifested in loss of visual field and other forms of visual deficit. There is a relatively poor correlation between level of intraocular pressure and subsequent tissue damage until the pressure is in a range of around 30 mm Hg or so. At the present time, the only way to tell with complete certainty whether or not an individual is predisposed to glaucoma damage is to wait until the person has glaucoma damage. Because such damage entails structural change, it is reasonable to suspect that the damaged individual then becomes predisposed to having more damage. Following up individuals to detect the earliest damage caused by glaucoma is expensive, time-consuming, and inconvenient. The existence of a test that will select those who are at greater risk for having glaucoma than others is a major step ahead, because it should facilitate the early diagnosis of the condition.

G.L. Spaeth, M.D.

Familial Glaucoma Iridogoniodysplasia Maps to a 6p25 Region Implicated in Primary Congenital Glaucoma and Iridogoniodysgenesis Anomaly

Jordan T, Ebenezer N, Manners R, et al (Inst of Ophthalmology, London; Southampton Gen Hosp, England)

Am J Hum Genet 61:882–888, 1997 3–12

Purpose.—Patients with familial glaucoma iridogoniodysplasia (FGI) have open-angle glaucoma related to developmental anomalies of the iris and irido-corneal angle. Affected families transmit juvenile-onset glaucoma as an autosomal dominant trait. A genetic-linkage study was performed in a large Caucasian family with FGI.

Findings.—The study included 71 family members belonging to a single, large branch originating in the fifth generation. Linkage analysis was performed in 46 family members, 24 of whom were affected by FGI. The 46 participants were examined for genetic linkage to microsatellite markers. Marker D6S967 mapping to chromosome 6p25 showed a peak score of 11.63 at a recombination fraction of 0. On haplotype analysis, the disease gene was localized to a 6.4 cm interval between D6S1713 and D6S1600. All patients with the characteristic iris appearance of FGI developed glaucoma before age 40 years; no patient with normal irides developed early glaucoma. A range of phenotypes was apparent, consistent with variable expressivity of the FGI gene.

Conclusions.—This genetic study links FGI to a 6.4 cm interval in the chromosome 6p25 region. This region has now been implicated in primary congenital glaucoma and iridogoniodysgenesis anomaly, as well as FGI. A common gene may be involved in all 3 conditions, or there may be a cluster of genes involved in eye development or function. The development of a mouse model of glaucoma should be a high research priority for pathogenetic and treatment studies.

► Frequently now, reports are published about newly-discovered relationships between how we manifest ourselves (our phenotype) and how we are formed (our genotype). In the field of glaucoma, relationships are being found between specific types of glaucoma and specific genetic characteristics. The excitement about these discoveries appears to be related primarily to two beliefs: first, that once we have understood our genetic make-up we will finally have the means of understanding who and what we are; and second, that "gene therapy" will permit the elimination of "bad genes," leading to a world that is almost completely free of disease. And indeed the new genetic discoveries are thrilling. But it is not likely that either of the above anticipated benefits will ever come to pass.

We are enormously complex creatures, and the way our genes interact with each other and with the environment to make us who we are will probably never be well understood, and will certainly never be fully understood. However, there will be important and valuable insights. We'll have a better sense of why it is that, according to the old adages, "Jack Sprat could eat no fat, his wife could eat no lean," or "One man's meat is another man's poison." It should be possible to make decisions about what will make us healthy and what will make us sick on a more rational basis.

The matter of gene replacement is even more unfathomable. Successful replacement of genes is proving far more difficult than most of us thought. The question is not just when but whether it will be possible to develop methods of splicing in new genes or taking out bad genes. But other, less dramatic approaches to gene therapy are not only proving possible but already finding application; for example, agents which selectively repress gene expression have been used. But again, deciding which genes to suppress and which to stimulate will not always be an easy choice; genes may well be beneficial in some settings and harmful in others, and the effects of altering the expression of a gene are not easily predictable.

Increasing the understanding of our genetic make-up may prove to be highly beneficial in determining who is at risk for developing a particular disease. This ability will be especially important where effective preventive therapies are already known, as is at least partially true with regard to glaucoma. It is not feasible to perform visual field examinations and to obtain optic disc photographs for every person every year. But if it is known that a person has, say, a 50% chance of developing optic nerve damage caused by glaucoma, in comparison to the normal 1% to 2% likelihood, then it becomes feasible to select those at high risk, to educate them, and to monitor them frequently enough that treatment can be started before troublesome symptoms develop.

G.L. Spaeth, M.D.

Chiropractic Care of a Pediatric Glaucoma Patient: A Case Study

Conway CM (Janesville, Wis)

J Clin Chiroprac Pediatr 2:155–156, 1997 3–13

Objective.—Infantile glaucoma is a rare but potentially disastrous condition. Surgical treatment with goniotomy is indicated, and may have to be repeated. There have been no published studies of the chiropractic management of glaucoma. The chiropractic care of an infant with congenital glaucoma is reported.

Case.—Girl, 17 months, was brought for chiropractic care. The infant was born with glaucoma, for which she had undergone 13 previous surgeries. She was prone to sinus infections, which led to severe eye infections requiring hospitalization. The patient was scheduled for adenoid surgery and had received systemic and topical steroids, antibiotics, and many other drugs. Examination revealed a high right shoulder with tension in the cervical paravertebral musculature and increased tonicity of the suboccipital muscles. Examination by Activator Methods showed right pelvic deficiency with right lateral atlas involvement. Adjustments were performed using the Activator Methods and Craniosacral techniques. Repeated adjustments were made over several months, with particular attention to the atlas and cervical spine. The chiropractor suspected birth trauma related to a short duration of labor. Dietary changes were made as well.

With 1 month of chiropractic care, the patient's intraocular pressure readings decreased from 21 to 17 mm Hg in the right eye and from 28 to 15 mm Hg in the left eye. Further reductions to 14 and 11 mm Hg, respectively, were achieved after 4 months. The scheduled adenoid surgery was canceled. At age 3 years, the patient's intraocular pressure was normal and she was free of all medications.

Discussion.—This article describes the benefits of chiropractic care for an infant with congenital glaucoma and recurrent sinus infections. The normalization of intraocular pressure achieved in this case is thought to result from the direct correlation of her cervical spine and its relationship to the CNS. The author calls for more study of the trauma of childbirth, its effects on the nervous system, and the potential for functional alterations in the newborn.

► Wow! Now it's possible to cure congenital glaucoma without the risk of surgery. Or is it? The author is apparently unaware that the signs of congenital glaucoma can disappear spontaneously. Occasionally infants are found to have cloudy corneas and elevated intraocular pressures in their early infancy and yet the cloudy corneas will clear spontaneously and the intraocular pressure will fall spontaneously with time. However, the case described by Conway is quite different. The axial lengths of the 2 eyes strongly suggest that the left eye had glaucomatous nerve damage of a significant degree. The difference in the intraocular pressures suggests that there was a real difference in the pressure between the two eyes. Yet, with no ocular treatment, the intraocular pressure in the left eye actually became lower than that in the right eye. Was there anything to the chiropractic treatment?

I rather doubt the author's suggestion that "the proposed mechanism of the normalization of her intraocular pressure . . . [was] the direct correlation of the cervical spine and its relationship to the central nervous system." However, it is becoming clear that physicians have been far too arrogant about the possible benefits of alternative or unconventional methods of therapy. We need to be far more open to the real possibility that some of these therapies are beneficial.

G.L. Spaeth, M.D.

Suggested Reading

Azuara-Blanco A, Spaeth GL: Methods to objectify reversibility of glaucomatous cupping. *Curr Opin Ophthalmol* 8:50–54, 1997.

► Almost 150 years ago von Jaeger described improvement in the appearance of the optic nerve when the eye became softer.[1] More recently, several authors, including Shin[2] and Raitta[3], have noted a high percentage of cases in which the optic disc shows an apparent improvement following lowering of intraocular pressure. The classic study done by Shiose years ago is strangely ignored.[4] He administered topical steroids to normal volunteers and noted that when the intraocular pressure rose, the disc became cupped and defects developed in the visual field. When the steroids were stopped, the intraocular pressure fell, the cup reverted to its previous appearance, and the visual field defects disappeared. The phenomenon of improvement in the appearance of the optic nerve following lowering of intraocular pressure is not rare. It is not a part of the mind-set of ophthalmologists, however, to look for such changes, and therefore such changes are not seen. Additionally, methods of examining the optic disc are still highly subjective, and objective methods, such as image analyzers, have limited resolution and a disturbing number of artifacts.

At present it has become customary to set "target pressures" as guidelines for what the ophthalmologist believes will be an intraocular pressure likely to be tolerated by the patient. The fact, however, is that there is still no evidence regarding how to go about setting a target pressure with accuracy. One study found that lowering pressure by approximately 30% appeared to be necessary in order to get a moderately reproducible improvement in the appearance of the optic disc.[5] But such a finding was noted in only about one third of patients.

Would improvement in the optic disc have been noted in other patients if the pressure lowering had been 40% or 50%? Is 30% really necessary in all patients? Are there some types of glaucomatous cupping in which apparent improvement in the optic disc simply does not occur? Is the likelihood for the disc to show an apparent improvement related to the stage of the glaucoma or the age of the patient? The answer to the last question is that the younger the patient and the earlier the glaucoma, the more likely the disc is to show an apparent improvement, but exceptions to this general guideline are numerous.

Is there any significance from the point of view of patient care to the phenomenon of apparent improvement in the optic disc? At least two issues come to mind here. The first has been studied by Burgoyne and others, and relates to the amount of damage the optic nerve can sustain before the damage is irreversible.[6] If one is to consider only the damage caused by intraocular pressure, then it is logical to conclude that at some level of intraocular pressure–induced stress to the connective tissue, the connective tissue is sufficiently stretched (or damaged), and even when the intraocular pressure is lowered the damage persists. Similarly, there is some amount of stress that an axon can withstand without dying, and, upon removal of the stress, the axon will recover to its normal state. Ophthalmologists must get past the "all or none" mentality of the healthy or a permanently damaged optic nerve. Axons are not necessarily either totally healthy or dead. There is a significant stage along the way when the axon is becoming sufficiently damaged, and when the supporting tissues are becoming damaged to the point that they will no longer return to their normal function. Perhaps the only way to determine the "point of no return" is to establish that point at which the disc no longer returns to its previous appearance. Similarly, comments could be made with regard to visual function. That is, the "point of no return" could be when lowering intraocular pressure or in any other means of treating glaucoma is no longer associated with an improvement in the visual function.

To date, the goal of most glaucoma specialists has been to prevent progressive deterioration of vision. It may well be that a more appropriate primary goal is to cause an improvement in the appearance of the optic nerve (or preferably visual function). Until an actual improvement has been seen, how can the ophthalmologist know that the intraocular pressure has been lowered adequately?

G.L. Spaeth, M.D.

References

1. von Jaeger E: *Ophthalmoskopischer Hand Atlas*. Vienna, Druck und Verlag der KK Hof und Staatsdruckerei, 1869, plates 7, 12, p 76.
2. Shin DH, Bielik M, Hong Y: Reversal of glaucomatous optic disc cupping in adult patients. *Arch Ophthalmol* 115:1599, 1989.
3. Raitta C, Tomita G, Vesti E, et al: Optic disc tomography before and after trabeculectomy in advanced glaucoma. *Ophthalmic Surg Lasers* 27:349–354, 1996.
4. Shiose Y, Ohmi Y, Kawase Y, et al: Glaucoma and the optic disease: I. Studies on the cup and pallor in the optic disc. *Jpn J Clin Ophthalmol* 32:51, 1978.
5. Katz LJ, Spaeth GL, Cantor LB, et al: Reversible optic disc cupping and visual field improvement in adults with glaucoma. *Am J Ophthalmol* 107:485–492, 1989.
6. Burgoyne CF, Quigley HA, Thompson HW, et al: Early changes in optic disc compliance and surface position in experimental glaucoma. *Ophthalmology* 102: 1800–1809, 1995.

Caprioli J: Criteria for success of surgical treatment of glaucoma. *Curr Opin Ophthalmol* 8:68–72, 1997.

▶ Caprioli makes the very important point that functional outcomes are of most significance in evaluating the success of surgical treatment for glaucoma. I would push that even a bit further by defining *functional* very broadly. The goal of glaucoma therapy is preservation or enhancement of the patient's health. The usual method of achieving that is by preventing the patients from getting further glaucoma damage, and the usual way of preventing further glaucoma damage is by lowering the intraocular pressure. But if the method of lowering intraocular pressure substitutes other problems, such as poor vision or an uncomfortable eye, the patient's health has not been enhanced or preserved.

Ophthalmology is an isolated specialty. About 50% of ophthalmologists, for example, do not ask patients what systemic medications they're taking. On the other hand, about 50% of family practitioners do not ask patients what eye drops they're taking. Unfortunately for ophthalmology and for our patients, we ophthalmologists have not had the kind of continuing interdisciplinary interchange that is typical of most of the other medical and surgical specialties. This isolation makes us even more likely to think of the patient in terms of an isolated eyeball. In the field of glaucoma, in which the control of intraocular pressure is central to accomplishing the immediate goal, it is easy to forget that the control of intraocular pressure is only one of the aspects of the method of achieving the *ultimate* goal: the preservation or enhancement of the patient's health.

G.L. Spaeth, M.D.

Gupta N, Weinreb RN: New definitions of glaucoma. *Curr Opin Ophthalmol* 8:38–41, 1997.

▶ Weinreb and his colleague Gupta write in this paper on one of the most critical issues facing all those who care for patients with glaucoma, specifically, "What is glaucoma?"

G.L. Spaeth, M.D.

McKinnon SJ: Glaucoma, apoptosis, and neuroprotection. *Curr Opin Ophthalmol* 8:28–37, 1997.

▶ It's easy to forget that new knowledge and new concepts don't just arise by themselves but are usually the result of a perceptive individual noting something or thinking something that other people have not noted or thought. The Romantic Period in history was obsessed with darkness and death, but since that time discussions of death have been, until recently, almost taboo. As medical practice became more powerfully able to keep people's hearts beating it became necessary to start making definitions of what really constituted life and what is meant to be "alive." Similarly, definitions of death, and of what is meant to be "dead," became common. Just what constitutes "death" is problematic. In the human organism individual cells such as red blood cells are dying constantly in huge numbers. They replenish themselves at about the same rate that they die. Other cells, such as some neurons, appear to die and not be replenished. By "die" I mean that they stop functioning and lose their spatial identity. Their parts are disseminated throughout the body. But while the individual cells are dying, the organism continues to live. Or, is the organism in a gradual, continuing process of dying? Is that process merely consummated when the heart stops beating or the brain stops metabolizing? In the field of glaucoma it has been clear since the disease was first recognized that people lost sight, that is, the sight "died." This loss of sight was attributed to a variety of causes, most recently to the death of the ganglion cells in the retina. Why is it that the ganglion cells die? Pathologists have considered this matter for over 100 years but only recently has there been concentrated attention. One of the individuals who deserves credit for this new look at why and how the ganglion cells die is Harry Quigley of the Wilmer Eye Institute at Johns Hopkins. The above mentioned article is by one of the new members who has joined Quigley's research group. Unfortunately, it does not bear abstracting very well, and the reader is encouraged to turn to the original article. It is beautifully written and will richly reward the reader with information, much of which will probably be new and all of which is important for those of us who have careers involved with preserving life.

One cautionary note, however, seems appropriate. It would be unfortunate if we fall into the same trap regarding how cells die in glaucoma that we've so frequently fallen into along the way, specifically, thinking in terms of a single mechanism. It seems virtually certain that there are many ways in which the neurons are damaged, and many ways in which they die. We need to learn more about the differences as well as the similarities.

G.L. Spaeth, M.D.

Schwartz B, Linner E, Araujo D: Rates of change of optic disc pallor of untreated ocular hypertensives, in Krieglstein GK (ed): *Glaucoma Update V.* Heidelberg, Kaden Verlag, 1995, pp 129–139.

▶ This article was published several years ago. However, it is being reviewed in this year's YEAR BOOK because it was published in a volume which was not widely read and deals with an issue which, to my way of thinking, is one of the most important aspects of consideration of glaucoma. Furthermore, it is an aspect which is almost totally ignored, to the extent that, to my knowledge, only two other centers have reported on the same issue. Airaksinen and Tuulonen in Finland have been interested in this concern,[1] as have we on the Glaucoma Service of the Wills Eye Hospital.[2] The issue to which I refer is the *rate* at which glaucoma gets worse.

One of the first questions that a physician must ask himself or herself when considering a patient with glaucoma is, "Does this patient have a condition which will cause blindness?" The question can also be phrased, "Considering this patient's presumed life expectancy, will this case of glaucoma get worse rapidly enough that it will cause visual impairment interfering with what this patient wants to do?" That is, an *essential* consideration of the patient with glaucoma is the *rate* at which the patient's vision is changing. Without an estimate of the rate of change, therapy cannot be rationally recommended. Nevertheless, as mentioned earlier, there has been almost no attention paid to methods designed to determine the rate of change of glaucoma. The reason for this absence of information relates to the difficulty in staging glaucoma. Does one consider change in the appearance of the optic disc in one eye or in both eyes? How is change in the optic disc to be monitored: increase in pallor, decrease in the width of the rim, frequency of disc hemorrhage? Does one consider change in visual field in one eye or in both eyes? Given the huge variability of visual field defects in different patients with glaucoma, and the huge variability of results in just one patient, how does one determine what really constitutes a deterioration of the field in the patient under consideration?

One only needs to be concerned about rate of change if one is able to make a reasonably accurate estimate of the number of days or years that the patient still has to live. Is this possible? Many ophthalmologists bridle at the thought of making such a determination. After all, they say, how can they tell how long a patient's actually going to live? The fact is, however, that they can come up with a reasonably accurate estimate of the patient's remaining life span. The life insurance companies, of course, have performed such estimates for many years, and without those estimates they would not be able to be profitable companies. Surely physicians can do as well as the nonmedical life insurance agent who asks the following questions: How old are your parents? If they have died, at what age did they die? Of what did your parents die? How old are your siblings? If they have died, how old were they when they died and of what did they die? What is your medical history? What medications do you take? What is your blood pressure? What is your weight and height? Do you smoke cigarettes? Have you smoked cigarettes in the past? How much do you drink? Do you use drugs other than alcohol? Do you participate in activities such as mountain-climbing, hand-gliding, or motorcycle racing? What is your occupation?

These questions or similar questions should be a part of every routine initial examination; they are not mysterious questions that deal with arcane issues.

What Schwartz, Linner, and Araujo showed in the above mentioned article was that the rate of increasing pallor of the optic disc was greater in the eyes of patients who went on to experience visual field loss than it was in the eyes of patients who did not have visual field loss. This is, of course, what one would expect. However, their article is an extremely important contribution because it brings attention to and provides information regarding the rate at which glaucoma changes.

G.L. Spaeth, M.D.

References

1. Airaksinen PJ, Tuulonen A, Alanko HI: Rate and pattern of neuroretinal rim area decrease in ocular hypertension and glaucoma. *Arch Ophthalmol* 110:206–210, 1992.
2. Spaeth GL, Fellman RL, Starita RL, et al: A new management system for glaucoma based on improvement of the appearence of the optic disc or visual field. *Trans Am Ophthalmol Soc* 183:268, 1985.

4 Cornea

Review of Cornea

by Peter R. Laibson, M.D.

Obtaining donor corneas for corneal transplantation is the function of the 101 eye banks in the United States. The Eye Bank Association of America (EBAA) sets the standards for these eye banks. It officially inspects them on a regular basis to maintain standards and to continue each eye bank's membership in the EBAA.

Standards for donor corneal tissue are continually reviewed by the EBAA, and this year some of these rules have changed. For instance, it is no longer necessary to test the donor tissue for the presence of syphilis, a rule that had been in place for many years.

There has been no upper age limit set by the EBAA for tissue use, although most surgeons prefer to use donor corneas as young as can be obtained from their eye bank. The endothelial cell count has been a gold standard. Corneal tissue is generally used as long as the cell count is over 2,000 cells/mm^2. What about using tissue from patients over 75 years of age with cell counts over 2,000 cells/mm^2? Most corneal surgeons would prefer not to use such corneas. Probst, Halfaker, and Holland[1] have suggested such tissue may be used if the cell count is satisfactory, (over 2,000 cells/mm^2) and other criteria are also satisfactory. This tissue could be used for older recipients. Their study on donor corneas also suggests that pseudophakic corneas are generally not suitable for transplantation. On the other hand, Johnston, Hasany, and Rootman[2] conclude that pseudophakic eyes could be used provided the endothelial cell counts are over 2,000 cells/mm^2. Perhaps the endothelium is healthier in Toronto than in Minneapolis. I generally use donor corneas up to 75 years of age and occasionally up to 80 (if the cell counts are over 2,000 cells/mm^2) for my patients who are undergoing corneal transplantation in the age group over 75. This provides me with corneal tissue that I feel to be quite adequate for patients in this age group. Many years ago Forster and Fine[3] actually found that older tissue provided clearer corneal transplants for longer periods than did some younger corneal donors. I still do not use tissue from pseudophakic eyes, although based upon Johnston's study, I will be taking a closer look at patients with endothelial cell counts over 2,000 cell/mm^2 who are pseudophakic.

Endophthalmitis after corneal transplantation is very uncommon, probably occurring in between 1 in 300 and 1 in 600 cases. Obtaining cultures from the rims of donor buttons has been done routinely for many years. Often rim cultures are found to be positive for bacterial or fungal growths days after the transplant, and there is no sign of infection. If the positive rim culture correlated with the organism causing the endophthalmitis, it would be a worthwhile procedure. Wiffen et al.[4] reviewed their rim cultures on 1,078 patients from 1981 to 1985 and found they were negative for the three cases of endophthalmitis that occurred. The rim cultures were positive in 209 (19.4%) of the 1,078 cases. They concluded that rim cultures were expensive and non-predictive of endophthalmitis. Rim cultures that are done for medicolegal purposes by some surgeons cannot be defended. We have stopped doing rim cultures for our donor buttons.

References

1. Probst LE, Halfaker BA, Holland EJ: Quality of corneal donor tissue in the greater-than-75-year age group. *Cornea* 16:507–511, 1997.
2. Johnston RH, Hasany S, Rootman DS: Endothelial cell analysis of corneas from donor eyes with an intraocular lens: A comparative study. *Cornea* 15:531–533, 1997.
3. Forster RK, Fine M: Relation of donor age to success in penetrating keratoplasty. *Arch Ophthalmol* 85:42–47, 1971.
4. Wiffen SJ, Weston BC, Maguire LJ, et al: The value of routine donor corneal rim cultures in penetrating keratoplasty. *Arch Ophthalmol* 115:719–724, 1997.

A Study of Topical Nonsteroidal Anti-inflammatory Drops and No Pressure Patching in the Treatment of Corneal Abrasions

Kaiser PK, and the Corneal Abrasion Patching Study Group (Cleveland Clinic Found, Ohio; et al)

Ophthalmology 104:1353–1359, 1997 4–1

Purpose.—Corneal abrasion is a very common problem that leads the patient to seek prompt medical attention. In most cases, the epithelial defect heals within 2 to 3 days. Only recently have some studies questioned the conventional treatment for corneal abrasions, namely antibiotics and pressure patching. A different approach to the treatment of corneal abrasions—1 drop of an ophthalmic nonsteroidal anti-inflammatory drug without pressure patching—was tested in a randomized, controlled trial.

Methods.—The study included 100 patients seen at a single center with noninfected, non-contact-lens-related corneal abrasions of less than 36 hours' duration. All patients were previously untreated and had a simple epithelial defect without stromal edema, loss, or infiltrate. All abrasions were smaller than 10 mm^2. All patients received cycloplegic drops and erythromycin or polymyxin B, without pressure patching. They were then randomized in double-masked fashion to receive either ketorolac tromethamine 0.5% ophthalmic solution or control vehicle drops. The patients were monitored by symptom evaluation, evaluation of the abra-

TABLE 1.—Cause of Corneal Abrasions

	No. (% of total)
Foreign body removal	31 (35)
Paper	8 (9)
Branch	7 (8)
Finger/toe	6 (7)
Hair brush/comb	5 (6)
Sand/stones	5 (6)
Nails/metal objects	5 (6)
Miscellaneous	4 (5)
Unknown	17 (19)

(Published courtesy of *Ophthalmology* from Kaiser PK, and the Corneal Abrasion Patching Study Group: A study of topical nonsteroidal anti-inflammatory drops and no pressure patching in the treatment of corneal abrasions. *Ophthalmology* 104:1353–1359, 1997.)

sion, and assessment of adverse events. Long-term complications were assessed after 3 to 8 months.

Results.—The final analysis included 78% patients, mean age 38 years, and 83% male. The most common cause of corneal abrasion was foreign body removal (Table 1). The 2 groups were well matched in age, sex, pain, and other variables. Nearly two thirds of patients had had previous corneal abrasions. The day after treatment, pain, photophobia, and foreign-body sensation were significantly lower in the ketorolac group than in the control group. The active treatment group were also quicker to resume their normal activities. Amount of tearing, healing time, and acuity changes were comparable in the 2 groups. Recurrent erosions occurred during follow-up in 2 patients in the control group and 1 patient in the ketorolac group.

Conclusions.—Ketorolac tromethamine 0.5% ophthalmic solution is a useful treatment adjunct for patients with noninfected, non-contact-lens-related traumatic corneal abrasions. This nonsteroidal anti-inflammatory drug is clearly effective in improving patient comfort, though the mechanism of this effect is uncertain. The authors present a recommended approach to treatment of corneal abrasions, including ketorolac drops (as needed for patient comfort), antibiotic ointment, no pressure patching, and perhaps a short-acting cycloplegic. Of course, fluorescein examination is needed to exclude other ocular diagnoses.

► Corneal abrasions are one of the most common problems an ophthalmologist sees on an emergency basis. In the past, an antibiotic ointment and patching, the ointment to prevent infection and the patching to enhance healing, was the treatment of choice. This is no longer the best way to treat corneal abrasions. Certainly, contact lens abrasions should not be treated with patching because of the fear for Pseudomonas, despite the use of an antibiotic (usually one that is not effective against Pseudomonas). Because of the discomfort and often pain with acute corneal abrasions, some ophthalmologists have treated these abrasions with bandage contact lenses. This too may cause problems such as a tight lens fit, or infection beneath the contact lens. The use of a topical nonsteroidal anti-inflammatory agent has been shown to be effective for photorefractive keratectomy and now this study shows the effectiveness of ketorolac tromethamine, which is one of the nonsteroidal anti-inflammatory drug group of approved ophthalmic drugs.

There were no complications with ketrorolac tromethamine use. Patients were more comfortable earlier and their corneal abrasions healed satisfactorily without delayed re-epithelialization or corneal infection.

The use of ketorolac tromethamine, mild cycloplegia, and antibiotics has proved to be effective in treating corneal abrasions. For contact lens abrasions, I would be a little more vigorous and use either one of the fluoroquinolones or an aminoglycoside, because of its effect against Pseudomonas, which is seen more often with contact lens corneal abrasions.

P.R. Laibson, M.D.

Use of Routine Antibiotic Sensitivity Testing for the Management of Corneal Ulcers

Kowal VO, Levey SB, Laibson PR, et al (Wills Eye Hosp, Philadelphia)

Arch Ophthalmol 115:462–465, 1997 4–2

Introduction.—The value of antibiotic sensitivity testing for patients with corneal ulcers has been questioned because many whose tests identify resistant organisms do well clinically after intensive topical antibiotic instillation. A prospective study of 32 consecutive patients with corneal ulcers and positive culture results examined the clinical importance of routinely obtained antibiotic susceptibility testing.

Methods.—All patients had been referred to the cornea service at Wills Eye Hospital between October 1, 1993, and May 31, 1994. Corneal scrapings were obtained for Gram's and Giemsa staining and for culture and antibiotic sensitivity testing. Initial treatment consisted of broad-spectrum empirical antibiotic therapy, administered every hour around the clock after smear and culture results were obtained. Daily modifications were made on the basis of clinical appearance, Gram's and Giemsa stain results, or organism identification. Clinicians were masked to sensitivity results unless they felt that a lack of this knowledge would compromise an individual patient's care.

Results.—Only 2 patients had sensitivity results checked when their corneal ulcer worsened or failed to improve. Ulcers healed in 15 patients after treatment with the initial empirical antibiotic therapy. Regimens were modified in 6 patients after stain or culture results were available, but the initial therapy improved their ulcers. Among the 11 patients whose ulcers did not respond to the initial empirical therapy, 7 ultimately improved with a change in therapy, and 4 did not improve. Sensitivity results in the 4 patients who failed to respond had indicated that the initial antibiotic therapy would be adequate.

Conclusion.—In this small patient sample, routine antibiotic susceptibility tests did not appear to provide clinically useful information for the management of most corneal ulcers. Culturing is important, however, because unusual infections that are inadequately treated by empirical therapy may be identified.

► The fact that this study of 32 consecutive patients referred to the Cornea Service at Wills Eye Hospital did not provide clinically useful information for the management of corneal ulcers further confirms our feeling that antibiotic sensitivity testing for the routine management of corneal ulcers is not warranted from the point of view of expense and usefulness in the management of these ulcers.

We definitely recommend culturing these patients because unusual organisms, such as *Acanthamoeba*, fungus, and microbacteria, may be involved in ulcers that seem to be routine bacterial ulcers. Certainly the whole question of when and when not to culture corneal ulcers is still evolving, but at Wills Eye Hospital we believe that small epithelial defects with infiltrates of less than 2 mm and limited to the nonvisual axis area of the cornea do not have to be cultured. Larger ulcers, those that are in the visual axis and those with hypopyon, routinely are cultured.

P.R. Laibson, M.D.

Intraoperative Mitomycin in Primary Pterygium Excision: A Prospective, Randomized Trial

Manning CA, Kloess PM, Diaz MD, et al (Wilford Hall Med Ctr, San Antonio, Tex; Univ of Texas, Houston)

Ophthalmology 104:844–848, 1997 4–3

Introduction.—Intraoperative mitomycin has been used safely and effectively in patients undergoing glaucoma-filtering procedures, but few studies have reported the benefits of this therapy in pterygia excision. The value of intraoperative mitomycin in pterygia surgery was examined in a prospective, randomized study, comparing it to the established methods of conjunctival autograft transplantation and postoperative mitomycin therapy.

Methods.—Between October 1992 and May 1994, 63 consecutive primary pterygia were excised in 56 patients. Follow-up was available for 50 patients (56 primary pterygia) randomly assigned to 1 of 3 treatment groups: group 1, conjunctival autograft; group 2, postoperative mitomycin (0.2 mg/mL 4 times a day for 7 days); and group 3, intraoperative mitomycin (0.4 mg/mL applied for 3 minutes). Patients in the mitomycin groups underwent pterygia excision using the bare sclera technique. Postoperative treatment consisted of neomycin-polymyxin-dexamethasone ointment for 4 weeks, followed by dexamethasone ointment tapered over 4 weeks. Patients were examined at postoperative days 1 and 7, then at 2, 6, and 12 months.

Results.—The 3 treatment groups were comparable in patient gender, age, and size of pterygia. Recurrence rates were 22.2% in group 1, 21.1% in group 2, and 10.5% in group 3. The difference between group 3 and groups 1 and 2 was not statistically significant. Only patient age had a significant association with recurrence; those older than 55 years had significantly fewer recurrences. All recurrences had developed by 6 months after excision of primary pterygia. There were only 2 complications, both in the postoperative mitomycin group.

Discussion.—Excision of the pterygium has a high rate of recurrence and associated morbidity. The most widely used techniques for the prevention of recurrence have been conjunctival autograft transplantation and postoperative mitomycin therapy. Relatively large cumulative doses of mitomycin are toxic and can cause vision-threatening complications when applied postoperatively. Intraoperative mitomycin can be delivered as a single, direct scleral bed application, resulting in a lower incidence of toxicity.

▶ The use of intraoperative mitomycin C and not postoperative mitomycin C is gathering momentum. This is a further study to indicate that when a comparison is made of postoperative application and intraoperative application, the recurrence rate is less for intraoperative application and also less for the patients with conjunctival autograft.

There still is concern about potential toxicity of the sclera and cornea with mitomycin C. For this reason, many surgeons still do conjunctival autografts, as the recurrence rate varies between 5% and 15% in this group, in many hands. The 22% recurrence rate stated by the authors in the conjunctival autograft group seems a little high, and if this did come down to 10%, it would be comparable to that with intraoperative mitomycin C. It is certainly easier to use intraoperative mitomycin C, but the long-term value of this compared to the conjunctival autograft for pterygium is not clearly established yet.

P.R. Laibson, M.D.

Aerosolization of Infectious Virus by Excimer Laser

Moreira LB, Sanchez D, Trousdale MD, et al (Univ of Southern California, Los Angeles)

Am J Ophthalmol 123:297–302, 1997 4–4

Background.—Excimer laser photorefractive keratectomy is used to correct refractive error and treat corneal opacities. Although levels of safety have been defined, the potential for aerosolization of infectious particles is unclear. There is concern regarding dissemination of infectious viral particles by the excimer laser plume and shock wave in patients with infectious viruses in their tears and corneal tissue, although infection may not be evident at the time of treatment. Herpes simplex virus, adenovirus, and HIV can be present in tear films and corneal cells before there are clinical signs of infection.

Methods.—To simulate virus-infected corneas, cell monolayers were infected with herpes simplex virus or adenovirus. The virus-infected petri dish was surrounded by other dishes with noninfected cell monolayers. Ablation with a 193-mm excimer laser was performed in the dish with the infected cell monolayers. The adjacent dishes were assayed for viral infection. The experiment was repeated 10 times.

Results.—There was viral spread of herpes simplex virus and adenovirus to the adjacent dishes. The likelihood of spread was affected by the titer of virus in the infected cell monolayers; a high titer of virus resulted in a higher spread of virus. Use of a vacuum aspiration system affected the direction of virus spread; dishes placed in the direction of the vacuum contained more virus. There was no virus spread when laser irradiation of the central infected dish was not performed.

Discussion.—These findings show that aerosolization of infectious virus can occur with photoablation with a large-diameter excimer laser beam. Vertical aerosolization of infectious viral particles may also occur, given the visible extension of the plume toward the vacuum nozzle. These findings may not apply to the clinical setting. The amount of virus used in this experiment exceeded the amount of virus normally found in human precorneal tear film or corneal tissue. Steps should be taken to reduce the risk of virus spread from patient to surgeon, staff, and other patients.

► Phototherapeutic keratectomy for herpes simplex virus corneal scars and herpes zoster, as well as adenovirus infections, has the potential for causing aerosolization of infectious viruses that can be spread to the surgeon and other personnel. This clinical study documents the potential for aerosolization of infectious virus particles with photo ablation of herpes simplex or adenovirus. Surgeons should take the precaution of using masks and gloves for phototherapeutic keratectomy of herpes simplex and adenovirus and adenovirus corneal scars.

Our experience at Wills Eye Hospital is not extensive in the use of phototherapeutic keratectomy for herpes simplex and adenovirus scars, and, from the literature one cannot find many cases of herpes simplex and adenovirus infection that have had phototherapeutic keratectomy for visual axis corneal scarring. Although the excimer laser ablation of cell monolayers infected with herpes simplex virus and adenovirus does not exactly mimic phototherapeutic keratectomy of corneal scars from herpes simplex and adenovirus infection, there still may be enough virus particles or partial viruses destroyed and aerosolized to warrant the surgeon taking precautions. We can't assure that there may not be remaining viral DNA there.

P.R. Laibson, M.D.

Herpes Simplex Virus Keratitis Among Patients Who Are Positive or Negative for Human Immunodeficiency Virus: An Epidemiologic Study

Hodge WG, Margolis TP (Univ of Calif, San Francisco; Univ of Ottawa, Ont)

Ophthalmology 104:120–124, 1997 4–5

Background.—Herpes simplex virus keratitis is common in patients with HIV infection and follows a similar clinical course as in patients who are immunocompetent. The literature shows that although herpes simplex virus infection is an AIDS-defining opportunistic infection, it is less common than other opportunistic infections in patients with AIDS.

Methods.—In a retrospective cohort study, patients were identified with epithelial or stromal herpes simplex virus keratitis and HIV infection. Control patients had herpes simplex virus keratitis, but were not HIV positive. Study patients were identified from 1,800 patient visits and control patients were identified from 48,200 patient visits. The medical records of all patients were reviewed.

Results.—There was no significant difference in incidence, lesion type, or location of herpes simplex virus keratitis between patients who were positive or negative for HIV infection. There was no differences in treatment time between the groups. The difference in recurrence rate between the 2 groups was statistically significant. In patients who were positive for HIV, the recurrence rate of herpes simplex virus keratitis was 2.48 times higher than in patients who were negative for HIV.

Discussion.—This is the first study to compare herpes simplex virus keratitis in patients who were positive and negative for HIV infection. It is unlikely that confounding factors affected the results because age, gender, race, systemic illnesses other than those related to HIV infection, and treatment regimen were controlled for in multivariate analysis. It is possible that other variables that could affect outcome were omitted from the analysis.

► Patients who are immunocompromised and are positive for HIV have a higher incidence of herpes zoster ophthalmicus than patients who are not HIV positive. This article indicates that the same is not true for herpes simplex virus infection. The authors, who work at San Francisco General Hospital, have access to a large group of HIV-positive patients. Their clinical impression was that HIV keratitis occurred infrequently in patients who were HIV positive, and this epidemiologic study proves their point. Why patients who are HIV positive have a higher incidence of herpes zoster and not herpes simplex infection is not clear.

The authors did find that the recurrence rate of herpes simplex virus keratitis was higher in patients who were HIV positive than those who were HIV negative. This, too, has no explanation at this time. Patients who have herpes zoster ophthalmicus and are seen by an ophthalmologist should usually be asked about their HIV status. This does not seem to be necessary for patients who have herpes simplex ocular infection. Patients who are HIV positive should also be warned about the possibility of herpes zoster infection and the signs and symptoms of the early onset of this disease.

P.R. Laibson, M.D.

Coexistent *Acanthamoeba* Keratitis and Herpetic Keratitis

Mathers WD, Goldberg MA, Sutphin JE, et al (Univ of Iowa, Iowa City; New York Eye and Ear Infirmary)

Arch Ophthalmol 115:714–718, 1997 4–6

Introduction.—*Acanthamoeba* keratitis may be difficult to diagnose, requiring corneal biopsy of the epithelium or stroma and specialized culturing methods. The introduction of clinical confocal microscopy has made it possible to visualize *Acanthamoeba* organisms on the corneal surface and increased the ease and frequency of diagnosis. A series of patients had both *Acanthamoeba* keratitis and concurrent herpes simplex virus (HSV) keratitis (herpetic keratitis).

Methods.—Diagnosis of *Acanthamoeba* organisms was made in 8 patients using confocal microscopy and epithelial biopsy with hematoxylin-eosin staining; biopsy of the stroma and epithelium was used in the remaining patient. Each patient was also identified as having evidence of HSV infection in the cornea, documented with viral cultures in 6 cases, immunologic stains in 2 cases, and in 1 by histopathologic examination for multinucleated giant cells in the corneal epithelium.

Results.—Potential predisposing conditions for the development of *Acanthamoeba* keratitis included previous use of contact lenses in 2 cases, previous corneal transplants in 2 cases, and a condition that could compromise epithelial function in 4 cases. Four of the 9 patients had a long history of presumed herpetic keratitis (23 years in 1 case) and 5 had clinical signs indicative of HSV infection. The length of time between the appearance of herpetic keratitis and the development of infection with *Acanthamoeba* organisms could not be determined in all cases. There was a wide variation in the relative severity of corneal disease, but most patients did not have seriously compromised visual acuity. Treatment for *Acanthamoeba* infections usually employed multiple drugs, and 7 of 9 patients appeared to have been cured. All patients received antiviral agents after HSV was detected.

Discussion.—Findings in this series of patients suggest that almost any condition that damages the surface epithelium, including HSV infection, can lead to *Acanthamoeba* keratitis. Patients with HSV that does not resolve quickly should be evaluated for *Acanthamoeba.*

► Diagnosing *Acanthamoeba* keratitis can be difficult at best. The pathologic findings frequently look like HSV infection, *Acanthamoeba,* or fungal keratitis. This is the first article to indicate that patients with HSV keratitis may also harbor *Acanthamoeba* organisms.

Tandem Scanning Confocal Microscope changes were positive for *Acanthamoeba* in 8 of 9 cases in this study, and all of them demonstrated the *Acanthamoeba* organism on epithelial scraping. This is the kind of evidence that is important to verify that Confocal Scanning microscopy is valid in diagnosing *Acanthamoeba*. In this article, only 2 of the 9 patients had a history of contact lens use, which is very different from the average patients with *Acanthamoeba*, for contact lens use is seen in the majority of patients.

For delayed healing of HSV corneal ulcers, we must look for *Acanthamoeba* now by epithelial scraping, and, if one has a research Confocal Microscope, by this technique as well.

P.R. Laibson, M.D.

Primary Varicella-Zoster Keratitis: Diagnosis by Polymerase Chain Reaction

Power WJ, Hogan RN, Hu S, et al (Harvard Med School, Boston)
Am J Ophthalmol 123:252–254, 1997 4–7

Introduction.—Polymerase chain reaction (PCR) is being used more and more to diagnose suspected infectious ocular pathology. A case of progressive corneal ulceration was described in which PCR made possible a previously unconsidered diagnosis.

Case Report.—Boy, 6 years, had a 1-week history of a red, painful eye. A corneal ulcer had been diagnosed at another facility,

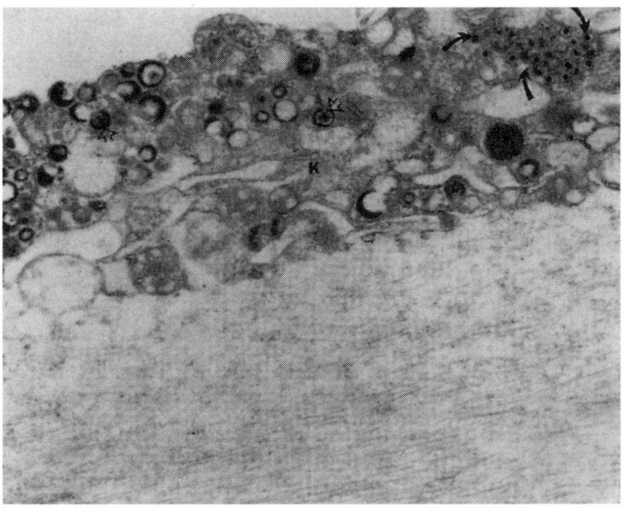

FIGURE 2.—This electron micrograph shows keratocytes (*K*) with capsids and core components of mature herpes particles. Trilaminar enveloped particles (*open arrows*) and an aggregate of capsids (*curved arrows*) are also visible; original magnification, (×46,500). (Courtesy of Power WJ, Hogan RN, Hu S, et al: Primary varicella-zoster keratitis: Diagnosis by polymerase chain reaction. *Am J Ophthalmol* 123:252–254, 1997.)

but it had worsened even after intensive antibiotic treatment. The boy had had 2 episodes of what was considered to be blepharo-conjunctivitis in the previous 6 months. Penetrating keratoplasty was performed, and the patient was discharged after 2 days. Five months later, the transplant was clear, compact, and had no signs of recurrent ulceration. The corneal specimen was examined by PCR and tested positive for varicella-zoster virus but negative for herpes simplex virus. A diagnosis of varicella-zoster keratitis with corneal perforation was made by PCR. Herpetic virus particles in the cornea were seen on examination by electron microscopy (Fig 2).

Discussion.—Primary varicella-zoster keratitis is rare, but it normally has a mild clinical course. It may manifest as infectious superficial keratitis, branching dendritiform lesions, or disciform keratitis weeks, or even months, after initial infection. This patient had a rare case of primary delayed varicella-zoster keratitis with progressive corneal ulceration and perforation. Polymerase chain reaction analysis of corneal buttons at the time of keratoplasty may be useful in diagnosing unresponsive corneal ulcers.

► The PCR has been used to diagnose unknown corneal diseases, particularly herpes simplex virus infection. Now this report shows its efficacy in diagnosing primary varicella-zoster virus in a patient who underwent an emergency corneal transplant for corneal ulcer where herpes zoster was not suspected. The patient was given hourly fluoroquinolones, and when a microperforation occurred, a corneal transplant was done. Examination of the corneal button by PCR was positive for varicella-zoster virus and negative for herpes simplex. This was confirmed by electron microscopy.

Although not available in all outpatient surgery centers or hospitals, PCR is a valuable technique for specifically diagnosing viral causes of corneal ulceration. It has been helpful in diagnosing herpes simplex virus, and now herpes zoster can be added to the list of diseases that may be detected from corneal specimens after corneal transplantation.

P.R. Laibson, M.D.

Amniotic Membrane Transplantation for Persistent Epithelial Defects With Ulceration

Lee S-H, Tseng SCG (Bascom Palmer Eye Inst, Miami, Fla)
Ophthalmology 123:303–312, 1997 4–8

Background.—Corneal epithelial defects can progress to ulceration and perforation, even after treatments such as tissue adhesive, conjunctival resection, lamellar keratoplasty, and penetrating keratoplasty. When there is poor visual potential, conjunctival flaps or tarsorrhaphy may be considered. One study reported that amniotic membrane transplantation had a 40% chance of restoring corneal clarity and epithelial phenotype in rabbits with a destroyed corneal and limbal surface. Based on these findings, the authors examined the question as to whether the preserved human amniotic membrane can be used as an alternative substrate to treat epithelial defects with ulceration.

Methods.—There were 11 consecutive patients with corneal ulcers and defects from various causes that had persisted for a mean of 17.5 weeks. Six patients were men; and the mean patient age was 69.9 years. Amniotic membrane transplantation was performed in 11 eyes. Human amniotic membrane was prepared using a previously described technique.

Results.—Ten patients healed within a mean of 3.9 weeks and had no recurrence during the 9 months of follow-up. One patient did not heal because of pre-existing corneal perforation resulting from severe rheumatoid arthritis. The transplanted amniotic membrane dissolved in 5 patients, 4 of whom remained healed (the exception was the patient with the corneal perforation).

Discussion.—Amniotic membrane transplantation can be considered before conjunctival flaps or tarsorrhaphy in cases of persistent epithelial defects and sterile ulceration that are unresponsive to conventional treatment. Amniotic membranes have been used as grafts for burned skin and conjunctival symblepharon; as a dressing for skin wounds and repair of omphaloceles; and as a substrate to prevent tissue adhesion in surgery of the head, abdomen, and pelvis. The thick basement membrane and avascular stromal matrix of the amniotic membrane may be critical to successful transplantation. Further research may reveal other indications for human amniotic membrane transplantation.

► The use of conjunctival flaps to close persistent corneal epithelial defects is a useful technique for problems that can lead to corneal perforation. Rather than using conjunctiva from the same eye or from the opposite eye (which requires bilateral surgery), amniotic membrane, usually obtained from cesarean section births, has recently been used for transplantation.

This article reports on 11 eyes of 11 consecutive patients with ulcers varying from neurotrophic to postinfection ulceration that were treated with amniotic membrane. Ten of the patients were satisfactorily treated.

There has been difficulty in obtaining amniotic membrane, but now there is a source in Miami Beach, Florida that may provide amniotic membrane on a commercial basis. The membrane is freeze dried and comes already pretested for of HIV, hepatitis, etc.

At a recent meeting of the Association for Research in Vision and Ophthalmology (ARVO), there were a number of posters concerning amniotic membrane use. It was interesting to note that the membrane can be used for transplantation on either side.

The amniotic membrane is an alternative substrate for closing epithelial defects and allowing the hosts own healing process to function when the defect is covered by alternate tissue. From this paper and the posters at ARVO, I have come to believe that this technique should be tried as an alternative to using scarce conjunctiva from the patient's same eye or operating on the fellow eye.

P.R. Laibson, M.D.

The Value of Routine Donor Corneal Rim Cultures in Penetrating Keratoplasty

Wiffen SJ, Weston BC, Maguire LJ, et al (Mayo Clinic and Found, Rochester, Minn)

Arch Ophthalmol 115:719–724, 1997 4–9

Introduction.—Routine donor rim cultures performed at the time of penetrating keratoplasty might yield information about microbial contaminants that could cause endophthalmitis. The costs and benefits of rim cultures in this setting have not been determined, however. Mayo Clinic records of patients who underwent penetrating keratoplasty were reviewed retrospectively for the value of routine donor rim cultures.

Methods.—Three-month follow-up data were available for all but 130 of 1,083 cases of corneal transplant performed at the Mayo Clinic between 1982 and 1995. Records were reviewed for donor corneal data, the documentation of positive cultures, clinical findings, the occurrence of endophthalmitis within 2 months of surgery, action taken in response to positive culture results, and the cost of cultures.

Results.—Donor rim culture results were available for all but 5 of the 1,083 consecutive transplantations performed during the study period. There were 3 (0.28%) cases of endophthalmitis and 1 case of suture abscess. In each of these cases, the results of rim cultures were negative. Donor rim cultures were positive in 209 (19.4%) cases. Action in response to positive cultures was documented in 17 (8.1%) of these cases. Actions taken usually involved antibiotic therapy. Only 1 of 17 patients had any unusual sign of ocular inflammation (conjunctivitis on the second postoperative day). The rate of positive cultures was increased for corneas stored in Optisol (20%), for corneas from cadaveric donors (20%), for corneas excised in situ (31.2%), and for corneas with a short storage time. The estimated average cost of routine rim cultures was $137 per donor cornea in 1994.

Conclusion.—Improvements in donor screening methods and eye bank procedures have contributed to a very low risk of endophthalmitis among patients undergoing penetrating keratoplasty. Routine donor corneal rim cultures at the time of surgery are an unnecessary expense because they have no predictive value and would have no clinical value in the management of endophthalmitis.

► We have been doing rim cultures at Wills Eye Hospital for many years. There have been many routine positive cultures resulting from *Staphylococcus* and *Streptococcus*, but none of them have correlated with endophthalmitis following penetrating corneal transplantation. I agree with the authors that it is not clinically valuable to do rim cultures when they are positive. Endophthalmitis rarely occurs, and when it does, it usually is not related to the rim culture being positive but rather to the bacteria related to the patient's lid margins or cul-de-sac. As of June 1997, we have stopped doing rim cultures during corneal transplantation.

P.R. Laibson, M.D.

Deep Lamellar Keratoplasty With Complete Removal of Pathological Stroma for Vision Improvement

Sugita J, Kondo J (Sugita Eye Hosp, Nagoya, Japan)

Br J Ophthalmol 81:184–188, 1997 4–10

Background.—Deep lamellar keratoplasty can significantly improve visual acuity and is comparable to penetrating keratoplasty. In deep lamellar keratoplasty, diseased corneal stroma are excised to Descemet's membrane, at least in the pupillary region. This procedure is indicated for eyes with preserved endothelial cell function and no epithelial or stromal edema.

Methods.—Deep lamellar keratoplasty was performed in 120 eyes in 106 patients. With the exception of 1 patient, there was no corneal epithelial or stromal edema. Just under half the patients were male; the age range was 8–86 years. After hydrodelamination (Fig 1), the stroma was excised, and only Descemet's membrane remained in the optical zone (Fig 3). Donor corneas were attached by suturing. Donor corneas were full or almost full thickness with Descemet's membrane removed, or were lathed to 0.4 mm in thickness from the endothelial side.

Results.—At a follow-up of 6 months or longer, the average postoperative visual acuity improved to 0.6 in 113 eyes with an average prospective

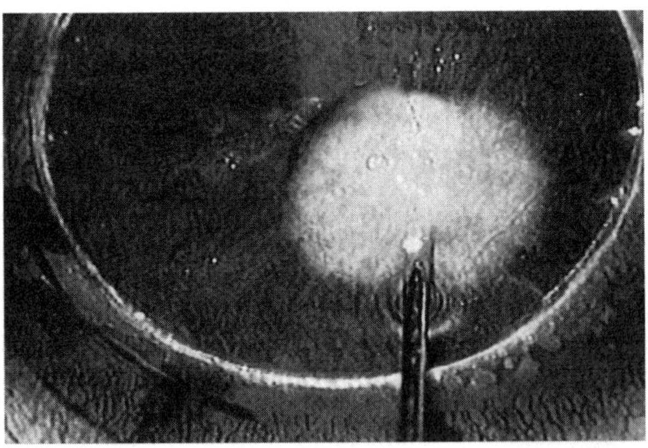

FIGURE 1.—Hydrodelamination. A solution injected into the normal stroma spreads evenly in all directions, and the remaining stroma whiten and swell. (Reprinted with permission of the BMJ Publishing Group, from Sugita J, Kondo J: Deep lamellar keratoplasty with complete removal of pathological stroma for vision improvement. *Br J Ophthalmol* 81:184–188, 1997.)

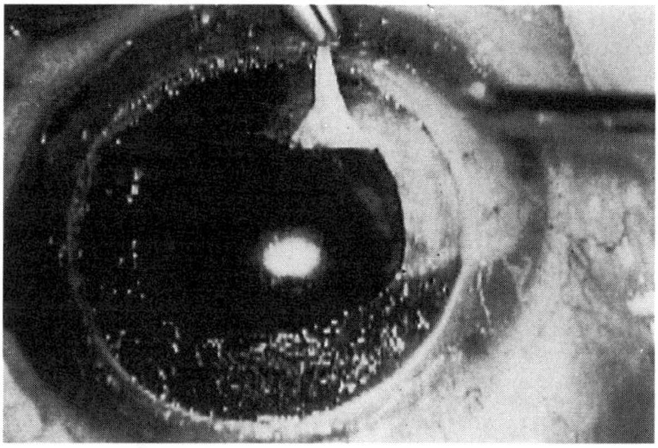

FIGURE 3.—Descemet's membrane is smooth and even, clearly distinguishable from the stroma. (Reprinted wih permission of the BMJ Publishing Group, from Sugita J, Kondo J: Deep lamellar keratoplasty with complete removal of pathological stroma for vision improvement. *Br J Ophthalmol* 81:184–188, 1997.)

visual acuity of 0.09. Specular microscopy showed average endothelial cell counts of 2,225/mm^2 at 1 month and 1,937/mm^2 at 24 months. Descemet's membrane was punctured during surgery in 47 of 120 eyes, but visual acuity and number of endothelial cells at 12 months in these eyes and in eyes that had not been punctured were similar. No postoperative endothelial rejection occurred. Restoration of visual acuity was good.

Discussion.—Deep lamellar keratoplasty allows endothelial cell counts to be maintained longer than penetrating keratoplasty, and results of deep lamellar keratoplasty are more consistent over time. Lamellar keratoplasty has numerous advantages as a keratoplasty, but because postoperative visual acuity is poor, it is primarily a therapeutic keratoplasty. Studies of deep lamellar keratoplasty indicate that it can significantly improve visual acuity while retaining the advantages of lamellar keratoplasty.

▶ The advantage of deep lamellar keratoplasty is the preservation of the host endothelium and the prevention of endothelial rejection. Most surgeons in the United States are not familiar with this technique, and their results with penetrating corneal transplants have generally been quite good. This is particularly true for keratoconus, in which the success rate for visual acuity, despite a 30% graft rejection is close to 100% for patients achieving 20/30 vision.[1]

For patients who have healthy endothelium, deep lamellar dissection can eliminate endothelial rejection because the host's own endothelium remains. In this study, specular microscopy revealed a healthy endothelial cell count despite puncturing of Descemet's membrane in almost 40% of the corneal transplants. Admittedly, when one gets down to Descemet's membrane, perforation of this thin remaining layer will be common; the authors' 39% perforation rate illustrates this point. Despite this, there was no difference in visual acuity or number of endothelial cells between eyes with and without Descemet's and endothelial perforation.

I cannot say that I will be attempting this technique in my keratoconus patients because our graft results are quite good, but in other diseases in which the deep stroma and endothelium appear normal, one should consider this technique for prevention of endothelial rejection. Admittedly, there will not be many cases that fall into this category, but if one does not think about new techniques they certainly are not going to be done. I believe that with the new microkeratomes now being developed, deep lamellar corneal transplantation will become more common in the future.

P.R. Laibson, M.D.

Reference

1. Silbiger JS, Cohen EJ, Laibson PR: The rate of visual recovery after penetrating keratoplasty for keratoconus. *CLAO J* 22:266–269, 1996.

Herpes Simplex Virus in Primary Graft Failure

Cockerham GC, Krafft AE, McLean IW (Armed Forces Inst of Pathology, Washington, DC)

Arch Ophthalmol 115:586–589, 1997 4–11

Introduction.—Primary failure of a corneal graft occurs infrequently, and no cause is identified in most cases. One recent study suggests that the presence of herpes simplex virus (HSV) in the donor is a potential cause. All cases of corneal graft failure on file at the Armed Forces Institute of Pathology from 1970 to 1995 were evaluated, and those determined to be primary graft failures were examined for the DNA of HSV type 1.

Methods.—Three (2.8%) of the 106 cases of graft failure met the definition of primary graft failure. These cases were examined microscopically and analyzed using polymerase chain reaction (PCR). Also retrieved and submitted for microscopic examination and PCR analysis were corneal buttons removed from patients with clinically suspected herpetic keratitis and from delayed regrafts that occurred 3 months to 23 years after the original graft.

Results.—The DNA from 2 of the 3 corneal buttons in cases of primary graft failure was amplifiable by PCR analysis. Both PCR analysis and Southern blot technique confirmed HSV type 1 in these 2 cases and in 2 of 3 control cases of clinically suspected herpetic keratitis. Of 4 corneal buttons from the late graft failures, 3 had DNA amplifiable by PCR analysis. All 3 were positive for HSV type 1. Acute inflammation with stromal necrosis was observed in the cornea from the first case of primary graft failure. The second case had loss of endothelium without inflammation.

Conclusion.—Primary graft failure is defined by the presence of a diffusely edematous penetrating corneal graft on the first postoperative day, failure to clear, and no identifiable cause. The incidence of primary graft failure in this series was 2.8%. Of the 3 corneal buttons, 2 were positive for HSV type 1 DNA, and no other factors associated with early graft failure appeared to be present in these cases. The seroprevalence of HSV type 1 in the general population is high. However, a larger study is needed to test the strength of the apparent relationship between HSV type 1 and primary graft failure.

► Primary graft failure, although very unusual, is devastating for the person who has the corneal transplant. This interesting article indicating the presence of herpes simplex virus, Type 1 in primary graft failures, warrants further investigation. Does primary graft failure occur because of herpes simplex virus in the donor button? If that is true, is it worthwhile for the small number of primary graft failures to go to the significant expense and time of doing PCR analysis on donor corneal buttons?

At this time I do not think it is worth the time and expense for such studies, but prospective studies of primary graft failure should evaluate this potential hazard for corneal transplantation. The Eye Bank Association of America is aware of this study and is organizing a prospective study to evaluate this potential problem.

P.R. Laibson, M.D.

Topical Aminocaproic Acid in the Treatment of Traumatic Hyphema

Crouch ER Jr, Williams PB, Gray MK, et al (Eastern Virginia Med School, Norfolk; Univ of Tennessee, Memphis)

Arch Ophthalmol 115:1106–1112, 1997 4–12

Introduction.—Up to 38% of patients with untreated traumatic hyphema will experience secondary hemorrhage within a few days after injury. Systemic therapy with the antifibrinolytic agent aminocaproic acid has been shown to reduce the incidence of rebleeding after hyphema. The role of topical aminocaproic acid in the management of traumatic hyphema was evaluated in a prospective, randomized trial.

Methods.—The multicenter study included 3 groups of patients with traumatic hyphema. Thirty-five were treated with topical aminocaproic acid, 0.2 mL of 30% aminocaproic acid every 6 hours; 29 were treated with systemic aminocaproic acid, 50 mg/kg orally every 4 hours; and 54, who refused participation in the trial, were left untreated. The patients underwent daily slitlamp examinations for grading of hyphema and corneal clarity. Visual acuity, applanation tonometry, and fundus indirect ophthalmoscopic findings were assessed as well. Mean follow-up was approximately 3 years.

Results.—Secondary hemorrhage developed in 22% of the untreated controls, compared with 3% in both of the aminocaproic acid-treated groups. A final visual acuity of 20/40 or better was reached by 43% of patients in the control group, compared with 86% of patients in the topical aminocaproic acid group, and 69% of those in the systemic aminocaproic acid group. The major causes of visual loss in the control group were corneal blood staining and optic atrophy, whereas causes related to ocular trauma predominated among aminocaproic acid-treated groups. Surgery for total hyphema was required by 5 of 5 patients in the control group versus 2 of 6 patients in the aminocaproic acid groups. Side effects such as nausea and vomiting or dizziness developed in 17% of patients in the systemic therapy group versus 3% of patients in the topical therapy group.

Conclusions.—For patients with traumatic hyphema, topical therapy with aminocaproic acid is safe and effective in the prevention of secondary hemorrhage. The topical approach is just as effective as systemic therapy in reducing the risk of secondary hemorrhage, but has no systemic side effects. Topical aminocaproic acid may be a useful outpatient treatment for patients with hyphemas occupying less than half of the anterior chamber.

▶ Recurrent bleeding, or secondary hemorrhage, is the most devastating effect of initial traumatic hyphema. To reduce this recurrent bleeding, the use of oral antifibrinolytic agents such as aminocaproic acid (Amicar) or tranexamic acid have been used orally. There are side effects to these medications and sometimes hospitalization is required with their use. The use of topical aminocaproic acid, now in gel form, seems to be as effective as oral aminocaproic acid, if Crouch et al.'s results are confirmed.

Presently, there is a double-blind study comparing topical aminocaproic acid and placebo, which this study does not do. A collaborative study involving 13 institutions is currently registering patients. Morton Goldberg, M.D. leads this group and he can be reached at the Wilmer Eye Institute for details about the cooperating centers. We await the results of the double-blind study, but in the meantime, use of topical aminocaproic acid is worthwhile, as this study shows.

P.R. Laibson, M.D.

5 Retina

Vitreous Substitutes

by Joseph I. Maguire, M.D.

Vitreoretinal surgery has undergone a continued technologic evolution since its inception with improved microsurgical technique, new procedures, and more sophisticated instruments that are smaller, less traumatic, and allow easier manipulation of intraocular structures. In addition, a multitude of vitreous substitutes, medications, and devices have been developed which allow increased flexibility in vitreoretinal surgical procedures and therapy for previously untreatable or difficult to treat conditions.

The expanded use of intravitreal antibiotics and antivirals have been highlighted by the Endophthalmitis Vitrectomy Study and work done leading to the approval of anti-cytomegalovirus retinitis medications with sustained release devices. Uses are being found for tissue plasminogen activator (t-pa) in severe postoperative inflammatory conditions and in dissolving subretinal hemorrhage associated with age-related macular degeneration. Still, the most commonly used intravitreal agents are the vitreous substitutes primarily used in the repair of retinal detachment. These include intraocular gases, silicone oil, and perfluorocarbon liquids.

Intraocular Gases

Intraocular gas is used primarily to tamponade retinal breaks and displace subretinal fluid or blood. Its use allows primary retinal detachment repair without scleral buckling, closure of macular holes, artificial pressurization of hypotonus eyes, retinal flattening with subretinal fluid removal during vitrectomy procedures, and displacement of submacular hemorrhage (with use of another intravitreal aid—t-pa). Like all gases, it will rise above a liquid medium and achieve a steady state with surrounding ambient gases. Different agents are available which have various half-lives and expansile properties.[1, 2, 3]

Air

Sterile air has no expansile abilities and is quickly reabsorbed within 5–6 days after introduction to the vitreous cavity. Short-term retinal tamponade, air-fluid exchange status after vitrectomy procedures, and reestablishment of normal intraocular pressure after significant drainage of subretinal fluid during retinal detachment repair are some of its common uses.

Sulfur Hexafluoride (SF-6)

Sulfur hexafluoride is an inert, colorless gas with a reabsorption rate of approximately 10–14 days. It has a high molecular weight and poor diffusion coefficient, allowing its greater intraocular longevity when compared to air. A 100% concentration of SF-6 gas will expand to roughly twice its volume within 4 days after injection and then slowly dissipate thereafter.[1] Intraocular pressure elevations can be seen within several hours of injection. A concentration of 18% SF-6 gas is nonexpansile. Complications of SF-6 injection include increased intraocular pressure, cataract, and transient corneal endothelial changes.

Perfluorocarbon Gases

Perfluoropropane (C3F8), Octa fluorocyclobutane (C4F8), and Perfluoro–butane (C4F10) are all fluorocarbon gases available for intraocular injection. Like SF-6 they are inert, colorless, and highly insoluble in water allowing long-term tamponade. However, their longer carbon chain backbone allows greater expansion with smaller volumes and a much slower rate of reabsorption resulting in longer tamponade.[2, 3] An injection of pure C3F8, for example, will expand 2–3 times its original volume within 3 days. A 12% concentration has been found to be nonexpansile. Reabsorption rates vary with the type of gas as well as clinical parameters such as aphakia, hypotony, and aqueous volume in contact with the gas bubble. A nonexpansile volume of C3F8 totally filling the vitreous cavity may last 2 months or more and may not significantly reduce its volume for up 2 weeks. As with other intraocular gases, intraocular pressure elevation and cataract and corneal changes are potential complications of perfluorocarbon gas use; careful monitoring is required.

Silicone Oil

The early use of intraocular silicone oil for retinal tamponade was championed by Paul Cibis 35 years ago, before the development of pars plana vitrectomy techniques.[4] At that time it was envisioned as a method to repair complicated retinal detachments, and this vision has been realized. Therefore, its major ability is in long-term retinal tamponade in advanced retinal detachment, where even long-term intraocular expansile gases prove inadequate.[5, 6] Unlike intraocular gas, silicone oil is a liquid polymer with no expansile properties, and it is not reabsorbed.

In its pure form, silicone oil is a clear, inert liquid with a high but variable viscosity which is dependent on polymer length. Although allowing diffusion of gas, it is immiscible in water and perfluorocarbon liquid, creating a readily visible miniscus during intraoperative use. Its refractive index is greater than that of water, approaches a vitreous refractive index, and therefore (unlike intraocular gas) allows easier intra- and postoperative evaluation of the retina. Its specific gravity (0.97) is slightly less than water and therefore (like oils) it floats. Although silicone oil's viscosity (a measure of flow resistance) is greater than that of gas, its buoyancy and surface tension are far less than that of intraocular gas, and therefore it exerts less retinal tamponade.[7] Its surgical utility resides in its long action.

Long-term silicone tamponade of the retina has been associated with protean complications. Ideally, silicone oil will be removed within several weeks to months. During that time, it is necessary to monitor the eye for glaucoma, emulsification, band keratopathy, optic neuropathy, development of cataract, migration into the anterior chamber, recurrence of proliferative vitreoretinopathy, droplet formation on silicone intraocular lenses, and migration through retinal breaks and into the subretinal space.[8] Because silicone oil needs additional surgical manipulation to be removed, it should be used only in more complicated vitreoretinal procedures in which the retina requires long-term tamponade, or the risk of recurrent detachment is high.

Perfluorocarbon Liquids

The introduction of perfluorocarbons is in my mind one of the most significant contributions to vitreoretinal surgery in the last decade.[9] Its use alone in the repair of giant tears has increased initial surgical success from no more than 50% to well over 90%! Perfluorocarbon liquids (PFCLs) were first investigated as artificial blood substitutes because of their ability to carry and exchange both oxygen and carbon dioxide.

Several physical properties make PFCLs an ideal temporary vitreous substitute for complicated retinal manipulations. Liquid perfluorocarbons are clear and inert, with a specific gravity almost twice that of water. As a result, they sink to a level below water unlike silicone oil, which floats. This allows displacement of subretinal fluid and retinal flattening in a posterior to anterior direction during their use. As a natural consequence, large rolled giant retinal tears can be returned to their correct anatomic position without the need for face down positioning of the patient during surgery.[10] Since PFCLs are heavier than water, all subretinal fluid is displaced forward and out of larger retinal breaks without the need for posterior retinotomies. Use of PFCLs also gives the surgeon an "extra hand," in that they stabilize posterior retina, thereby allowing counter traction while peeling membranes in eyes with proliferative vitreoretinopathy.[9, 10]

The tamponading effect of PFCLs is greater than that of silicone, but the viscosity of the latter is less, thereby allowing easy injection and removal through small bore needles. Unlike silicone oil or intraocular gases, perfluorocarbons are not well tolerated longterm by the retina; their utility is intraoperative manipulation of the retina and subretinal fluid not long-term tamponade.[11] Since they are immiscible in both water, gas and silicone oil, PFCLs can be readily visualized during surgery and used with all three.

References

1. Sabates WI, Abrams GW, Swanson DE, et al: The use of intraocular gases: The results of sulfur hexafluoride gas in retinal detachment surgery. *Ophthalmology* 88:447–454, 1981.

2. Lincoff H, Coleman J, Kressig I, et al: The perfluorocarbon gases in the treatment of retinal detachment. *Ophthalmology* 90:546–551, 1983.
3. Lopez R, Chang S: Longterm results of vitrectomy and perfluorocarbon gas for treatment of severe proliferative vitreoretinopathy. *Am J Ophthalmol* 113:424–428, 1992.
4. Cibis P, Becker B, Okun E, et al: The use of liquid silicone oil in retinal detachment surgery. *Arch Ophthalmol* 68:590–599, 1962.
5. Leaver P, Grey R, Gamer A: Silicone oil injection in the treatment of massive preretinal retraction: II. Late complications in 93 eyes. *Br J Ophthalmol* 63:361–367, 1979.
6. Silicone Study Group: Vitrectomy with silicone oil or perfluoropropane gas in eyes with severe proliferative vitreoretinopathy: Results of a randomized clinical study. *Arch Ophthalmol* 110:780–792, 1992.
7. Petersen J: The physical and surgical aspects of silicone oil in the vitreous cavity. *Graefes Arch Clin Exp Ophthalmol* 225:452–456, 1987.
8. Haut J, Ullem M, Chemmet M, et al: Complications of intraocular injections of silicone combined with vitrectomy. *Ophthalmologica* 180:29–35, 1980.
9. Chang S: Low viscosity liquid fluorochemicals in vitreous surgery. *Am J Ophthalmol* 103:38–43, 1987.
10. Chang S, Lincoff H, Zimmerman NJ, et al: Giant retinal tears: Surgical techniques and results using perfluorocarbon liquids. *Arch Ophthalmol* 107:761–766, 1989.
11. Chang S, Sparrow J, Iwamoto T, et al: Experimental studies of tolerance to intra vitreal perfluoro–octane liquid. *Retina* 11:367–374, 1991.

Hydroxychloroquine and Visual Screening in a Rheumatology Outpatient Clinic

Grierson DJ (Royal Infirmary, Glasgow, Scotland)
Ann Rheum Dis 56:188–190, 1997 5–1

Background.—Hydroxychloroquine is routinely used for the management of connective tissue and skin disorders. The College of Ophthalmologists has suggested that ophthalmic monitoring of these patients is not necessary unless their daily dose exceeds 6.6 mg/kg of lean body weight or their cumulative dose exceeds 200 g. To determine whether this recommendation is valid, 10 years of ophthalmic screening of patients taking hydroxychloroquine was evaluated.

Study Design.—After baseline visual examination, 758 patients receiving hydroxychloroquine were monitored every 6 months for corrected visual acuity, central field screening with red Amsler grid, slit-lamp examination, and retinoscopy.

Results.—Of the 758 patients, 272 had a cumulative hydroxychloroquine dose in excess of 200 g. None of the patients had impaired visual acuity resulting from retinal toxicity. Twelve patients reported visual disturbance, which was related to ocular muscle imbalance in 4 patients. Ten patients reported defects on the red Amsler grid test, but none was related to retinal toxicity. Corneal drug deposits developed in 7 patients, which cleared when drug dose was reduced.

Conclusions.—The results of this study support the suggestion of the College of Ophthalmologists that patients receiving less than a daily dose of 6.5 mg/kg or a cumulative dose of 200 g of hydroxychloroquine do not require regular ophthalmic examinations.

Incidence of Hydroxychloroquine Retinopathy in 1,207 Patients in a Large Multicenter Outpatient Practice

Levy GD, Munz SJ, Paschal J, et al (Kaiser Permanente Med Ctr, Bellflower, Calif; Kaiser Permanente Med Ctr, Anaheim, Calif; Kaiser Permanente Med Ctr, Bakersfield, Calif; et al)

Arthritis Rheum 40:1482–1486, 1997 5–2

Background.—The College of Ophthalmologists has suggested that routine ophthalmic monitoring of patients receiving hydroxychloroquine is not necessary unless the daily dose exceeds 6.5 mg/kg of lean body weight or the cumulative dose exceeds 200 g. To determine whether this recommendation is valid, a large group of patients receiving hydroxychloroquine was examined.

Study Design.—A retrospective chart review was performed of the 1,556 patients in 11 Southern California Kaiser Permanente Medical Care Program centers who had prescriptions for hydroxychloroquine filled from 1991 to 1993. Of those patients, 1,207 had documented ophthalmic screening.

Findings.—Of the 1,207 patients who were screened, 21 charts indicated potential hydroxychloroquine toxicity. From among these patients, 1 with definite toxicity and 5 with probable toxicity were identified. All these patients had received greater than 6.5 mg/kg of lean body weight of hydroxychloroquine per day. The incidence of hydroxychloroquine retinal toxicity in patients treated with less than 6.5 mg/kg/ day was 0.

Conclusions.—Hydroxychloroquine-treated patients with normal renal function and a daily dosage of less than 6.5 kg/mg do not require routine ophthalmic screening. Patients with higher daily doses, long-term hydroxychloroquine therapy, or renal dysfunction may require ophthalmic screening.

► Any first-year resident would likely be able to tell you the consequences of chloroquine toxicity on the retina, i.e., pigmentary changes with bulls-eye maculopathy. The side-effect potential of plaquenil (hydroxychloroquine) is clearly different. This difference appears to result from the added hydroxyl group, which limits penetration of the blood-retina barrier.

Previous standards of care called for a biannual dilated fundus examination with all manner of various ancillary testing. Proposed baseline and follow-up evaluation included fluorescein angiography, visual field testing, red object visual field testing, Amsler grids, color vision, and electrophysiology. Most of the above carry a significant cost and have an unproven benefit in a drug reaction that is unusual.

These 2 separate studies (Abstracts 5–1 and 5–2), 1 prospective and the other retrospective, both come to similar conclusions: (1) retinal toxicity from hydroxychloroquine as normally administered is very rare; and (2) regular ophthalmic screening is not indicated if the daily dose is less than 6.5 mg/kg. In Grierson's report, a cumulative dose greater than 200 g, especially in years 5–10 of treatment, should lead to re-evaluation annually. Levy and colleagues are more liberal and recommend yearly evaluation only if the dose is greater than 6.5 mg/kg or the patient has been treated longer than 10 years. Neither report demonstrates a benefit of ancillary testing in the absence of baseline funduscopic findings.

J.I. Maguire, M.D.

Use of Polymerase Chain Reaction Assays of Aqueous Humor in the Differential Diagnosis of Retinitis in Patients Infected With Human Immunodeficiency Virus

Danise A, Cinque P, Vergani S, et al (San Raffaele Scientific Inst, Milan, Italy)
Clin Infect Dis 24:1100–1106, 1997 5–3

Background.—Infectious retinopathy is a common complication of HIV infection. Polymerase chain reaction (PCR) assay of aqueous or vitreous fluids may be useful for diagnosing infectious retinopathy in HIV-infected as well as immunocompetent patients. The diagnostic value of PCR assay of aqueous humor from HIV-infected patients with a clinical diagnosis of retinitis and an initially unclear ophthalmoscopic presentation was evaluated.

Methods.—Eight hundred twenty patients evaluated at 1 center underwent ophthalmoscopic examination of the retina. Thirteen percent were diagnosed as having infectious retinitis, based on characteristic ophthalmoscopic findings. In 15 patients, PCR assays were performed to detect cytomegalovirus (CMV), varicella-zoster virus (VZV), herpes simplex virus (HSV), and *Toxoplasma gondii* DNA in aqueous humor.

Findings.—In 11 patients, VZV, CMV, and *T. gondii* retinitis were definitively diagnosed based on the evolution of the ophthalmoscopic findings and treatment response (Table 3). Findings were positive for CMV DNA, and negative for HSV, VZV, and *T. gondii* DNA in all 5 patients with CMV retinitis. One of 2 patients with ZVZ retinopathy had VZV DNA. Three of 4 patients with *T. gondii* retinitis had positive *T. gondii* DNA findings.

Conclusions.—Polymerase chain reaction assay of aqueous humor is useful for diagnosing retinitis of unclear origin in most patients. For appropriate treatment decision making, a PCR assay of aqueous humor should be done in all patients in whom an etiologic diagnosis of retinitis is difficult to determine.

► At a recent meeting, one of my retinal colleagues was asked what the three most common opportunistic infections of the retina and choroid were in the HIV-infected population. His answer was, tongue-in-cheek: CMV, CMV, and CMV. His point was that cytomegalovirus should always be the leading

TABLE 3.—Ophthalmoscopic Findings, PCR Results, and Final Diagnoses for the 15 HIV-infected Patients With Retinitis of Unclear Origin at Presentation

Group	Patient no.	Sex/age (y)	Ongoing treatment*	Affected eye	Retinal signs: Necrosis	Retinal signs: Detachment	Retinal signs: Hemorrhages	Cotton-wool spots	Vitreal reaction	Posterior-pole involvement	Peripheral retinal involvement	PCR on aqueous humor: Positive for:	PCR on aqueous humor: Negative for:	Medical treatment	Response to treatment, or clinical outcome	Final diagnosis of retinitis (etiology)
A	1	M/32	None	R	Y	N	N	N	N	Y	N	CMV	VZV, HSV, *T. gondii*	Ganc	Y	CMV
	2	M/33	None	R	Y	N	N	N	N	Y	N	CMV	VZV, HSV, *T. gondii*	Ganc	Y	CMV
	3	M/29	None	R	Y	Y	Y	N	N	N	Y	CMV	VZV, HSV, *T. gondii*	Ganc	Y	CMV
	4	M/43	None	R	Y	N	Y	N	N	N	Y	CMV	VZV, HXV, *T. gondii*	Ganc	Y	CMV
	5	M/46	None	L	Y	N	N	N	N	N	Y	VZV†	CMV, HSV, *T. gondii*	Acyc	Y	VZV
	6	F/35	None	R	Y	N	Y	N	Trace	N	Y	*T. gondii*	CMV, VZV, HSV	PRM + SDZ	Y	*T. gondii*
	7	M/35	None	R	Y	N	N	N	N	Y	N	*T. gondii*	CMV, VZV, HXV	PRM + SDZ	Y	*T. gondii*
	8	M/34	None	L	Y	N	N	N	N	N	Y	*T. gondii*	CMV, VZV, HSV	PRM + SDZ	Y	*T. gondii*
	9	M/37	None	L	Y	N	Y	N	N	Y	N	None	CMV, VZV, HSV, *T. gondii*	Acyc	Y	VZV
	10	M/33	PRM + Cm‡	L	Y	N	N	N	N	Y	N	None	CMV, VZV, HSV, *T. gondii*	PRM + Cm	Y	*T. gondii*
	11	M/45	TMP-SMZ§	R	Y	N	N	N	N	Y	N	None	CMV, VZV, HSV, *T. gondii*	PRM + Cm + Ganc	Y	None
B	12	M/59	None	R	N	N	Y	Y	N	Y	N	None	CMV, VZV, HSV, *T. gondii*	None	Impr	None
	13	M/30	None	L	N	N	Y	Y	N	Y	N	None	CMV, VZV, HSV, *T. gondii*	None	Impr	None
	14	M/26	None	L	N	N	Y	Y	N	Y	N	None	CMV, VZV, HSV, *T. gondii*	None	Impr	None
	15	M/35	None	L	N	N	Y	Y	N	N	Y	CMV	VZV, HSV, *T. gondii*	Ganc	Y	CMV

Abbreviations: Acyc, acyclovir; *Cm*, clindamycin; *CMV*, cytomegalovirus; *Ganc*, ganciclovir; *HSV*, herpes simplex virus type 1 or 2; *Impr*, improvement; *L*, left; *N*, no; *PRM*, pyrimethamine; *R*, right; *SDZ*, sulfadiazine; *TMP-SMZ*, trimethoprim-sulfamethoxazole; *VZV*, varicella-zoster virus; *Y*, yes.

*Ongoing treatment or prophlyaxis with antiviral drugs active against herpesviruses or with antiparasitic drugs.

†A second aqueous humor sample, obtained after 3 weeks of treatment, was VZV DNA–negative.

‡Pyrimethamine, 75 mg daily; clindamycin, 600 mg 4 times daily (orally).

§Trimethoprim, 160 mg; sulfamethoxazole, 800 mg (daily orally).

(Courtesy of Danise A, Cinque P, Vergani S, et al: Use of polymerase chain reaction assays of aqueous humor in the differential diagnosis of retinitis in patients infected with human immunodeficiency virus. *Clin Infect Dis* 24:1100–1106, 1997.)

differential diagnosis point in any presumed primary retinitis in this patient group. Toxoplasmosis, lymphoma, lues, and other herpes-related retinitis (i.e., HSV and HZV) are also worthy considerations, but less common. Initial descriptions of CMV retinitis, with its "prairie fire" or "blood and cottage cheese" appearances, have been modified greatly, due to the development of increasingly effective and divergent antiviral agents. This change in the clinical appearance of CMV retinitis is, at least in part, responsible for rare diagnostic confusion.

The authors of this review found only a very small percentage of patients whose source of retinitis was in doubt: 15 of 820. Previously, options of diagnostic vitrectomy, retinal biopsy, viral culture, and viral antigen studies all had problems with either reliability, rapidity, or degree of invasiveness. This report shows the real potential of PCR assays through an aqueous sample alone. Although the number of sampled eyes was small, and the end point for judged correctness was treatment effect, the sensitivity and specificity of the test were impressive.

J.I. Maguire, M.D.

Management of Varicella Zoster Virus Retinitis in AIDS

Moorthy RS, Weinberg DV, Teich SA, et al (Associated Vitreoretinal and Uveitis Consultants, Indianapolis, Ind; Northwestern Univ, Chicago; Mount Sinai Med Ctr, New York, et al)

Br J Ophthalmol 81:189–194, 1997 5–4

Introduction.—Varicella zoster virus retinitis (VZVR) in patients with AIDS (also known as progressive outer retinal necrosis) is a clinically distinct necrotizing retinitis syndrome caused by the varicella zoster virus. Most of these patients become blind. Medical therapies of 20 consecutive patients with AIDS and VZVR from 6 centers were evaluated to determine the long-term clinical course and visual outcomes.

Methods.—Medical records were reviewed for clinical characteristics at initial evaluation. Final visual acuities were evaluated in patients treated with acyclovir, ganciclovir, foscarnet, or a combination of foscarnet and ganciclovir.

Results.—The median follow-up was 6 months for the 20 patients, who had a mean age of 37.5 years. At initial evaluation, 14 patients (70%) had bilateral disease. Fifteen patients (75%) had previous or concurrent extraocular manifestations of VZVR infection. Median visual acuities were 20/40 at baseline and hand movements at final evaluation. At final evaluation, there was no light perception in 19 of 39 eyes (49%). Rhegmatogenous retinal detachments occurred in 27 eyes (69%). Visual acuity was significantly better at final evaluation in patients treated with a combination ganciclovir and foscarnet therapy or ganciclovir alone, compared with patients treated with acyclovir or foscarnet.

Conclusion.—The long-term visual outcome may be improved in patients with VZVR with aggressive medical treatment and appropriate medications. Acyclovir seems to be ineffective in treating VZVR in patients with AIDS. This report represents the second largest series, longest follow-up, and first analysis of visual outcomes based on medical treatment in patients with VZVR and AIDS.

► Progressive outer retinal necrosis (PORN) is a herpes zoster–related retinitis in patients with AIDS. Although it shares many characteristics of the acute retinal necrosis syndrome (ARN), its progression is unrelenting in many eyes, and it has an exceptionally grim visual prognosis because of its poor response to IV acyclovir. On our Retina Service at Wills Eye Institute, we have witnessed the catastrophic progression of this necrotizing retinitis and its ability to cause total bilateral loss of vision within weeks of presentation.

This report is important because it allows us to benefit from the experience of others and take a more aggressive treatment posture from the outset with these eyes, via the use of ganciclovir and combination therapy with ganciclovir and foscarnet. The study also reviews the importance of correct diagnosis of PORN and ARN to prescribe correct treatment. Progressive outer retinal necrosis should be thought of first in those individuals seen with bilateral retinitis and a history of HIV infection and previous cutaneous herpes zoster infection. The retinitis is deep and usually peripheral, with minimal associated vitritis. Healing perivascular changes can give a "cracked mud" appearance and retinal detachment is a frequent later complication.

J.I. Maguire, M.D.

Ganciclovir-loaded Polymer Microspheres in Rabbit Eyes Inoculated With Human Cytomegalovirus

Veloso AAS Jr, Zhu Q, Herrero-Vanrell R, et al (Harvard Med School, Boston)
Invest Ophthalmol Vis Sci 38:665–675, 1997 5–5

Introduction.—The most common cause of visual loss in patients with AIDS is cytomegalovirus (CMV) retinitis. Ganciclovir prevents replication of CMV DNA, but its short half-life requires frequent intravitreous injections to maintain a therapeutic level. An implantable sustained release device is available that can be placed in the vitreous cavity for several months. This device is not biodegradable and must be replaced, using a large incision, every 6–8 months. Microspheres of biodegradable poly(DL-lactide-co-glycolide) (PLGA) loaded with ganciclovir were used in rabbit eyes inoculated with human CMV to determine whether disease progression could be controlled.

Methods.—Human CMV (HCMV) was inoculated 4 days after rabbits underwent gas compression vitrectomy. Rabbit eyes were injected 2 days later with either ganciclovir-loaded microspheres or blank microspheres. Eyes were inspected for 14 days and vitritis, retinitis, and optic neuritis were graded to separate early HCMV-induced disease sequelae from later nonspecific host inflammatory responses. Biodegradation and tissue rejection were observed for 8 weeks in rabbits injected with ganciclovir-loaded microspheres.

Results.—Vitritis was reduced from days 3 to 14 and retinitis and optic neuritis were decreased from days 3 to 9 in eyes injected with ganciclovir-loaded microspheres. Vitritis increased from days 3 to 7, retinitis increased from days 3 to 9, and optic neuritis increased from days 3 to 14 in eyes that were injected with blank microspheres. Immunofluorescence of HCMV antigens were observed in control eyes but not in treated eyes. Histopathologic analysis indicated minimal focal disruption of the retinal architecture in treated eyes. Disorganization of the normal retinal architecture was seen in control eyes. There were no clinical or histopathologic indications of adverse tissue reaction in treated eyes at 8-week follow-up.

Conclusion.—The progression of fundus disease was controlled using ganciclovir-loaded microspheres in HCMV-inoculated rabbit eyes.

► Fifteen years ago, patients with AIDS and CMV retinitis were blind in 3 months and dead in one half year. Today, because of progress in the identification, understanding, and treatment of HIV infection and related complications, the longevity of patients with AIDS has significantly increased. This makes the identification of eyes at risk for CMV retinitis and their aggressive treatment imperative.

Current approved anti-CMV therapy includes ganciclovir, foscarnet, and cidofovir. Most patients receive IV management, but this has significant systemic risk, requires time-consuming daily dosing, and fails to prevent extension of disease for more than several months. The recent development of local therapy with ganciclovir sustained-release intravitreal devices has been of tremendous benefit. However, these devices require a large surgical wound and are not biodegradable. Replacement is required every 6–8 months.

The development of an injectable, biodegradable source of anti-CMV treatment would have the benefit of high intravitreal drug concentrations without the greater risk and visual morbidity of a more extensive surgical procedure requiring the insertion of a large inert drug source. With the introduction of better antiretroviral systemic treatments leading to increased life span in patients with AIDS, the importance of safer long-term local drug delivery systems is obvious.

J.I. Maguire, M.D.

Incidence of Retinopathy and Associated Risk Factors From Time of Diagnosis of Insulin-dependent Diabetes

Klein R, Palta M, Allen C, et al (Univ of Wisconsin, Madison; Med College of Wisconsin, Milwaukee)

Arch Ophthalmol 115:351–356, 1997 5–6

Introduction.—It is not known whether early glycemic control in insulin-dependent diabetes is more beneficial in preventing retinopathy than control achieved later in the course of diabetes. The prevalence of retinopathy and its relationship to glycemic control from the time of diagnosis was evaluated at baseline and at 4 years in a geographically defined, unselected population of young children, adolescents, and young adults in Wisconsin.

Methods.—Of 598 patients identified at baseline, 188 had fundus photographs taken. Photographs were gradable in at least 1 eye in 185 patients. Blood samples were evaluated for glycosylated hemoglobin, and 24-hour urine samples were obtained for determination of creatinine concentration during routine clinical visits.

Results.—At diagnosis, the prevalence of retinopathy was 1.3%. At 4 years' follow-up after diagnosis, retinopathy was observed in 5.1% of the cohort overall and in 9.7% of patients age 15 years or older. Patients with a mean glycosylated hemoglobin level of 12% or higher were 3.2% times as likely to have retinopathy at 4-year follow-up after controlling for age, compared with those with a mean glycosylated hemoglobin level of less than 12%.

Conclusion.—Age and glycemic control were important determinants in the risk of the development of retinopathy. Patients younger than 15 years and those with early glycemic control had a lower incidence of retinopathy.

► Data from several recent prospective trials, including the Diabetes Control and Complication Trial, have clearly demonstrated the reduced risk of retinopathy progression in juvenile insulin-dependent diabetics. This report amplifies certain inferences made in other studies, namely, the definitive impact of immediate tight glycemic control in newly diagnosed insulin-dependent diabetics. The risk of retinopathy development is over 3 times greater in subjects with higher glycosylated hemoglobin levels. Interestingly, the age of the subjects was also significant, with the risk of diabetic retinopathy progression over 4.5 times greater in persons over the age of 15 years, even when adjusted for glycosylated hemoglobin levels.

J.I. Maguire, M.D.

Natural History and Clinical Management of Central Retinal Vein Occlusion

Clarkson JC, for the Central Vein Occlusion Study Group (NIH, Bethesda, Md)

Arch Ophthalmol 115:486–491, 1997 5–7

Objective.—Clinical guidelines for the practical management of patients with central retinal vein occlusion (CRVO) were developed from a study of the natural history of CRVO, which was part of the prospective Central Vein Occlusion Study.

Methods.—Between August 1988 and August 1992, 725 patients (728 eyes), 53% male, with CRVO from 9 ophthalmic practices were examined at 4-month intervals for as long as 56 months. Iris neovascularization (INV), angle neovascularization (ANV), neovascular glaucoma, and visual acuity were measured. Risk factors for INV and ANV were identified.

Results.—Patients in the Central Vein Occlusion Study were more likely to be male and older than age 65 years. Visual acuity at inception was an important predictor of acuity at the end of the study. Of the patients entering the study with 20/40 vision or better, 65% had similar visual acuity at the end of the study. In patients with visual acuities ranging from 20/50 to 20/200, 19% improved, 44% were unchanged, and 37% worsened by the end of the study. Approximately 80% of patients entering the study with visual acuities less than 20/200 did not improve. Visual acuity and the amount of capillary nonperfusion seen with fluorescein angiogram studies were significant predictors of INV and ANV. Neovascularization should be treated by panretinal photocoagulation (PRP) at the first sign and should be observed every 2–4 weeks. Because, in rare cases, neovascularization can develop first in the angle, gonioscopic examinations should be conducted with an undilated pupil. Grid pattern photocoagulation should be considered for patients younger than 65 years who have perfused macular, but not ischemic, edema and who have a visual acuity of 20/50 or worse.

Conclusion.—Visual acuity is an important predictor of final acuity for CRVO patients with good and poor acuity. Patients with intermediate acuity have variable outcomes. Close follow-up to watch for INV and ANV is necessary, and prompt PRP treatment at the earliest sign reduces the complications resulting from neovascular glaucoma.

► Previous reports from the Central Vein Occlusion Study Group have reviewed the benefits of laser treatment in patients with ischemic central vein occlusions (CVO) who have anterior segment neovascularization. The group has also shown the lack of benefit of lasers for perfused macular edema in individuals older than the age of 65 years and had identified risk factors for secondary neovascularization. The current study outlines recommended management guidelines for eyes with CVO.

Visual acuity remains an important predictor of final acuity and anterior segment neovascularization. In summary:

1. Eyes with good initial vision (better than 20/40) have a good chance of maintaining excellent vision.
2. Eyes with poor initial acuity have a poor long-term visual prognosis.
3. Eyes with intermediate vision have variable outcomes.
4. The risk of secondary anterior segment neovascularization was 16% in the study group. Risk factors for secondary neovascularization were initial poor vision and capillary nonperfusion on fluorescein studies.
5. Eyes with a higher risk for anterior segment neovascularization should be observed monthly for the first 6 months after development of CVO.
6. Examinations should be conducted with an undilated pupil and should include gonioscopy.
7. Panretinal photocoagulation should be instituted when anterior segment neovascularization is first noted, not prophylactically.
8. The role of grid laser treatment in perfused macular edema involving individuals younger than the age of 65 years is unclear and may have a benefit.

J.I. Maguire, M.D.

Occult Choroidal Neovascularization in Age-related Macular Degeneration: A Natural History Study

Stevens TS, Bressler NM, Maguire MG, et al (Univ of Wisconsin-Madison; Johns Hopkins Univ, Baltimore, Md; Univ of Pennsylania, Philadelphia, et al)

Arch Ophthalmol 115:345–350, 1997 5–8

Introduction.—Prospectively collected information on the natural course of the morphology of subfoveal choroidal neurovascularization (CNV) is rare. Morphologic changes were observed in the visual acuity of eyes with occult CNV that did not meet eligibility criteria for participation in a macular photocoagulation trial of laser treatment.

Methods.—Eyes of 40 patients were followed for changes in size of lesion, development of classic CNV, change in vision, and development of subretinal fibrosis. Patients were symptomatic and eyes had poorly demarcated CNV associated with age-related macular degeneration.

Results.—During a follow-up of 9–12 months, 32% of occult CNV lesions increased more than twice their baseline size. In 52% of eyes without CNV at baseline, classic CNV developed during follow-up. There was a median loss of 2.5 lines in visual acuity. Subretinal fibrosis developed more frequently and more visual acuity was lost in eyes with classic CNV, subretinal blood, or both at baseline evaluation.

Conclusion.—Eyes with occult CNV lesions may have a highly variable course. The presence of subretinal blood or a component of classic CNV may affect the prognosis for further vision loss.

► This paper suffers from several deficiencies readily detailed by the authors. One is its small patient population in which more than 20% of the subjects were lost in a short follow-up. However, it makes many interesting contributions regarding the behavior of certainly the most common form of exudative age-related macular degeneration (ARMD), i.e., eyes with poorly demarcated subfoveal occult neovascularization.

Presently, less than 25% of evaluated eyes with exudative ARMD can be treated with laser in part because of the high incidence of foveal occult CNV. Many investigative trials—including those with low-dose radiation, photodynamic therapy, and submacular surgery—are now underway to evaluate the efficacy of therapy directed to eyes with this set of problems. However, good prospective natural history data are still lacking.

Stevens and colleagues point out clearly that these data do not include eyes with extrafoveal occult CNV; nonetheless, their efforts uncover some interesting findings. These include the substantial growth of occult changes during the study period, the greater tendency to disciform scar formation in those eyes with associated blood but not in those eyes with occult CNV alone, the approximate 50% of eyes with occult CNV in which areas of classic CNV develop within 1 year, and the smaller median amount of visual loss when compared with eyes with discrete subfoveal choroidal CNV. Overall, this small population of eyes with subfoveal poorly demarcated CNV shows a rather variable course and cautions against uncontrolled new treatment trials.

J.I. Maguire, M.D.

Risk Factors for Choroidal Neovascularization in the Second Eye of Patients With Juxtafoveal or Subfoveal Choroidal Neovascularization Secondary to Age-related Macular Degeneration

Maguire MG, for the Macular Photocoagulation Study Group (NIH, Bethesda, Md)

Arch Ophthalmol 115:741–747, 1997 5–9

Introduction.—Epidemiologic studies have identified a number of risk factors for age-related macular degeneration (ARMD) and for choroidal neovascularization (CNV). A follow-up study of 670 patients with CNV secondary to ARMD was conducted to confirm previously reported risk factors for the development of CNV in the fellow eye; to examine characteristics of the pericentral macula that may influence the risk for development of CNV; and to determine whether the presence of occult CNV in the first eye affects the development of CNV in the fellow eye.

Methods.—Study participants were enrolled in the Macular Photocoagulation Study trials of laser photocoagulation for new juxtafoveal CNV, new subfoveal CNV, or recurrent subfoveal CNV secondary to ARMD. Patients were classified according to systemic hypertension status. Follow-up for development of CNV in the fellow eye was scheduled for 3 and 6 months after enrollment and at 6-month intervals thereafter for up to 5 years. Color photographs were taken, and fluorescein angiography was performed at follow-up visits.

Results.—Complete information on development of CNV in the fellow eye within 5 years was available for 408 (61%) patients. Gradings of the central macular zone were available for 485 patients and of the pericentral macular zone for 333. Among those with no classic or occult CNV in the fellow eye, CNV developed in 35% within 5 years. The cumulative incidence rate at 5 years was 42%, and the incidence was higher for those with (49%) than without (33%) definite hypertension (relative risk [RR], 1.7). Also independently associated with an increased risk of developing CNV were the following 3 characteristics of the central macula of the fellow eye: (1) the presence of 5 or more drusen, (2) focal hyperpigmentation, and (3) 1 or more large drusen (RR 2.1, 2.0, and 1.5, respectively). The estimated 5-year incidence rates for CNV in the second eye ranged from 7% for patients with no risk factors to 87% for those with all 4 risk factors. Variables not strongly associated with development of CNV were characteristics of the pericentral macula. Occult CNV in the first eye did not influence the development of CNV or the type of CNV in the fellow eye.

Conclusion.—Both the presence of systemic hypertension and certain characteristics of the central macula of the fellow eye increase the risk for development of CNV. Patients with high risk may be candidates for preventive interventions.

► Age-related macular degeneration (ARMD) is the leading cause of severe central visual loss in the Western world. The increase in life expectancy over the last half century and the maturing of the baby boom generation ensures greater focus on this widespread condition. At present, laser photocoagulation benefits only a minority of patients, thus stimulating interest in the development of investigational therapies such as radiation, antiangiogenesis factors, photodynamic therapy, submacular surgery, and prophylactic use of laser of drusen. To determine which individuals might be more appropriate for enrollment these protocol studies, assessment of relative risk is imperative.

The Macular Photocoagulation Study expands on previous work outlining ocular and systemic risk factors for the development of choroidal neovascular membranes in the second eye of patients with juxtafoveal or subfoveal choroidal neovascularization caused by ARMD. Five or more drusen, focal hyperpigmentation, and 1 or more large drusen in the contralateral central macula, and systemic hypertension are all independent risk factors that confer increased risk of CNV. Estimated 5-year incidence rates of CNV ranged from 7% in eyes with no risk factors to nearly 90% in eyes with all 4 risk factors. These data are helpful not only in identifying patients at risk for appropriate counseling but also in allowing for better selection of individual eyes for investigational studies.

J.I. Maguire, M.D.

Inhibition of Angiogenesis by Tissue Inhibitor of Metalloproteinase-3

Anand-Apte B, Pepper MS, Voest E, et al (Univ Med Ctr, Geneva; Harvard Med School, Boston; Strangeways Research Lab, Cambridge, England)

Invest Ophthalmol Vis Sci 38:817–823, 1997 5–10

Background.—Sorsby's fundus dystrophy is a dominantly inherited form of blindness caused by mutations in the tissue inhibitor of metalloproteinase-3 (TIMP-3) gene. Choroidal neovascularization is a prominent

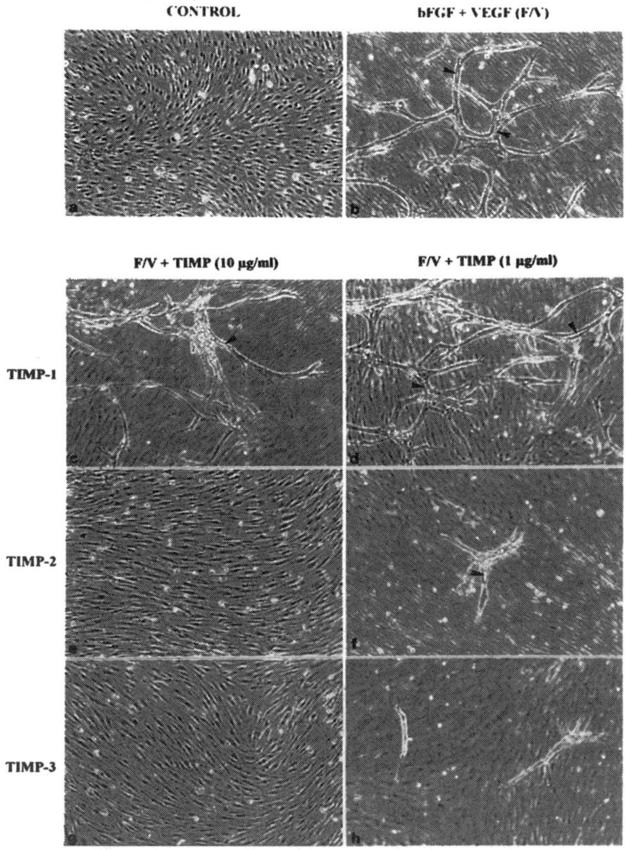

FIGURE 3.—Tissue inhibitor of metalloproteinase-2 (YIMP-2) and tissue inhibitor of metalloproteinase-3 (TIMP-3) inhibit endothelial cell invasion and tube formation in vitro. Confluent monolayers of bovine microvascular endothelial cells on 3-dimensional collagen gels were cotreated with basic fibroblast growth factor (bFGF) (10 ng/mL) and vascular endothelial growth factor (VEGF) (30 ng/mL) for 4 days. This results in the formation of cell cords within the gel, which can be observed by phase contrast microscopy by focusing beneath the surface monolayer (**b**). In control (untreated) cultures, the cells form a monolayer on the surface of the gel (**a**). Invasion by coadded by bFGF and VEGF was inhibited by TIMP-2 (**e, f**) and TIMP-3 (**g, h**) but not by TIMP-1 (**c, d**). TIMPs were added at 1 µg/mL (**d, f, h**) and 10 mg/mL (**c, e, g**). Arrowheads indicate translucent slit-like lumina. Magnification = 100×. (Reproduced by permission of the Association for Research in Vision and Ophthalmology, from Anand-Apte B, Pepper MS, Voest E, et al: Inhibition of angiogenesis by tissue inhibitor of metalloproteinase-3. *Invest Ophthalmol Vis Sci* 38:817–823, 1997.)

characteristic of this condition. The possible role of TIMP-3 protein in the regulation of angiogenesis was investigated.

Methods and Findings.—A modified Boyden chamber assay was used to examine chemotaxis of endothelial cells toward vascular endothelial growth factor (VEGF) and basic fibroblast growth factor (bFGF). Endothelial cells were placed in the upper chamber and allowed to migrate through an 8 μm pore polycarbonate membrane toward VEGF or bGFG in the lower chamber. The cells were then incubated with varying amounts of TIMP-3 during the assay to determine the ability of TIMP-3 to inhibit chemotaxis. Treatment with VEGF and bFGF resulted in invasion of the gel and formation of tubelike structures. Tissue inhibitors of metalloproteinases 1, 2, and 3 were then added to the culture specimens, and their effect on invasion was noted. An in vivo chorioallantoic membrane (CAM) assay using methylcellulose discs containing bFGF with or without TIMP-3 was performed. New blood vessel induction was examined with a stereomicroscope. Chemotaxis of vascular endothelial cells toward VEGF and bFGF was inhibited by TIMP-3. In addition, collagen gel invasion and capillary morphogenesis in vitro were inhibited, as well as bFGF-induced angiogenesis in the CAM assay in vivo (Fig 3).

Conclusions.—These data show that TIMP-3 inhibits some of the endothelial cell responses to physiologic angiogenic agents. It inhibits migration and prevents invasion and tube formation by endothelial cells in a 3-dimensional collagen matrix. A CAM assay confirmed that this inhibition of activity was relevant to angiogenesis in vivo. However, TIMP-3 has no discernible effect on endothelial cell proliferation.

► Sorsby's fundus dystrophy has several similarities to age-related macular degeneration including the breakdown of matrix materials within Bruch's membrane and the near certain development of choroidal neovascularization (CNV). The identification of a genetic locus responsible for the development of this entity makes it important as a learning tool for the mechanism of CNV development in other maculopathies including age-related macular degeneration.

In this report, the authors define how tissue inhibitor of metalloproteinase-3 (TIMP-3) inhibits the angiogenic properties of known angiogenic factors such as vascular endothelial growth factor (VEGF) and fibroblast growth factor (bFGF) in vitro. In vivo, the development of CNV requires multiple interactions from basement membrane degradation to endothelial cell proliferation, migration, and organization to form viable capillaries. The exact mechanism of TIMP-3's influence in this process is unknown but incontrovertible and may serve as a tool in our better understanding of exudative age-related maculopathy.

J.I. Maguire, M.D.

Interferon Alfa-2a Is Ineffective for Patients With Choroidal Neovascularization Secondary to Age-related Macular Degeneration: Results of a Prospective Randomized Placebo-controlled Clinical Trial

Guyer DR, and the Pharmacological Therapy for Macular Degeneration Study Group (Manhattan Eye, Ear & Throat Hosp, New York; et al)
Arch Ophthalmol 115:865–872, 1997 5–11

Background.—Age-related macular degeneration is the leading cause of blindness in the United States. The majority of patients with exudative maculopathy cannot be successfully treated with laser therapy. Interferon α-2a is an effective antiangeogenic agent. The safety and efficacy of this interferon for the treatment of choroidal neovascularization secondary to age-related macular degeneration was examined in a prospective, multicenter trial by the Pharmacological Therapy for Macular Degeneration Study Group.

Methods.—A randomized, placebo-controlled, parallel, multicenter, double-blind trial was performed at 45 ophthalmic centers. The study group consisted of 481 patients with clinical signs of exudative age-related macular degeneration. These patients were randomly allocated to 4 treatment groups, placebo or 1.5, 3.0, or 6.0 million international units (MIU) of interferon (Roferon-A). Visual acuity testing, clinical examination, fluorescein angiography, and indocyanine green angiography were performed. The primary clinical end point was loss of visual acuity at 1 year.

Results.—At 1 year, 38% of those in the placebo group and 50% of those in the combined treatment groups had lost at least 3 lines of visual acuity. At the highest treatment dosage, placebo appeared to be a better treatment than interferon. Signs of interferon-associated retinopathy were associated with the higher doses of interferon used in this study.

Conclusions.—This large case series demonstrates that interferon α-2a has no benefit greater than placebo for the treatment of choroidal neovascularization secondary to age-related macular degeneration. At higher doses, it may be associated with poorer visual outcome than placebo.

► The treatment of age-related macular degeneration (ARMD) has seen an explosion of investigative treatment protocols over the past 5 years. This is not surprising when one considers the demographics of our current population and the dire predictions regarding the state of Medicare and Social Security as the Baby Boomers reach retirement age. Certainly, we will be dealing with an ever-increasing threat to the welfare of our aging society from ARMD just on the basis of pure numbers of people at risk. Currently, laser is the only proven beneficial treatment for exudative ARMD, but a woefully inadequate one. The uses of investigative treatments including radiation, submacular surgery, photodynamic therapy, and pharmacologic treatment are natural outgrowths of photocoagulation's weakness.

If one mixes a large population of patients with a common condition making a significant impact on their lives, and the condition has a less than satisfactory therapy, a vacuum is created into which all manner of proposed treatments will be drawn. This creates opportunity for both real scientific medical investigation and also abuse. As physicians, we must constantly be aware of the inherent difficulties with individual case reports and case series that have no control population or randomization. It is disturbing to see the increasing amount of physicians quoted outside of peer-reviewed journals, in all forms of popular media, regarding such treatment. This has the tendency to sensationalize and mislead our patients. The use of interferon alfa-2a was initially reported as an effective treatment for many cases of ARMD and occupied our attention for several years in professional meetings and literature. Members of the Pharmacologic Therapy for Macular Degeneration Study Group should be commended for their rapid and scientific study of this treatment and their unambiguous finding that it is not beneficial.

J.I. Maguire, M.D.

Laser Photocoagulation for Persistent Central Serous Retinopathy: Results of Long-term Follow-up

Burumcek E, Mudun A, Karacorlu S, et al (SKK Okmeydani Hosp, Istanbul, Turkey)

Ophthalmology 104:616–622, 1997 5–12

Background.—Central serous retinopathy (CSR) is characterized by serous detachment of sensory retina in the posterior pole. It often occurs in otherwise healthy young men with type A personality. On angiography, 1 or more focal leaks can be seen at the level of the retina pigment epithelium. Although the serous detachment frequently disappears spontaneously in 3–4 months, CSR may persist. The effect of laser photocoagulation in patients with persistent CSR was investigated.

Methods.—Thirty-eight patients with 45 affected eyes in which CSR did not resolve after 4 months of observation were offered laser photocoagulation. Fourteen patients with 16 affected eyes declined this treatment and served as a control group. Argon green laser photocoagulation was performed on 9 of the remaining eyes, dye-yellow laser photocoagulation in 12, and dye-orange laser photocoagulation in 8. The patients were observed for a mean 4.8 years.

Findings.—Compared with untreated eyes, treated eyes had a shorter duration of serous detachment and better final best-corrected visual acuity (BCVA). Seven untreated eyes and none of the treated eyes had a recurrence during follow-up.

Conclusions.—Direct laser photocoagulation of the leakage sites for persistent CSR is effective and safe. This treatment shortens the duration of serous detachment, improves final BCVA, and reduces the incidence of recurrence.

▶ Fortunately, most cases of idiopathic central serous chorioretinopathy (CSR) resolve without intervention within 4 months of their appearance.

Unfortunately, a small percent of eyes progress to a chronic stage with varying degrees of pigment epitheliopathy and visual loss. Previous reports regarding the utility of laser photocoagulation in this condition have pointed to its ability to limit the length of an individual episode but not affect final visual outcome or future recurrence. This paper supports a different analysis and lends support to more aggressive treatment of persistent CSR in individuals with retinal involvement greater than 4 months' duration. Laser photocoagulation was deemed successful in shortening episodes of CSR while improving best corrected visual acuity and reducing recurrence rate when compared to controls.

J.I. Maguire, M.D.

Parabulbar Anesthesia for Primary Vitreoretinal Surgery

Sharma T, Gopal L, Parikh S, et al (Sankara Nethralaya, Madras, India)

Ophthalmology 104:425–428, 1997 5–13

Introduction.—Parabulbar anesthesia (sub-Tenon) is an alternative technique of local anesthesia that can be performed under direct observation, thus helping avoid the risk of globe perforation. This approach has not been evaluated regarding onset of anesthesia, volume of anesthetic mixture, need for local or systemic supplementation, or grading of its efficacy. The efficacy and safety of parabulbar anesthesia was analyzed in patients undergoing primary vitreoretinal surgery.

Methods.—There were 3 stages to parabulbar anesthesia administration: (1) orbicularis oculi injection, (2) subconjunctival injection, and (3) sub-Tenon irrigation. Anesthesia effects were graded on a scale of 0 (inadequate anesthesia or akinesia) to 5 (adequate anesthesia and akinesia without supplementation). Of 100 patients undergoing primary vitreoretinal surgery, vitrectomy was performed in 93 patients without buckling and 4 patients had an encircling band; 3 had scleral buckling. The mean surgical time was 89.38 minutes.

Results.—Most patients underwent pars plana vitrectomy and associated procedures (Table 1). Adequate anesthetic effect was achieved within 1–2 minutes in 94% of patients and within 3–5 minutes in the remaining 6% of patients. The anesthetic mixture volume was below 10 mL in 92% of patients. No supplementation was required in 69% of patients with grades 4–5 anesthesia. Thirty-one percent of patients with grades 1–3 anesthesia required local supplementation for either inadequate anesthesia, inadequate akinesia, or both. No ocular or systemic complications were observed. Early onset of anesthesia was significantly correlated with adequate anesthesia throughout the procedure.

Conclusion.—Parabulbar anesthesia may be considered a safe and effective approach to local anesthesia in patients undergoing primary vitreoretinal surgery.

TABLE 1.—Vitreoretinal Surgical Procedures

Procedures	No. of Patients
Vitrectomy and associated procedures	87
Lensectomy + vitrectomy + gas/silicone oil, endolaser	4
Scleral buckling	4
Vitrectomy + encircling and associated procedures	2
Lensectomy + vitrectomy + endolaser	2
Lensectomy + vitrectomy + encircling + silicone oil injection + IOFB removal + endolaser	1
Lensectomy + vitrectomy + encircling + gas + endolaser	1

Abbreviation: IOFB, intraocular foreign body.
(Published courtesy of *Ophthalmology*, from Sharma T, Gopal L, Parikh S, et al: Parabulbar anesthesia for primary vitreoretinal surgery. *Ophthalmology* 104:425–428, 1997.)

► Advances in anterior segment microsurgical technique with better instrumentation and foldable lenses allowing small self-sealing wounds have, in turn, facilitated the move to less invasive anesthesia. More and more we are seeing cataract surgery with topical treatment alone. The advantages are clear; safer delivery of anesthetic with less cost and more rapid patient recovery.

In vitrectomy procedures, minimal manipulation of external ocular structures and small surgical incision size allow parabulbar injection. This technique gives both adequate anesthesia and akinesia while avoiding the risks of globe penetration or orbital and optic nerve injury. Drug delivery is easily supplemented in longer cases. We will often use a technique similar to the authors' in eyes we think are at higher risk for inadvertent needle penetration. In the managed care era, effective and safe techniques with less cost and more rapid patient turnover will become the standard.

J.I. Maguire, M.D.

Removal of Retained Lens Fragments After Phacoemulsification Reverses Secondary Glaucoma and Restores Visual Acuity

Vilar NF, Flynn HW, Smiddy WE, et al (Univ of Miami, Fla)
Ophthalmology 104:787–792, 1997 5–14

Background.—The rate of dropped nuclei or retained lens fragments after phacoemulsification procedures is reported to be about 3 in 1,000. It is inversely correlated with the individual surgeon's patient volume. Removing retained lens fragments by pars plana vitrectomy generally restores good visual function and reverses many complications. The effect of vitrectomy on secondary glaucoma and visual acuity outcomes in patients with retained lens fragments after phacoemulsification is reported.

Methods and Findings.—One hundred twenty-six patients undergoing vitrectomy for retained lens fragments after phacoemulsification during a 3-year period were included in the retrospective analysis. Glaucoma was

TABLE 1.—Clinical Features of Patients With Retained Lens Fragments on the Initial and Final Examination: No. of Patients (%)

	Initial Examination (N = 114)*	Final Examination (N = 126)
Glaucoma (IOP ≥ 30 mmHg)	42 (36.8)	4 (3.2)
Visual acuity ≤ 20/200	76 (66.6)	25 (19.8)
Retinal detachment†	11 (9.6)	11 (8.7)

*Twelve patients had phacoemulsification and vitrectomy on the same day, precluding an initial examination.
†Newly diagnosed retinal detachment occurred in 11 eyes before or during vitrectomy and in 11 eyes after vitrectomy.
(Published courtesy of *Ophthalmology*, from Vilar NF, Flynn HW, Smiddy WE, et al: Removal of retained lens fragments after phacoemulsification reverses secondary glaucoma and restores visual acuity. *Ophthalmology* 104:787–792, 1997.)

defined as an intraocular pressure of 30 mmHg or more. Thirty-seven percent of 114 patients had glaucoma before vitrectomy, and 3.2% of 126 had it after vitrectomy. The rates of persistent glaucoma did not differ, regardless of the intervals between cataract surgery and vitrectomy. Visual acuity was 20/40 or better in 11.4% of the patients before vitrectomy and in 59.5% after vitrectomy. The rates of visual acuity of 20/40 or better were also similar for all intervals (Tables 1 and 2).

Conclusions.—Vitrectomy for removal of retained lens fragments decreases secondary glaucoma and results in favorable outcomes in visual acuity. Early vitrectomy is generally recommended for eyes with increased intraocular pressure. However, outcomes are also favorable when vitrectomy is delayed.

► The evolution of cataract surgery to small incisional technique with phacoemulsification has increased the incidence of retained nuclear fragments in the posterior segment related to capsular tears. Although cortical remnants usually resolve on their own, nuclear fragments often result in the development of secondary uveitis, intraocular pressure elevation, corneal edema, and phacoanaphylaxis. This report highlights the use of pars plana vitrectomy in the removal of retained lens fragments and its ability to restore vision and ameliorate pressure elevation and secondary uveitis. Timing of vitrectomy in this study did not significantly alter endstage intraocular pressure or final visual acuity. Retinal detachment remains a significant risk both before and after surgery at rates almost approaching 20% in eyes with

TABLE 2.—Glaucoma* Prevalence [No. (%)] in the 3 Time Intervals Between Phacoemulsification and Vitrectomy

	≤1 Week (N = 49)	>1 Week to ≤4 Weeks (N = 39)	>4 Weeks (N = 38)
Initial examination (before vitrectomy)	16 (32.6)	10 (25.6)	16 (42.1)
Final examination (after vitrectomy)	2 (4.1)	1 (2.5)	1 (2.6)

*Glaucoma was defined as an intraocular pressure of at least 30 mmHg.
(Published courtesy of *Ophthalmology*, from Vilar NF, Flynn HW, Smiddy WE, et al: Removal of retained lens fragments after phacoemulsification reverses secondary glaucoma and restores visual acuity. *Ophthalmology* 104:787–792, 1997.)

retained nuclear material. Anterior segment surgeons are cautioned to act conservatively with posteriorly migrating lens material and avoid the use of maneuvers with instruments that can promote vitreoretinal traction, vitreous hemorrhage, macular edema, and corneal decompensation. A staged approach with vitrectomy at a later date is preferable to overzealous maneuvers at the time of cataract surgery.

J.I. Maguire, M.D.

The Management of Giant Retinal Tears Using Perfluoroperhydrophenanthrene: A Multicenter Case Series

Kertes PJ, and the Vitreon Collaborative Study Group (Louisiana State Univ, New Orleans)

Ophthalmology 104:1159–1165, 1997 5–15

Background.—Giant retinal tears are retinal breaks that are at least 90 degrees in circumference. They are more common in males and are associated with trauma and myopia. High-grade proliferative vitreoretinopathy often complicates treatment. Perfluorocarbon liquids, such as perfluoroperhydophenanthrene (Vitreon), are low viscosity, heavier-than-water liquids, which are inert, optically clear, and immiscible with blood or water. They can be used for atraumatic manipulation of the retina. The experience of the Vitreon Collaborative Study Group with intraoperative and adjunctive postoperative use of Vitreon in the treatment of giant retinal tears was evaluated.

Study Design.—A multicenter, prospective case series study of 162 eyes of 161 patients with retinal detachments secondary to giant retinal tears was performed from 1989 to 1994. Patients were observed for at least 6 months after surgery. The surgery included a complete 3-port pars plana vitrectomy followed by membrane dissection or retinotomy. Perfluoroperhydrophenanthrene was injected over the optic nerve to flatten the retina. Endophotocoagulation or cryopexy was used to manage the flap edge. Perfluoroperhydrophenanthrene was left in 16 eyes for extended retinal tamponade.

Results.—Four eyes were considered irreparable. Retinal reattachment was achieved in the remaining 158 eyes. This attachment was retained in 147 eyes at the most recent follow-up. The most common postoperative complications were recurrent retinal detachments in 49.4%, cataract formation, macular pucker, corneal decompensation, and hypotony. About half of these patients had improvement in their Snellen acuity score of at least 1 line. Hypotony, macular detachment, history of cataract surgery, tear extension of greater than 180 degrees, and higher grade proliferative vitreoretinopathy were all predictive of poor visual outcome. In those eyes in which Vitreon remained after surgery, it was well tolerated and the outcomes were similar to the rest of the group.

Conclusions.—This large case series demonstrates that the perfluorocarbon liquid, Vitreon, is safe and effective in the management of giant retinal tears. It may also be useful for extended post-operative retinal tamponade.

► The development of perfluorocarbon liquids is, in my opinion, one of the most significant vitreoretinal developments of the last 10 years. Its physical properties of low viscosity, a specific gravity close to water, optical clarity, and immiscibility with water—as well as silicone oil—make it an ideal tool for retinal manipulation, especially in the setting of retinal detachment secondary to giant retinal tears.

Retinal detachment from giant retinal tears previously had a significant failure rate at initial surgery because of retinal rolling and slippage. This occurs from the absence of anterior support with large tears. Previous surgical techniques often called for inversion of the patient in a prone position and performing air-fluid exchange to unroll and flatten the retina. This required the surgeon to assume a position below the patient, often while sitting on the floor. Retinal tacks, retinal sutures, and silicone oil manipulation were alternate methods of repair, but carried risks of bleeding and additional intraoperative damage.

At present, the use of heavier than water vitreous substitutes allows retinal flattening and repositioning with minimal manipulation and at the operating microscope in a standard operating position. Despite this, the incidence of redetachment is high, nearly 50% in this study. Proliferative vitreoretinopathy continues to be a major consequence of giant retinal tear development even with perfluorocarbon liquids. However, anatomical reattachment, visual acuity, and stabilization are tremendously improved with their use and they are now the standard of care.

J.I. Maguire, M.D.

Laser Treatment in Eyes With Large Drusen: Short-term Effects Seen in a Pilot Randomized Clinical Trial

Sternberg P, for the Choroidal Neovascularization Prevention Trial Research Group (Emory Univ, Atlanta, Ga)
Ophthalmology 105:11–23, 1998 5–16

Introduction.—Large or soft drusen disappear with various forms of laser treatment. Because such drusen are strong risk factors for the development of exudative age-related macular degeneration (AMD) in fellow eyes of patients with 1 eye already affected, and in eyes of patients without exudative AMD, there has been great interest in investigating whether laser treatment decreases the incidence of neovascular AMD and the accompanying loss of vision. There has been concern that the potentially preventive laser treatment may cause visual field abnormalities, the development of choroidal neovascularization (CNV), or geographic atrophy. The effects of laser treatment in reducing the area of drusen were evaluated. The short-term safety of the laser treatment was evaluated.

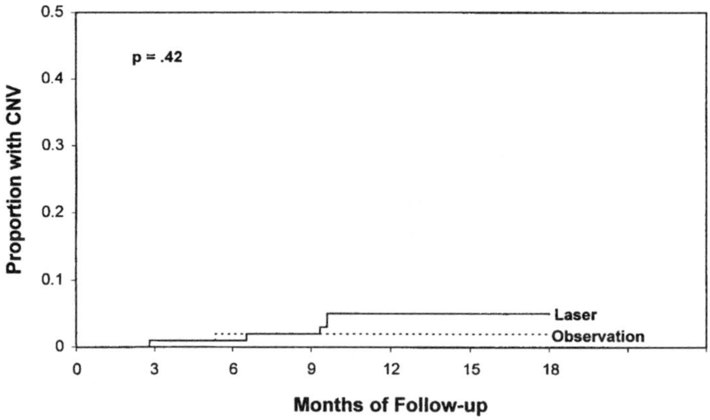

FIGURE 5.—Estimated proportion of eyes in the Bilateral Drusen Study in which choroidal neovascularization (*CNV*) developed by treatment group and months of follow-up. (Courtesy of the Choroidal Neovascularization Prevention Trial Research Group: Laser treatment in eyes with large drusen: Short-term effects seen in a pilot randomized clinical trial. *Ophthalmology* 105:11–23. Copyright 1998, published courtesy of *Ophthalmology*.)

Methods.—There were 312 eyes of 156 patients in the Bilateral Drusen Study and 120 eyes of 120 patients in the Fellow Eye Study. The patients in the Bilateral Drusen Study did not have exudative AMD but had more than 10 large drusen (greater than 63 μm) in each eye. In the Fellow Eye Study, 59 eyes were assigned to laser treatment and 61 eyes were assigned to observation. The patients in the Fellow Eye Study had exudative AMD in 1 eye and more than 10 large drusen in the other eye. Eighty-five percent of eyes had 210 laser burns, 100 μm in diameter in a pattern of 3 rows. A second treatment was applied with 24 laser burns in a circular pattern of 2 rows surrounding the macular drusen nasal to the fovea in a mirror

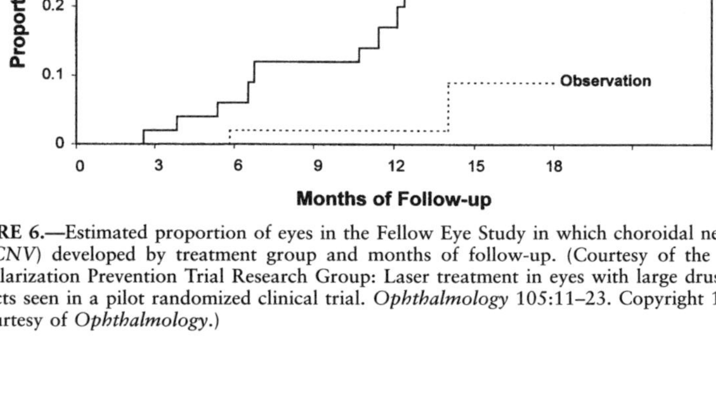

FIGURE 6.—Estimated proportion of eyes in the Fellow Eye Study in which choroidal neovascularization (*CNV*) developed by treatment group and months of follow-up. (Courtesy of the Choroidal Neovascularization Prevention Trial Research Group: Laser treatment in eyes with large drusen: Short-term effects seen in a pilot randomized clinical trial. *Ophthalmology* 105:11–23. Copyright 1998, published courtesy of *Ophthalmology*.)

image of the first treatment when the area of drusen had not been reduced by 50% or more in 6 months

Results.—In 14 of 156 treated eyes and in 2 of 156 observed eyes, CNV developed in the Bilateral Drusen Study (Fig 5). The proportions were 2 of 61 observed eyes and 10 of 59 treated eyes in the Fellow Eye Study (Fig 6). In treated and observed eyes in the Bilateral Drusen Study, changes in visual acuity were similar through 18 months. However, more visual acuity was lost in the observed eyes in the Fellow Eye Study than in the treated eyes. In treated and observed eyes in each study, changes in contrast threshold were similar.

Conclusions.—The short-term incidence of CNV may be increased by laser treatment to high-risk fellow eyes. More observation is necessary to determine long-term effects in fellow eyes and effects in patients with bilateral drusen. Because of an increased short-term incidence of choroidal neovascular development, the study suspended further treatment of laser prophylaxis to contralateral eyes in the Fellow Eye Study.

► Age-related macular degeneration is a continual frustration because of a dearth of effective treatment regimens. Currently, laser remains the only proven effective therapy for exudative maculopathy. However, it is a decidedly inadequate one benefiting perhaps 10% of all eyes afflicted with "wet" changes. Into this treatment vacuum steps laser treatment for drusen and a host of pilot studies, including that by the Choroidal Neovascularization Prevention Trial Research Group, aimed at evaluating prophylactic photocoagulation in eyes with non-exudative disease. I am pleased that such a group exists and that it has undertaken a randomized pilot study. Clearly, an attempt to pre-empt exudative changes with their overall horrible visual results is a viable concept in high-risk eyes.

In this trial, there are 2 separate groups, 1 with bilateral drusen alone and the other with a unilateral disciform process. Although many studies have quantified risk of CNV in the contralateral eye of individuals with unilateral disciforms, there is still no single good natural history study that assesses long-term risk of CNV in eyes with bilateral nonexudative disease alone; some estimates predict a less than 5% risk over a 10-year period. This study has suspended further treatment of laser prophylaxis to contralateral eyes with unilateral CNV because of increased short-term risk of CNV development. However, the bilateral drusen treatment group continues. In this arm of the trial, the mean age is 71 years. The question is whether such a treatment is necessary at all in a group at small risk over their remaining life, especially if the potential for creating increased risk is present.

J.I. Maguire, M.D.

Decision-making in the Treatment of Subfoveal Neovascularization in Age-related Macular Degeneration: An Analysis From the Patient's Perspective

Bernstein PS, Seddon JM (Massachusetts Eye & Ear Infirmary, Boston)

Retina 16:112–116, 1996 5–17

Introduction.—The leading cause of new blindness among the elderly is age-related macular degeneration. Recently updated findings from the Macular Photocoagulation Study have determined specific clinical situations from which prompt photocoagulation of subfoveal membranes is recommended in patients with age-related macular degenerations. Because of the potential immediate decrease in visual acuity induced by the laser treatment, many ophthalmologists in clinical practice still do not recommend photocoagulation for many of their patients. Little is known regarding patient attitudes toward this controversial treatment of exudative age-related macular degeneration. Whether subfoveal neovascular membranes caused by age-related macular degeneration should be treated was analyzed from the patient's perspective.

Methods.—There were 68 patients with age-related macular degeneration who were surveyed with 5 hypothetical clinical scenarios to measure their preferences for the immediate visual loss induced by laser therapy compared with the potential long-term benefits of laser photocoagulation. The questions assessed the patient's willingness to trade an immediate decrease in visual acuity in the only seeing eye vs. the retention of good reading vision for 1 year followed by a severe loss of vision; the ability to drive as a measure of visual function; the willingness to have laser treatment when vision remains normal in the unaffected eye; and prompt treatment with a substantial risk of immediate visual loss in the only seeing eye vs. deferral for 6 months with a risk of progression to an untreatable lesion.

Results.—Despite the risk of immediate visual loss, patients strongly preferred laser intervention. The laser treatment outcome was preferred over the natural course of the disease on all 5 questions.

Conclusions.—When ophthalmologists are making clinical recommendations to patients with subfoveal exudative macular degeneration, they may suggest that according to a survey, a substantial number of patients preferred laser treatment instead of no treatment.

▶ The debate continues regarding treatment of foveal choroidal neovascularization in the setting of age-related macular degeneration. My personal feeling is that if a hypothetical patient survey is needed to find support for a therapy, then it must be one with overall poor practical results. If the Oregon Plan for the triage of health care dollars was in force, I believe sincerely that foveal ablation would be one of its first casualties. As always, there are individual exceptions. In patients with large disciform scars, especially those with extramacular extension, I will treat subfoveal lesions if vision is less than 20/100. However, the severe visual limitations of this therapy, the high risk of recurrence, and the health care dollars involved direct me to recommend it rarely.

J.I. Maguire, M.D.

Suggested Reading

Wright AF: Gene therapy for the eye. *Br J Ophthalmol* 81:620–623, 1997.

► "Preventative medicine at its pinnacle" would be an apt descriptor of gene therapy. For all of us in medical care, the environment vs. hereditary argument is a weighty issue. We constantly advise our patients on the benefits of diet, exercise, and the avoidance of certain behaviors or practices which directly increase our risk in contracting certain diseases. Despite exemplary behavior, however, we are still at the mercy of those who came before and left us their genetic patterns.

The increasing sophistication of genetic analysis and the location of specific loci for certain conditions is the first step in our future ability to eliminate these sequences and thus modify or eliminate disease states. Currently, specific defects have been found in 20 of 87 mapped genes known to be involved in hereditary retinal disease. This is exciting, a first step in a homology similar to that of Koch's postulates. Instead of identifying an organism, we identify the responsible genetic sequence. Then, removal of that sequence tests the validity of it as the source of the problem.

The development of technology and our abilities to easily, safely, and permanently remove, disable, or modify a particular disease-causing sequence will be the focus of future research.

J.I. Maguire, M.D.

6 Oculoplastic Surgery

Adopting New Technology

by Robert B. Penne, M.D.

New technology and products are presented daily in modern medicine. The difficulty is in determining which technology is adequately tested and proven for adoption into your practice. Even though most new treatments have a background of research and controlled use, there is always doubt about safety efficacy until a product has been time tested on a large population.

For a practicing ophthalmologist, there is a fine line between waiting until a new technology is well tested and the fear of falling behind in providing the most modern technology for your practice. The modern era of advertising has encouraged the introduction of new technology. Advertising the use of the newest techniques will attract public interest; however, these techniques may not always be the very best for our patients. Companies producing new technology will push their newest product to establish a share in the marketplace. This may add pressure to try a new technology.

In choosing articles for the YEAR BOOK, one aim is to introduce readers to new technology. An attempt is made to introduce the more promising changes in the articles reviewed over the year. A paper will only provide a single view on the new technology. I then try and give my view on the usefulness of this new technology.

Over the past year, there have been a number of changes introduced in oculoplastics. These include advances in skin resurfacing, new implants, lacrimal surgery, and changes in treating orbital vascular lesions, among others. What changes have I made in my practice? None of these changes represent any experimental technology. Rather they are adoption of technology or techniques that have been shown to be safe and effective and fill a need in my practice.

The first change I have made is the use of balloon dacryoplasty for the treatment of partial nasolacrimal duct obstruction. This is not a new procedure and has been done by radiologists since 1986. The technology of a balloon introduced through the external lacrimal system has been available for nearly 2 years. Despite this, the exact success rate and the type of obstruction (partial vs. complete) on which this should be used are being studied. This is certainly a good example of a technology introduced before all the indications for use were determined. At Wills Eye Hospital, we are studying this for use in partial nasolacrimal duct obstruction, and we feel success will be in the 70% rate. These results are not yet long-term. This technique does offer a good chance of successfully treating a partial obstruction without cutting.

The entire area of treatment for lacrimal obstruction continues to evolve. All technology is compared to the standard dacryocystorhinostomy with a success rate in the low 90%. Balloon dacryoplasty may ultimately be a procedure that can be done in the office, which would certainly make the lower success rate more acceptable.

The second change I made in my practice relates back to a new technology released in 1990. The hydroxyapatite implant was introduced in 1990 and rapidly became the accepted implant for enucleation and evisceration. Implantation was followed by optional peg placement 6–9 months later to try and improve motility. Since then a porous polypropylene implant, which has a motility peg system, has been introduced and is also widely used. There has been little written to either prove or disprove the motility improvement with either peg system. What has recently become evident in my practice is that only a small percent of patients go on to peg placement, and there can be complications associated with them. Pegs definitely have a higher maintenance requirement for patients. I find most of my patients are happy with the motility they achieve with a porous implant and do not encourage them to proceed with peg placement unless their motility is very poor or they are very motivated. I am also looking closely at my choice of implants and doing more eviscerations except in traumatic cases.

No single source or person can predict what technology will prove successful and should be adopted. As you read the selected papers, keep in mind that there are only two opinions being expressed, mine and the author's. If this stimulates your interest in a particular new method, then a personal review of the literature will allow you to fairly and completely judge its value for your own practice.

Relation Between Signs and Symptoms of Dry Eye in the Elderly: A Population-based Perspective

Schein OD, Tielsch JM, Munõz B, et al (Johns Hopkins Univ, Baltimore, Md)
Ophthalmology 104:1395–1401, 1997 6–1

Objective.—Routine tests for dry eye, or Sjögren's syndrome include the Schirmer test or the rose bengal test. The generalizability of these methodologies is limited because dry eye is heterogeneous in etiology and pathophysiology, and clinical research has been confined to clinic-based populations. Results of the first population-based study on the relation of dry eye symptoms, Schirmer test, and rose bengal tests in the United States are explored.

Methods.—A dry eye symptom evaluation was completed in 1993 by 2,420 community-dwelling individuals (58% women, 26% black), age 65–84, living in Salisbury, Maryland. Symptoms and prevalence were recorded by age-group, sex, and race. Rose bengal and Schirmer tests were performed on those with 1 or more symptoms. Associations between test results and frequency of symptoms and demographic characteristics were compared statistically.

Results.—No symptoms were reported by 41% of patients, 1 or more symptoms rarely or sometimes by 45%, and 1 or more symptoms often or all the time by 14%. There were no significant differences between any of the groups. The average Schirmer test score in the lower scoring eye was 12.4. The average rose bengal test score in the higher scoring eye was 1.4, although 57% had a rose bengal score of 0, and 42% had a score of ≥1. There were no differences between any of the groups with respect to symptoms or test scores. Those with more frequent symptoms tended to have more rose bengal staining. Sensitivities for the individual rose bengal and Schirmer tests never exceeded 30%, and the 2 methods had little overlap.

Conclusion.—This population-based study showed that the rose bengal and Schirmer tests had little overlap and low sensitivity for the detection and classification of individuals with dry eye.

► The conclusion of this study is that there is little relationship between those patients with complaints consistent with dry eyes and those found on clinical basis (Schirmer and rose bengal testing) to have dry eyes. This certainly makes one wonder if these tests really have any value in making this diagnosis.

Successful identification and management of patients with dry eyes cannot be done with a single test but requires a complete evaluation, as with most ocular conditions. Schirmer and rose bengal testing are only a part of the evaluation for dry eyes. This may be the real point that can be taken from this study. Why some patients appear clinically to have dry eyes but exhibit few symptoms, whereas others have complaints without signs, is less than clear. This study simply verifies with statistical backing the clinical variability we all deal with in our practice. Dry eyes, although often viewed as a trivial disease, offers significant challenge in its correct diagnosis and in the proper long-term treatment.

An extension of these results would be the wide variability patients have in response to the treatment of dry eyes. We all have patients who have little response to any treatment yet on clinical examination, these patients appear similar to patients who have a good response to treatment. All these factors, which have a tremendous amount of subjective variability, show why studies on dry eyes or blepharitis treatment are so difficult.

R.B. Penne, M.D.

Periorbital and Orbital Cellulitis in the *Haemophilus influenzae* Vaccine Era

Barone SR, Aiuto LT (New York Univ, Manhasset)

J Pediatr Ophthalmol Strabismus 34:293–296, 1997 6–2

Objective.—Since the introduction of *Haemophilus influenzae* type b vaccines in 1985, the incidence of periorbital and orbital infections by the organism has declined dramatically. Characteristics of children with periorbital and orbital infections in the era of *H. influenzae* vaccines are defined.

Methods.—Medical records of 106 patients, average age 56 months, with periorbital cellulitis, and 28 patients, average age 92 months, with orbital cellulitis, hospitalized between 1985 and 1995 were reviewed.

Results.—Of the 133 patients tested 5, had a positive blood culture, and 2 cultures grew *H. influenzae* type b. No cultures after July 1987 grew *H. influenzae* type b. Sinusitis was diagnosed in 38 of 47 (81%) patients with periorbital cellulitis who underwent a radiographic evaluation and in 96% of patients with orbital cellulitis. Abscesses developed in half of the patients with orbital cellulitis.

Conclusion.—*H. influenzae* type b is no longer the primary causative agent for periorbital and orbital cellulitis. Clinicians should look for organisms that can cause sinusitis in children with periorbital and orbital cellulitis.

► The choice of antibiotic coverage for orbital cellulitis has long included the need to cover *H. influenzae* in children. This was a concept that was drilled into our heads during our training as residents and fellows. Since the introduction of a vaccine for *H. influenzae* in 1985, the need to cover for this bacteria as a significant pathogen in orbital cellulitis has decreased. This study looks at *H. influenzae* as a cause of orbital cellulitis and finds that the organism now appears to be almost nonexistent in children with orbital cellulitis.

This seems like a significant change for the management of orbital cellulitis. In reality, we use the broadest spectrum of antibiotics aimed at the sinus organisms because we rarely know the actual organism until later in treatment. In doing so, most choices of broad-antibiotics cover *H. influenzae* as well. Thus, the actual choice of antibiotics is not altered at this time. However, the intellectual approach to this disease in children has taken a significant turn. The concept of vaccines like this certainly gives us hope for the improvement of treatment, or even eradication of infections, in the future.

R.B. Penne, M.D.

Outcome of Orbital Myositis: Clinical Features Associated With Recurrence

Mannor GE, Rose GE, Moseley IF, et al (Moorfields Eye Hosp, London)
Ophthalmology 104:409–414, 1997 6–3

Background.—Most cases of orbital myositis respond to timely systemic therapy. However, recurrent or persistent episodes may require long-term therapy, sometimes including chemotherapy, radiation therapy, or surgery. The clinical features of patients with acute nonrecurrent and recurrent orbital myositis were analyzed.

Methods.—The study included 26 patients with orbital myositis, as defined by specific clinical criteria. Each patient's clinical, laboratory, and radiologic data were analyzed. The radiologist who reviewed the CT scans was unaware of the patients' clinical findings or outcome. Fisher's exact test was used to determine the frequency of various clinical and radiologic parameters among the 20 patients with a single, acute episode of orbital myositis and the 6 patients with recurrent episodes.

Results.—Factors associated with recurrent orbital myositis included male sex, lack of proptosis, eyelid retraction, and horizontal extraocular muscle (EOM) movement. Other factors linked to recurrent episodes were multiple or bilateral EOM involvement, muscle tendon sparing, and failure to respond to systemic corticosteroids or nonsteroidal anti-inflammatory drugs. Five of 6 recurrent episodes required systemic corticosteroid therapy, 4 required radiation therapy after EOM biopsy, and 2 required surgery for permanent EOM restriction.

Conclusions.—Factors associated with recurrent orbital myositis are identified. A treatment algorithm is presented for patients with orbital myositis, starting with up to 3 weeks of treatment with a nonsteroidal anti-inflammatory drug such as ibuprofen. Patients who do not respond to this treatment or in whom recurrent disease is likely should receive prednisone for 1–4 weeks, sometimes longer. Early systemic steroids may be considered for patients with characteristics associated with recurrent disease.

► Treatment of orbital myositis is often initiated with oral prednisone. This treatment has the advantage of prompt resolution of pain and discomfort, often in 48–72 hours. Prednisone does have the real risk of side effects even in young healthy patients. This paper suggests the initiation of treatment with nonsteroidal anti-inflammatory medication in these patients. The study identifies a subgroup of patients at risk of recurrent disease and suggests treating these patients initially with oral steroids. Recurrent disease is treated with oral prednisone and orbital radiation is suggested as the third line of treatment.

This approach has the advantage of using a medication with less potential side effects, which is certainly desirable. What is less clear is how quickly the symptoms resolve with the use of nonsteroidal medication. This is not directly stated in the study. If it takes 1–2 weeks for symptoms to resolve, that is a disadvantage. There also needs to be a concern that slower treatment could make recurrence more likely. This did not seem to be the case in this study.

The observation that sparing of the muscle tendon is not diagnostic of thyroid-related ophthalmopathy has been noted before but is restated here and is important to remember. This study showed an 18% incidence of muscle tendon sparing in myositis.

The use of nonsteroidal medication in orbital myositis appears to have merit in patients not known to be at risk of recurrent disease. I will be more likely to give patients a trial of nonsteroidal anti-inflammatory treatment before starting oral prednisone. I still feel that patient selection is important in the use of this mode of treatment.

R.B. Penne, M.D.

The Prevalence and Implications of Ocular Hypertension and Glaucoma in Thyroid-associated Orbitopathy

Cockerham KP, Pal C, Jani B, et al (Walter Reed Army Med Ctr, Washington, DC; Alleghent Gen Hosp, Pittsburgh, Pa; Case Western Univ, Cleveland, Ohio)

Ophthalmology 104:914–917, 1997 6–4

Background.—The prevalence of ocular hypertension in patients with thyroid-associated orbitopathy (TAO) has not been well documented. Its prevalence in one population of patients with TAO was established to determine the incidence of progression to glaucomatous damage and to identify potential risk factors for progression.

Methods and Findings.—The records of 500 consecutive patients with TAO seen at 1 center between 1985 and 1995 were reviewed. Twenty-four percent had an intraocular pressure (IOP) between 22 and 30 mm Hg. The affected patients were 86 women and 34 men, mean age 55 years. Mean follow-up was 4 years. Seven patients were classified as having suspected glaucoma based on increased but nonprogressive cup-to-disk ratios or nonprogressive, atypical visual field changes in the presence of increased IOP. Two patients had progressive visual field abnormalities and cupping. The duration of active orbital involvement was the only factor studied that was associated significantly with progression to glaucomatous damage. Mean TAO duration was 3 years in patients with ocular hypertension, 8 years for those with suspected glaucoma, and 12 years for patients with glaucomatous damage.

Conclusions.—In this study, progression to glaucomatous damage was correlated only with a prolonged duration of active TAO in association with ocular hypertension. Patients with chronic TAO need special attention and close follow-up to prevent optic nerve damage.

▶ The significant number of thyroid-associated orbitopathy patients with elevated intraocular pressure is not surprising in a disease where inflammation and scarring cause elevated intraorbital pressure and impingement of tissues on the globe. The development of increased intraocular pressure in upgaze in thyroid-associated orbitopathy patients has long been recognized. Often the intraocular pressure varies greatly with eye position or even slight squeezing by the patient when the pressure is checked. My experience has been similar to that in this study in that despite elevated intraocular pressure, glaucoma develops in only a few of these patients. In addition, lowering a patient's intraorbital pressure with orbital decompression will not always alter the course of glaucoma in the patient with both diseases.

Visual field changes developed in only 2 of the study patients. What is missing in this study is good definition of the severity of the thyroid-associated orbitopathy. If the patients with optic nerve compression were not included because they had field changes from optic nerve compression, this likely eliminated some of the more advanced cases of thyroid-associated orbitopathy. Nowhere is there an attempt to quantitate the severity of disease. Did most of these patients have large muscles and tight orbit or were the muscles slightly enlarged with minimal orbital tightness? Certainly, these are two different populations that may have different outcomes.

This paper is of value in pointing out that all thyroid patients should be monitored for elevated pressure and if present, investigated. However, not every patient with elevated pressure needs anti-glaucoma treatment. This adds to the argument that glaucoma is not simply a disease of elevated intraocular pressure causing nerve damage.

R.B. Penne, M.D.

Optic Nerve Avulsion

Foster BS, March GA, Lucarelli MJ, et al (Harvard Med School, Boston)
Arch Ophthalmol 115:623–630, 1997 6–5

Background.—In optic nerve avulsion, the optic nerve is forcibly disinserted from the retina, choroid, and vitreous. In addition, the lamina cribrosa is retracted from the scleral rim. The current paper characterizes the presentation, role of diagnostic imaging, and course in patients with optic nerve avulsion.

Methods and Findings.—The records of 6 patients with optic nerve avulsion seen at one center between 1991 and 1995 were reviewed. Initially, their visual acuity ranged from 20/100 to no light perception. Computed tomography and/or MRI were done in all patients and B-scan US in 4. One patient underwent color Doppler US to assess optic nerve vasculature. In 1 patient, CT suggested an optic nerve avulsion. Neuroimaging in the other 5 patients, including MRI, did not show avulsion. During follow-up, visual acuity was unimproved in 4 patients, improved from no light perception to bare light perception in 1, and improved from 20/100 to 20/25 in 1.

Conclusions.—Final visual outcome in patients with optic nerve avulsion appears to depend on initial postinjury visual acuity. Neuroimaging,

B-scans, and Doppler US were usually not useful for establishing the presence of optic nerve avulsion. However, they may be of value for assessing comorbid conditions.

▶ Fortunately, optic nerve avulsion is a rare condition, though its recognition is important. This diagnosis can be made visually if the fundus view is clear. The difficult cases are those with vitreous or anterior segment blood that obscures the view. There is no treatment for an avulsion. Other traumatic optic nerve injuries may be treated with high dose steroids or optic canal decompression. To try and avoid unnecessary high dose steroids or surgery it is important to establish the diagnosis if possible. This study looked at cases from 1991 to 1995 and concluded that MRI, B-scan, and Doppler ultrasonography were of little value in establishing the diagnosis of optic nerve avulsion. One problem with studying these cases is the relatively small numbers of cases available to study. Even the most recent cases are now 2 years old. A lot of changes in MRI technology have taken place. With the significant improvements that have been and will be made in orbital MRI technology, I feel that MRI will offer more help in making this diagnosis in the future.

R.B. Penne, M.D.

Complications of Hydroxyapatite Orbital Implants: A Review of 100 Consecutive Cases and a Comparison of Dexon Mesh (Polyglycolic Acid) With Scleral Wrapping

Oestreicher JH, Liu E, Berkowitz M (Univ of Toronto)

Ophthalmology 104:324–329, 1997 6–6

Background.—Implant exposure is the most widely discussed complication of hydroxyapatite orbital implants. Other complications, less significant but often troublesome, are not as well described. All complications of the first 100 hydroxyapatite orbital implants performed by 1 surgeon were reported, and those associated with scleral wrapping and with Dexon mesh wrapping were compared.

Methods and Findings.—Mean follow-up was 9.6 months. Complications were classified as soft-tissue problems, eyelid problems, and prosthesis and peg problems. Although many minor complications occurred (Table 3), the rate of exposure was only 3%. None of the implants was lost. The complications associated with Dexon mesh wrapping were comparable to those associated with scleral wrapping. However, more posterior implant placement was needed to avoid exposure in the Dexon-wrapped group.

Conclusions.—The various minor complications associated with the use of hydroxyapatite implants can be easily addressed without compromising the appearance or health of the implant. With longer term studies verifying current results, Dexon mesh will be very useful when donor tissue needs to be avoided.

TABLE 3.—Complications Encountered with Hydroxyapatite Ocular Implant

	Dexon (n = 32)	Evisceration (n = 6)	Sclera (n = 62)	Total (n = 100)
Soft tissue problems				
Exposure	3 (9.4)	0	0	3
Thinning of conjunctiva	2 (6.3)	0	4 (6.5)	6
Persistent pain/discomfort	0	0	2 (3.2)	2
Discharge	2 (6.3)	1 (16.7)	14 (21.0)	16
Tissue overgrowth	0	0	17 (27.4)	17
Pyogenic granuloma	2 (6.2)	0	6 (9.7)	8
Inclusion cyst	0	0	2 (3.2)	2
Symblepharon	0	0	3 (4.8)	3
Papillary reaction	0	0	1 (1.6)	1
Eyelid problems				
Ptosis	2 (6.3)	2 (33.3)	12 (19.4)	16
Surgical repair	0	0	2 (3.2)	2
Lid laxity	3 (9.4)	2 (33.3)	17 (27.4)	22
Surgical repair	0	0	6 (9.7)	6
Formix insufficiency	1 (3.1)	0	9 (14.5)	10
Chalazion	0	0	1 (1.6)	1
Prosthesis and peg problems				
Mild enophthalmos	1 (3.1)	0	1 (1.6)	2
Mild hypo-ophthalmos	1 (3.1)	1(16.7)	10 (16.1)	12
Insufficient vascularity	1 (3.1)	0	5 (8.1)	6
Peg extrusion/sleeve protrusion	0	1 (16.7)	10 (16.1)	11
Poor peg positioning	0	1 (16.7)	4 (6.5)	5
Redrilling	0	1 (16.7)	1 (1.6)	2
Broken peg	0	0	2 (3.2)	2

Note: Values in parentheses are percentages.

(Published courtesy of *Ophthalmology*, from Oestreicher JH, Liu E, Berkowitz M: Complications of hydroxyapatite orbital implants. *Ophthalmology* 104:324–329, 1997.)

▶ This article reviews in detail all complications associated with 100 cases of hydroxyapatite implants. Included are enucleations, eviscerations, and secondary implants. An important contribution is the listing of even relatively minor complications in this study. This then serves as a good reference for the potential problems that can be encountered with the use of hydroxyapatite implants.

Hydroxyapatite appears to be well tolerated and these results confirm this. One surprising statistic was that 71% of patients underwent drilling of their motility peg after hydroxyapatite implant. This is greater than in most studies and certainly higher than in my practice. The real reason is stated in the study. In Canada, patients pay for the implant themselves. Once they decide to spend the extra money on the hydroxyapatite implant, they will likely follow through with the motility peg. It is a waste of resources to put more costly hydroxyapatite implants in so many patients who never proceed on to drilling. However, in a health care system where patients don't pay for the care directly, the cost is often not a factor.

One real advance with the motility peg has been the introduction of the teflon sleeve that is screwed in the implant after drilling. The peg can then be placed into the sleeve. In my practice, this has made peg problem much less common. It is not clear which type of peg system was used in these patients. The fact that peg complications were less in later cases could be the result of surgical evolution, as suggested by the author, or secondary to the use of the sleeved peg in the later cases.

There are now more series outlining the complications seen with hydroxyapatite implants. This knowledge is just in time for the introduction of the Medpor motility peg. The Medpor implant itself is less expensive than the hydroxyapatite implant and has been used for a number of years without the peg. The success of this and the complications will take time to evaluate just as with the hydroxyapatite implant.

R.B. Penne, M.D.

Complications of Motility Peg Placement for the Hydroxyapatite Orbital Implant

Edelstein C, Shields CL, De Potter P, et al (Thomas Jefferson Univ, Philadelphia)

Ophthalmology 104:1616–1621, 1997 6–7

Background.—The hydroxyapatite ocular motility implant can achieve natural movement of ocular prosthetics. The best movement results are achieved when a peg is used to couple the implant to the artificial eye. There have been no reports of complications associated with this procedure. Complications of hydroxyapatite motility peg placement and associated risk factors were reviewed.

Patients.—The study included 47 patients undergoing hydroxyapatite motility peg placement over a 5-year period. Peg extrusion occurred in 26% of cases, nonspecific conjunctivitis in 6%, an audible click in 6%, temporary excessive conjunctival edema in 4%, and temporary excessive pain after surgery in 4%. However, no patient had infection, persistent pain, persistent edema, or a discharge at the peg site. Peg extrusion occurred a median of 52 months after placement. The only factor significantly related to peg extrusion was age older than 50 years. Peg extrusion rate was 32% with nonsleeved pegs versus 0% for sleeved pegs. Patient sex, previous ocular surgery or radiotherapy, giant papillary conjunctivitis, time from enucleation to peg placement, and implant vascularization on MRI scanning had no effect on peg extrusion. Twelve patients had extrusion of a nonsleeved peg. Five of these 8 patients underwent placement of a sleeved peg, 1 had another nonsleeved peg placed, and 6 were left without a peg.

Conclusions.—The only common complication of hydroxyapatite motility peg placement is peg extrusion. Extrusion is less likely to occur when a sleeved peg system is used. Patients who benefit the most from hydroxyapatite peg placement are those with personal or professional reasons to desire an excellent cosmetic result.

► Attempts to couple the prosthesis with the orbital motility after enucleation have been made for many years. None of these past attempts has been successful. The latest has been the hydroxyapatite implant. With widespread use since 1990, this implant appears far superior to other attempts but is not without problems.

The largest problem was extrusion of the motility peg, which occurred in 26% of implants. All of these were in nonsleeved pegs. This nonsleeved peg was the original system, but it has been replaced by sleeved motility pegs. Thus, 2 different pegging systems were used in this group of patients. The study included only 9 patients with sleeved pegs. None of these had extrusions. However, this is a small number and the follow-up time for these patients was only half that for the patients with nonsleeved pegs. The real question to someone considering peg placement is how the sleeved pegs did, because that is the system currently available. The answer is very well, but the sample size is very small, so more data is needed.

One interesting complication of hydroxyapatite implants was a 47% incidence of giant papillary conjunctivitis(GPC) in these patients. This incidence seems to be high but is something I note often in my practice. GPC seems more common with hydroxyapatite implants than with old acrylic ball implants, but I know of no data on this. A higher incidence of GPC could be due to different prosthesis material, better movement of the prosthesis, or other unknown factors. There was no comment on GPC after peg placement in this article. I find GPC continues to be as much or even more of a problem after peg placement. I also have noted that even without GPC there is often increased discharge after peg placement.

Motility after implantation of either hydroxyapatite or Medpor implants is often very good. Peg placement may improve motility but often not dramatically. For this reason and because of a perceived general increase in the need for care and maintenance of the prosthesis, I am drilling fewer pegs in my patients these days.

R.B. Penne, M.D.

Floppy Eyelid Syndrome and Obstructive Sleep Apnea

McNab AA (Royal Melbourne Hosp, Australia)

Ophthal Plast Reconstr Surg 13:98–114, 1997 6–8

Background.—Floppy eyelid syndrome (FES), presenting as a unilateral or bilateral chronic papillary conjunctivitis, is a condition that usually affects middle-aged obese men. It is characterized by a lax, floppy upper eyelid that is easily everted. The laterality of the condition corresponds to the side on which the patient usually sleeps. Some authorities have suggested that FES is associated with obstructive sleep apnea (OSA). The current review includes 17 newly reported patients and 79 previously reported patients.

Floppy Eyelid Syndrome and OSA.—In addition to the classic presentation, patients may also have upper lid ptosis, lash ptosis or trichiasis, lower lid ectropion or entropion, or corneal complications. Eight patients were assessed for OSA in addition to FES, and 20 patients known to have

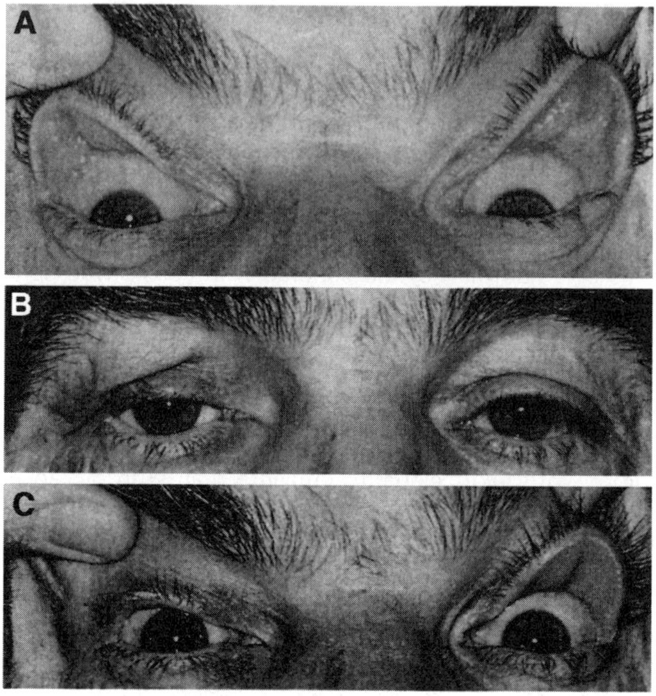

FIGURE 7.—Case 12. **A**, bilateral FES a year after 17 mm right upper lid wedge. **B,C**, two weeks after a further 15 mm wedge excision. (Courtesy of McNab AA: Floppy eyelid syndrome and obstructive sleep apnea. *Ophthal Plast Reconstr Surg* 13:98–114, 1997.)

OSA were evaluated for FES and other possibly associated ocular features. All 8 patients in the former group had OSA. In the latter group, 1 patient was found to have FES, and 2 had features of early asymptomatic FES. Normal tension glaucoma was discovered in 1 patient with FES and OSA (Fig 7).

Conclusions.—The performance of sleep studies should be considered for patients with FES. With simple screening of patients with OSA, FES may be detected and late corneal complications avoided.

► Floppy eyelid syndrome has become a better-recognized syndrome to most ophthalmologists and one that is quite treatable. Whether this is some abnormality of the lids that has yet to be identified or is from years of mechanical rubbing is not clear. This article provides a valuable reference to the manifestations of floppy eyelid syndrome and also outlines the associated systemic problems. Recognizing the possibility of sleep apnea in these patients and getting them proper evaluation can be of great service to patients. Although sometimes not taken seriously, sleep apnea is a life threatening condition for select patients. Even people with less severe disease can spend much of their life nonfunctional because of the problem. Likewise patients with sleep apnea need to be screened for eyelid problems.

My experience with treatment of the ocular manifestation of floppy eyelid syndrome is that they usually require surgical treatment. Lubrication will improve symptoms somewhat but these patients usually remain symptomatic. Trying a shield or patch at night to prevent eyelid eversion often doesn't work because the same rubbing that occurs at night to cause the problem causes the patch or shield to be dislodged. Patients often become impatient and frustrated with these treatments. I always suggest a trial of lubrication and eye patching or shielding before surgical correction. Eyelid tightening works well for these patients—lower lids with a tarsal strip and upper lids with a pentagon resection. Some only need upper lid surgery, others will require all 4 lids. Attempts to minimize the mechanical stretching at night may slow this recurrenc[illegible] important to get patients to understand these symptoms can recur as the lids stretch further.

R.B. Penne, M.D.

Functional Eyelid Surgery
Meyer DR (Albany Med College, NY)
Ophthal Plast Reconstr Surg 13:77–80, 1997 6–9

Background.—Insurers are increasingly demanding evidence of functional impairment to justify many elective ophthalmic procedures, including cataract surgery and strabismus and ophthalmic plastic surgery. Although physicians, as patients' advocates, are often in an adversarial role with insurers, physicians need to be aware of the responsibility that insurers have for their membership. "Functional eyelid surgery" is discussed in the current paper.

Functional Eyelid Surgery.—The purpose of functional reconstructive surgery is to restore normalcy to a structure damaged by trauma, infection, inflammation, degeneration, neoplasia, or congenital conditions. Consequently, the result of such surgery is functional improvement. By contrast, cosmetic surgery aims to improve the appearance of tissues or structures that are histologically and functionally normal. Functional reconstructive surgery of the eyelids, face, and other visible parts of the body may improve appearance as well as function. Obviously, cosmetic surgery is not expected to improve function, since there was no functional impairment before surgery.

Currently, there are no national standards providing specific criteria for determining functional indications for ptosis repair and related surgeries. Existing editorials and consensus statements are somewhat ambiguous about the magnitude of ptosis severity and/or visual field loss or other criteria that constitute indications for functional surgery. In general, available recommendations state that upper-lid blepharoplasty or ptosis surgery is indicated if the eyelid position results in a visual field defect. In practice, insurers have different specifications on the amount of visual field loss that must exist for upper eyelid surgery to be considered functional.

▶ The definition of functional eyelid surgery is very difficult to determine. Dr. Meyer points out much of the difficulty concerning the definition. Functional impairment occurs in many eyelid conditions with ptosis being the one most often debated. It's important to realize that like everything else in medicine, the point at which ptosis becomes a functional problem varies greatly among patients. This then makes any single definition of a functional deficit from ptosis invalid for a part of the population. However we are nowhere close to even having a consensus on a definition that everyone will accept. Thus, both patient and physician are unsure what is a covered service and what is considered cosmetic. Most insurers will at least make this determination prior to surgery. To add even more to this difficulty, Medicare will not even preapprove ptosis surgery in most areas. They reserve the right to not cover the procedure after it has been done. Yet there is no universal definition of the amount of deficit present to make ptosis functional. There is little wonder that patients are confused about functional and cosmetic eyelid surgery. It appears no one really knows the correct answer. Without a true definition, insurers can approve or deny at will.

I agree with Dr. Meyer that a universal definition of ptosis is desirable. Whether this would result in more or fewer covered cases, it would certainly make it easier for patients and physicians to understand the indications for ptosis surgery. I am hopeful that this goal can be achieved in the near future by physicians and then the insurers may follow.

R.B. Penne, M.D.

Dacryocystorhinostomy With Intraoperative Mitomycin C

Kao SCS, Liao CL, Tseng JHS, et al (Natl Taiwan Univ, Taipei)

Ophthalmology 104:86–91, 1997 6–10

Background.—Dacryocystorhinostomy (DCR) is considered a very successful procedure for treating epiphora. Obstruction of the common canaliculus and osteotomy site closure are the 2 most common causes of DCR failure. Inhibiting fibrous tissue growth and scarring by the application of antiproliferative agents over the anastomosed flaps and osteotomy site would reduce the failure rate. The effects of intraoperative mitomycin C on osteotomy site size after DCR were studied.

Methods.—Fifteen eyes with primary acquired nasolacrimal duct obstruction in 14 patients were assigned randomly to a mitomycin C or control group. The operative procedures in both groups were identical, except that, in the treatment group, a piece of neurosurgical cottonoid soaked with 0.2 mg/mL mitomycin C was applied to the osteotomy site. The cottonoid was removed transnasally after 30 minutes. Nasoendoscopic assessment was performed immediately after surgery and at 1, 3, and 6 months in both groups.

Findings.—The success rate in the mitomycin C group was 100% and in the control group, was 87.5%, respectively. One patient in the control group had recurrent epiphora. Two patients in the control group (25%) had septo-osteotomy adhesion, compared to none in the treatment group. At 6 months, the mean final surface area of the osteotomy was 27 mm^2in the treatment group and only 10.83 mm^2 in the control group. Although the 2 groups did not differ in osteotomy surface area immediately after surgery, the difference was significant at 6 months.

Conclusions.—The intraoperative use of mitomycin C effectively maintains a larger osteotomy size. This may improve the success rates associated with traditional DCR.

► Mitomycin C offers an interesting adjunct to DCR surgery, especially in patients prone to scarring. The use of mitomycin C has become widespread in glaucoma surgery to inhibit scarring, and DCR surgery is similar in that we are trying to maintain a fistula while the body heals a surgical wound. Whether this is as effective in routine DCR surgery remains to be answered. However, a patient with failed DCR surgery because of scarring would seem to be especially appropriate for use of mitomycin C.

This is a small study of 15 patients and really looks at osteotomy size rather than success or failure of the DCR itself. The results show a significantly larger size of the osteotomy at 6 months in patients who received mitomycin C. This suggests that mitomycin C inhibits healing. Whether the difference continues out to 1 and 2 years after surgery remains a question. The ultimate proof of success is in the patency of the DCR at 2 years' time.

The use of mitomycin C raises a number of concerns about potential side effects. These adverse effects must be weighed against the benefits in deciding if mitomycin C is helpful. Dacryocystorhinostomy is already at least 90% successful for routine surgery. Thus, the most improvement possible would be 10%. A large study is needed to determine the percent improvement and the incidence of side effects. More likely mitomycin C will find its usefulness for previously failed DCRs. If use in these patients shows promise without adverse effects, then the potential for more widespread use may be realized.

R.B. Penne, M.D.

Obstructed Nasolacrimal Duct System in Epiphora: Long-term Results of Dacryocystoplasty by Means of Balloon Dilation

Janssen AG, Mansour K, Bos JJ (De Tjongerschans Hosp, Thialfweg, The Netherlands; Univ of Groningen, The Netherlands)

Radiology 205:791–796, 1997 6–11

Introduction.—When epiphora results from obstruction of the lacrimal drainage system, the treatment is usually surgical, with dacryocystorhinostomy. Recent reports have described the use of nonsurgical dacryocystoplasty using fluoroscopically guided balloon dilation. However, there

TABLE 6.—Association Between Initial Success and Obstruction

Obstruction	Initial Success	Initial Failure	Total
Complete	24	3	27
Partial	72	1	73
Total	96	4	100

(Reprinted courtesy of the Radiological Society of North America, from Janssen AG, Mansour K, Bos JJ: Obstructed nasolacrimal duct system in epiphora: Long-term results of dacryocystoplasty by means of balloon dilation. *Radiology* 205:791–796, 1997.)

are few follow-up data on this procedure. The long-term results of balloon dacryocystoplasty for patients with epiphora caused by nasolacrimal duct obstruction are reported.

Patients.—The experience included 100 eyes of 84 patients with complete or incomplete obstruction of the lacrimal sac and duct. The patients were 59 females and 25 males, mean age 61 years. The dacryocystoplasty procedures were performed using a catheter with a 3 mm diameter balloon, without stent placement. With follow-up of 5–48 months, patency rates were evaluated by Kaplan-Meier analysis.

Outcomes.—Dacryocystoplasty had a long-term primary patency rate of 70%. The procedure initially failed or reobstruction occurred during follow-up in 11 cases. Dacryocystoplasty was successfully repeated in 10 of these, for a long-term secondary patency rate of 81%. The chances of success were unrelated to the length of the obstruction or the duration of symptoms before the procedure. However, success rates were significantly higher for patients with incomplete versus complete obstructions (Tables 6 and 7).

Conclusions.—For patients with epiphora caused by obstruction of the nasolacrimal ducts, balloon dacryocystoplasty gives good long-term results. The procedure is safe and simple and can be repeated if necessary. Dacryocystoplasty may become the initial treatment of choice for this indication. If initial or repeat dacryocystoplasty failed or if dacryocystoplasty were contraindicated—such as by anatomic malformations of the lacrimal duct or bony canal—surgical dacryocystorhinostomy would be performed.

TABLE 7.—Association Between Long-term Success and Obstruction

Obstruction	Long-term Success	Long-term Failure*	Total
Complete	16	11	27
Partial	62	11	73
Total	78	22	100

*Four initial failures and 18 reobstructions.

(Reprinted courtesy of the Radiological Society of North America, from Janssen AG, Mansour K, Bos JJ: Obstructed nasolacrimal duct system in epiphora: Long-term results of dacryocystoplasty by means of balloon dilation. *Radiology* 205:791–796, 1997.)

► Nonsurgical treatment of dacryostenosis has been attempted tor years. Yet the standard for treatment remains the open dacryocystorhinostomy (DCR). Since 1990, there have been multiple articles in the radiology literature describing balloon dilation of the lacrimal system for treatment of dacryostenosis. This article looks at the success in 100 eyes treated over 4 years.

This method is performed under fluoroscopy and involves passing the balloon from a nasal approach over a wire in the lacrimal system. There are no tubes placed in the system. Both partial and total lacrimal obstructions were treated in this study. Follow-up was 548 months. Overall long-term success was 70%, which is fairly good compared to other nonsurgical attempts. When patients with complete obstructions were excluded, the long-term success was 85%, which is very good. Standard DCR success is in the range of 92%.

The success of this technology led to the exploration of similar technology that could be used without fluoroscopy and that would be accessible to nonradiologists. The introduction of a lacrimal probe with a balloon on the end made this technology available to ophthalmologists. We now have the technology to pass a balloon from the punta into the lacrimal duct, blow up the balloon, and dilate the system. The technology is fairly straightforward. However, the long-term results are still unknown. At Will's Eye Hospital, we have results in the range of 70%. However, the numbers are still small and the results not long-term. We also treat only partial obstructions and place silicone tubing in the lacrimal system for 5–6 weeks.

This approach, especially to treating partial obstructions, holds promise. Whether it becomes the standard of care or just another failed attempt at achieving the success of a DCR without surgery remains to be seen.

R.B. Penne, M.D.

Transcanalicular Neodymium:YAG Laser for Revision of Dacryocystorhinostomy

Patel BCK, Phillips B, McLeish WM, et al (Univ of Utah, Salt Lake City)
Ophthalmology 104:1191–1197, 1997 6–12

Objective.—External dacryocystorhinostomy (DCR) is the treatment of choice for nasolacrimal duct (NLD) obstruction. With the advent of laser technology, laser-assisted DCR would appear to be a less invasive method for revision DCR. Results of a prospective study to assess the efficacy of transcanalicular laser-assisted revision dacryocystorhinostomy (TCLARDCR).

Methods.—Between May 1991 and January 1994, 24 TCLARDCR procedures were performed on 21 patients (8 males), age 7–89 years, who had undergone 1 or more unsuccessful external DCR procedures within the previous year. Obstruction was caused by acquired NLD obstruction in 17 patients, trauma in 3, previous radical maxillectomy and radiation therapy for malignancy of the nose and paranasal sinuses in 2, Wegener's granulomatosis in 1, and Down syndrome in 1. Patients were monitored for 5–34 months.

> *Technique.*—The procedure was performed with the aid of a video endoscope. A fiberoptic contact probe attached to a Nd:YAG laser was advanced to the obstruction and used to fashion an internal ostium at power settings of 3–7 W and 0.5 seconds. Soft tissue adhesions were removed, and a suction probe removed the smoke. When the opening was sufficiently enlarged so that a Bowman's probe could be inserted through the upper and lower canaliculus, a nasal examination was conducted and a middle turbinectomy was performed. The upper and lower canaliculus were stented.

Results.—The average duration of surgery was 78.2 minutes. Stent removal occurred at 1–30 weeks after surgery. Seven patients accidentally lost stents before 12 weeks. Surgery was successful in 11 (46%) patients. Three patients had partial relief.

Conclusion.—Given the 85% success rate of conventional DCR, TCLARDCR, with a 46% success rate, does not compare well. TCLARDCR also is more expensive.

► Multiple different approaches continue to be tested to try and avoid an external incision in DCR surgery. This concept is by no means new; however, the approaches have always been less successful. Both transcanalicular laser surgery as well as transnasal surgery with and without laser have been tried. The problem has been a lower success rate for this surgery when compared with traditional external DCR surgery.

This study seems to agree with other papers that these alternative approaches have a lower success rate. The authors in this study looked at failed previous DCR patients. These patients don't need a new bony ostium made, which should be an advantage with laser. However, these patients already have failed a previous surgery, which may mean they are at greater risk to fail a second time. The reasons for failure are outlined in the paper. The common factor in all the "internal" approaches is the creation of a smaller ostium and less complete removal of tissue. These may be the reasons they fail.

It is important to realize this study wasn't looking at primary DCR surgery, but the general theme for primary and secondary surgery using an internal or transcanalicular approach is similar. They just do not seem to work as well. Until these alternative approaches to DCRs can come close to the success rate of external DCR, it is unlikely that they will become widely used. Even then, the cost of equipment, the learning curve, and the long surgical times may make most surgeons unlikely to abandon an old but successful technique.

R.B. Penne, M.D.

Anatomy and Physiology of Eyelash Follicles: Relevance to Lash Ablation Procedures

Elder MJ (Moorfields Eye Hosp, London)

Ophthal Plast Reconstr Surg 13:21–25, 1997 6–13

Background.—The anatomy and physiology of the follicles of the human eyelashes are not well understood. Such understanding is important to lash ablative procedures. The anatomy of eyelash follicles was studied.

Methods and Findings.—Histologic specimens of the upper and lower lids from 10 patients were analyzed. The dimensions of the follicles were a mean 1.8 mm for the upper lid depth and 0.9 mm for the lower lid depth. Mean bulb widths on the upper and lower lids were 188 and 132 µm, respectively. Mean shaft widths were 205 and 158 µm. The upper lid had 41% active follicles, compared to only 15% in the lower lid.

Conclusions.—The anatomy of the follicles on the upper and lower lids differs significantly. To completely contact 95% of all follicles on the upper lid, an electrolysis needle needs to be inserted 2.4 mm. For the lower lid, it would be inserted 1.4 mm. A beam width of less than 200 µm for the lower lids and a width of less than 250 µm for upper lids, are needed to treat similar depths by argon laser ablation. The greater proportion of actively growing upper lid follicles explains why eyelashes on the upper lid are longer.

▶ Ablation of aberrant lashes Is a relatively common procedure with variable results. This study looks at the anatomy and growth of lash follicles to assist in more successful treatment of aberrant lashes. Any treatment of eyelashes is often accompanied by a percentage of regrowth, which is much of the frustration associated with these procedures.

Good recommendations are made for depth of treatment and the differences between upper and lower lids. The long period of follicular inactivity in eyelash growth and its implication for lash treatment was interesting. Because a lash may be inactive for 4–9 months, the article suggests that true success for eyelash ablation procedures may not be known for up to 1 year.

What is not studied in this article is the effect of eyelid inflammation and scarring on eyelash anatomy and growth. Many of the patients treated with aberrant lash have them as a result of scarring from trauma or eyelid inflammation. Pemphigoid, Stevens-Johnson syndrome, and chronic blepharitis are the more common reasons for eyelid inflammation and scarring to result in aberrant lashes. The association of this scarring and inflammation with these aberrant lashes makes treatment much more difficult and recurrence more likely. When a patient is seen with aberrant lashes from a lid laceration, success is usually quite good. Patients with aberrant lashes with pemphigoid or other conjunctival scarring disease are a different story. Successful treatment of lashes is much more difficult to achieve and has a shorter duration in these patients. It is possible that there is some change in the direction of the follicle because of scarring, which makes complete treatment with a straight needle or laser less successful. The entire growth cycle of the follicle may be changed in some way and the stimulation to growth of new lashes may be enhanced.

This article gives a good anatomical basis for proper treatment of aberrant lashes in normal eyelids. It is important to emphasize the need to look for evidence of conjunctival scarring disease in patients with aberrant lashes. Diagnosis and treatment of these diseases will often make eyelash control easier. Treatment of eyelashes, especially in patients with conjunctival scarring disease, can often be long and frustrating for the patient and physician. Recognizing this and discussing this with the patient before starting treatment is helpful.

R.B. Penne, M.D.

Accuracy of Clinical Diagnosis of Cutaneous Eyelid Lesions
Kersten RC, Ewing-Chow D, Kulwin DR, et al (Univ of Cincinnati, Ohio)
Ophthalmology 104:479–484, 1997 6–14

Background.—Previous research on cutaneous eyelid lesions has been retrospective in design and has involved multiple contributing surgeons. The accuracy of the clinical diagnosis of benign, premalignant, and malignant cutaneous eyelid lesions and whether all clinical diagnoses require histopthologic confirmation were studied prospectively.

Methods and Findings.—Eight hundred sixty-four eyelid lesions were biopsied during an 85-month period. Of the 153 clinically thought to be malignant, 91.5% proved to be malignant on histopathologic assessment. Histologic evaluation showed that 16 of the 19 lesions thought to be

TABLE 1.—Distribution of Specific Diagnoses of Clinically Malignant Eyelid Lesions and Correlation With the Final Histopathologic Diagnosis

Clinical Diagnosis	Final Histopathologic Diagnosis
Basal cell ca (n = 143)	128 Basal cell ca
	2 Squamous cell ca
	1 Sebaceous ca
	7 "Papillomas"
	2 Nevi
	1 Hydrocystoma
	1 Fibrous myxoma
	1 Sebaceoma
Squamous cell ca (n = 7)	4 Squamous cell ca
	1 Basal cell ca
	1 Sebaceous ca
	1 Lichenoid keratosis
Malignant melanoma (n = 1)	Malignant melanoma
Eccrine mucinous ca (n = 1)	Eccrine mucinous ca
Sebaceous ca (n = 1)	Sebaceous ca

Abbreviation: ca, carcinoma.
(Published courtesy of *Ophthalmology*, from Kersten RC, Ewing-Chow D, Kulwin DR, et al: Accuracy of clinical diagnosis of cutaneous eyelid lesions. *Ophthalmology* 104:479–484, 1997.)

TABLE 3.—Distribution of the Clinically Benign Eyelid Lesions and Distribution of the Unsuspected Malignant Histopathologic Diagnoses that Masqueraded as Clinically Benign Lesions

Clinical Diagnosis	Malignant Histopathologic Diagnosis
Papillomas (n = 304)	5 Basal cell ca 1 Squamous cell ca
Epidermal inclusion cysts (n = 154)	2 Basal cell ca
Melanocytic nevi (n = 87)	1 Basal cell ca 1 Non-Hodgkin lymphoma
Hydrocystomas (n = 75)	2 Basal cell ca
Chalazion (n = 22)	None
Molluscum contagiorum (n = 6)	None
"Other" benign (n = 29)	1 Adenoid cystic ca
"Unknown" benign (n = 15)	None

Abbreviation: ca, carcinoma.
(Published courtesy of *Ophthalmology*, from Kersten RC, Ewing-Chow D, Kulwin DR, et al: Accuracy of clinical diagnosis of cutaneous eyelid lesions. *Ophthalmology* 104:479–484, 1997.)

premalignant processes clinically actually were premalignant. Of the remaining 3, 2 were benign and 1 malignant. Of the 692 lesions thought to be benign clinically, 13 (1.9%) were found to be malignant histopathologically. These included 10 basal cell carcinomas and 1 squamous cell carcinoma, 1 non-Hodgkin's lymphoma, and 1 adenoid cystic carcinoma. Three of the clinically benign lesions (0.4%) were found to be premalignant histopathologically. The 13 malignancies missed included lesions clinically diagnosed as papilloma, epidermal inclusion cyst, melanocytic nevus, hydrocystoma, and trichoepithelioma. Of the 153 lesions thought to be malignant clinically, 6 that were highly suggestive of malignancy on clinical assessment were initially diagnosed as benign on histopathologic assessment. Results of repeat biopsy of all 6 of these lesions verified the suspected malignant diagnosis (Tables 1 and 3).

Conclusions.—Malignant eyelid lesions may mimic a number of different clinically benign conditions. All excised eyelid lesions should undergo histopathologic confirmation, as clinical assessment is not 100% accurate. However, strong clinical suspicion of malignancy signals a need for repeat biopsy if the initial histopathologic findings do not concur.

► The question of whether to biopsy all lesions that are removed from the eyelid is often asked. There is a significant cost involved with evaluating all benign lesions and can this cost be justified? This study looks at all eyelid lesions excised or biopsied over an 85-month period by 1 experienced oculoplastic surgeon. The conclusion is similar to other studies that there is some error in the clinical accuracy of diagnosing skin lesions. This then suggests that all lesions should be biopsied after excision.

The percentage of malignant lesions labeled as benign was low at 1.9%; however, this represented 13 cases. The authors estimated that the cost of detecting these malignant lesions was $2,699 per lesion. What this cost means I'm not sure; however, I do think this study suggests that routine lesions should be biopsied. The surgeon was an experienced oculoplastic surgeon who deals with skin lesions daily. This is an important factor to note because the rate of error for someone less experienced in eyelid lesions would likely be higher.

R.B. Penne, M.D.

Laser Microsurgery for Superficial T1–T2 Basal Cell Carcinoma of the Eyelid Margins

Bandieramonte G, Lepera P, Moglia D, et al (Istituto Nazionale per lo Studio e la Cura dei Tumori, Milan, Italy; Ospedale Fatebenelzatelli e Oftalmico, Milan, Italy; Univ of Milan, Italy)
Ophthalmology 104:1179–1184, 1997 6–15

Objective.—Basal cell carcinoma (BCC) is the most common malignancy in white populations and represents 75% of head, primarily eyelid, cancers. Treatment can create functional impairment or disfigurement. Technical and clinical effectiveness of carbon dioxide laser removal and posterior tumor-margin vaporization of superficial BCC of the eyelid are discussed.

Methods.—Three carbon dioxide surgical lasers mounted on an operating microscope were used to remove 18 T1 tumors and 9 T2 tumors of the eyelid margin in 26 patients (12 women), age 30–81 years. Cosmetic, functional, and clinical results were evaluated at 1 month and at 3-month intervals thereafter. Surgeries were performed on an outpatient basis using local anesthesia and lasted an average of 15 minutes.

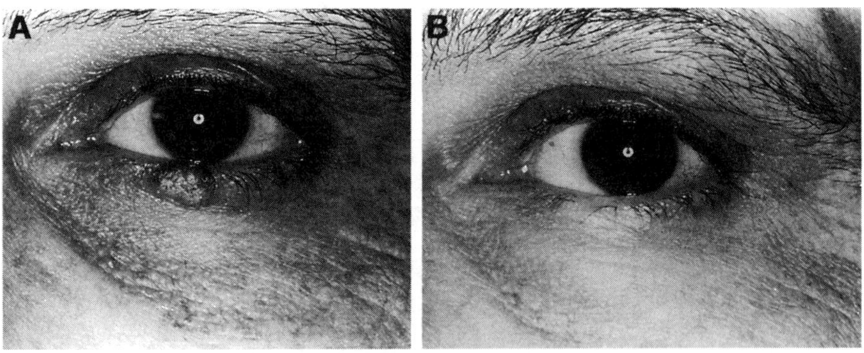

FIGURE 2.—A, Basal cell carcinoma (T2) of the lower eyelid margin in a 55-year-old man. The lesion extended to the intermarginal space but without involvement of the conjunctival border. Combined laser surgery (excision plus lateral and deep vaporization) was performed. The adjunctive vaporization contributed to the completeness of the removal and to the cosmetic modeling of the wound. B, Healing of the lid 3 weeks after the treatment. Despite a little alopecia and light skin hypopigmentation, cosmetic outcome was satisfactory. (Courtesy of Bandieramonte G, Lepera P, Moglia D, et al: Laser microsurgery for superficial T1–T2 basal cell carcinoma of the eyelid margins. *Ophthalmology* 104:1179–1184, 1997. Published courtesy of *Ophthalmology*.)

Results.—There were no significant intraoperative or postoperative complications. Median healing time was 10 days. All patients without scarring had good or excellent cosmetic and functional results (Fig 2). Alopecia was limited when it occurred. One patient had a recurrence at 22 months. He was retreated and is disease-free 51 months after treatment. Three patients had adjuvant radiation therapy and are disease-free.

Conclusion.—Carbon dioxide laser treatment of BCC of the eyelid is safe and effective and clinically successful after a reasonably long follow-up period. There was 1 recurrence that was successfully retreated.

▶ Use of a laser in medicine implies a better, more advanced form of treatment to many people. For this reason, laser surgery is sometimes used as a marketing tool in advertising medical care. This paper looks at the use of a laser in the treatment of BCC. In evaluating this treatment, the potential advantages and disadvantages must be carefully weighed.

Treatment of BCC with laser surgery offers the potential advantage of better hemostasis when removing the tumor. Most lasers have some degree of cauterization associated with the cutting. The degree of cauterization can be varied as desired. This form of treatment seems to give good cosmetic results. There was careful patient selection for this technique, with no patient who had a tumor invading the lid margin or with indistinct borders being selected. Thus, the smaller, easier to treat BCC tumors were selected for treatment. This would seem to be a subset of patients who would have better cosmetic results.

The main disadvantage is the lack of good margins for pathologic evaluation. The thermal damage caused by the laser results in an area of tissue that cannot be evaluated for basal cell. Thus, complete excision cannot be ensured. This is an important point because without pathologic guidance for the extent of the excision, the surgeon may leave residual BCC, which can recur years later in the orbit or on the lid. This is the same criticism of radiation and cryotherapy for BCC treatment, and I think it is a valid one. As mentioned, the technique is not used if the tumor reaches the conjunctiva or is full thickness eyelid. These are then less extensive tumors, which is important in reviewing the results and in considering its use. Patients were monitored for an average of 6 years, with only 1 recurrence in 24 cases. If these results hold up for the long term, they are good. However, these small, carefully selected cases likely have a good prognosis with any technique.

This approach offers an interesting alternative for BCC treatment, but until larger studies are done to confirm these results, I believe that the lack of good surgical margins for tumor control makes this technique less than ideal.

R.B. Penne, M.D.

Predictability of Magnetic Resonance Imaging in Differentiation of Orbital Lymphoma From Orbital Inflammatory Syndrome

Cytryn AS, Putterman AM, Schneck GL, et al (Washington Hosp Ctr, Washington, DC; Univ of Illinois at Chicago; Stonybrook Health Science, New York; et al)

Ophthal Plast Reconstr Surg 13:129–134, 1997 6–16

Background.—Differentiating between orbital lymphoma and orbital inflammatory syndrome (OIS) may be difficult, since their clinical and radiographic features often overlap. The value of MRI in differentiating between these entities was investigated.

Methods.—Twenty-two patients with 25 affected orbits underwent MRI before biopsy. The MRI signal characteristics of all tumors were evaluated to determine whether MRI would add specificity to radiographic diagnosis, with a focus on the signal intensity of each tumor on T1- and T2-weighted images.

Findings.—Twelve eyes were diagnosed as having orbital lymphomas. In 75% of these, the tumors appeared hyperintense to fat on T2-weighted images, becoming brighter relative to their appearance on T1-weighted images. In 85% of the 13 orbital infiltrates with OIS, the tumors appeared isointense to fat on T2-weighted images, becoming slightly darker or unchanged compared with their appearance on T1-weighted images. Tumor density and homogeneity were comparable in all lesions and not useful for further differentiating between lymphoma and OIS. Moderate enhancement with gadopentetate dimeglumine occurred in all but 1 tumor and was also not useful for further differentiation.

Conclusions.—Orbital lymphoma and OIS can usually be distinguished by their signal intensity on T2-weighted images. Although MRI assessment cannot replace orbital biopsy, it may better identify patients needing tissue diagnosis and be a useful adjunct to biopsy, particularly when the histopathologic diagnosis is questionable.

▶ The search for an orbital imaging test that will positively identify orbital tissue and eliminate the need for orbital biopsy continues. The authors offer some valuable observations about the characteristics of orbital inflammatory disease vs. orbital lymphoma. These two conditions make up a large percentage of orbital disease and they often appear similar on imaging. The differences seen with MRI imaging are present in most cases; however, these differences are not absolute. Therefore, we must still rely on orbital biopsy.

When looking at tissue, pathologists often cannot agree on where along the spectrum of lymphoid lesions a lesion sits despite many studies. It is not surprising then that an imaging test is not definitive for these orbital lesions. The information here is helpful in that if the MRI is consistent with inflammation one may be more willing to try steroid therapy again after a flare than if the lesion appears lymphoid. Likewise, if these differences prove consistent a lesion suggesting lymphoma may require biopsy without a steroid trial. The bottom line for now is that patients still require biopsy for definitive diagnosis if the clinical response is not that of orbital inflammation.

R.B. Penne, M.D.

The Role of Second-Intention Healing in Periocular Reconstruction

Lowry JC, Bartley GB, Garrity JA (Mayo Clinic and Found, Rochester, Minn)

Ophthal Plast Reconstr Surg 13:174–188, 1997 6–17

Objective.—Second-intention healing often results in remarkable cosmetic and functional outcomes. The role of second-intention healing in periocular reconstruction is discussed and a comprehensive review of published reports, an assessment of outcomes in a cohort of patients treated by this technique, and recommendations and guidelines for appropriate applications in selected patients are presented.

Methods.—Records of 59 patients (28 women), age 44–85, who underwent periorbital tumor excision without closure from 1986 through 1994 were reviewed. The Mohs excision technique was used in 37 patients, and frozen-section control was used in 22. Patients were monitored for an average of 19 months and for as long as 8 years.

Results.—Tumors were located in the medial canthal area in 32 patients, the lower eyelid in 20, the upper eyelid in 4, the glabella in 2, and the nasojugal fold in 1. The eyelid margin was involved in 5 patients and the canalicular system in 3 (Fig 2, A). Defects ranged in size from 3 × 3 mm to 22 × 27 mm and healed in 2–6 weeks, depending on depth and size. Functional and cosmetic results were acceptable in 83% of patients (Fig 2, F). Wound management was focused on maintaining a moist, occluded environment to stimulate granulation and epithelialization. Exposed bone and cartilage must be monitored for and protected against drying out, necrosis, and osteomyelitis, and lacrimal injuries should be repaired. Com-

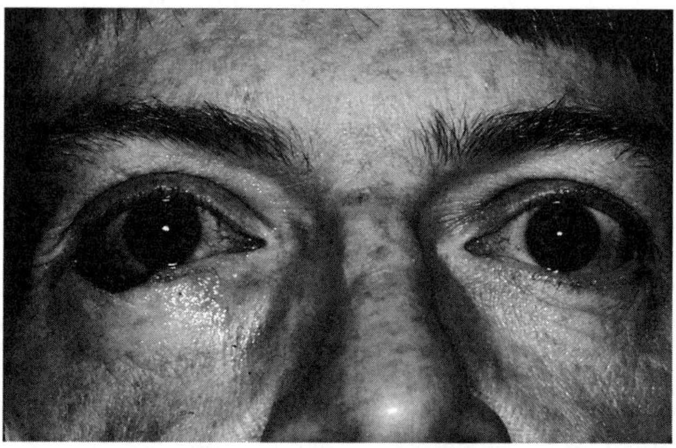

FIGURE 2, A.—Case 10. Right lower eyelid defect after Mohs excision of basal cell carcinoma. (Courtesy of Lowry JC, Bartley GB, Garrity JA: The role of second-intention healing in periocular reconstruction. *Ophthal Plast Reconstr Surg* 13:174–188, 1997.)

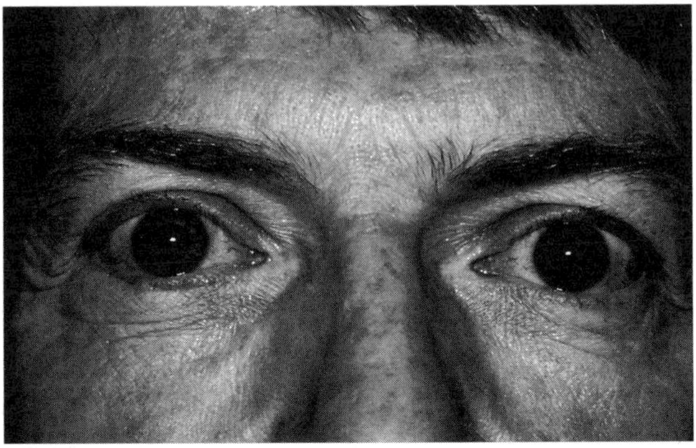

FIGURE 2, F.—Case 10. Despite a small defect in the lateral portion of the right lower eyelid margin, the functional and aesthetic results were acceptable to the patient. (Courtesy of Lowry JC, Bartley GB, Garrity JA: The role of second-intention healing in periocular reconstruction. *Ophthal Plast Reconstr Surg* 13:174–188, 1997).

plications can include tissue distortion, eyelid malposition, wound contraction, infection, pain, bleeding, and hypertrophic granulation and scarring. Optimal cosmetic outcome is largely dependent on wound location, size, and depth; skin color and texture; age; and, to an important extent, the patient's expectations and acceptance of treatment. Cosmesis continues to improve for 6–12 months. Candidates for delayed wound healing should be selected carefully.

Conclusion.—Delayed wound healing is a safe and effective technique in selected patients and gives acceptable cosmetic and functional results in 83% of patients.

► Allowing wounds to heal on their own is a technique that was abandoned long ago in favor of our present-day reconstructive techniques. Few people these days have much experience with allowing surgical wounds to heal by second-intention. The general feeling has become that more reconstructive surgery, even if extensive, is always better. That approach may not always be best. This technique like any other has merit but needs to be used in the proper case. This paper explores the potential use of second-intent healing after tumor removal and discusses when it may be useful.

Patient selection is very important. The accepting patient must be selected, and wounds in concave areas of the body tend to have the best results. If grafts and flaps are used and the reconstructive results are poor, the patient usually feels everything was done and is more accepting. If the wound is left open to heal and the results are poor, the patient and surgeon are more likely to feel the result could have been better if reconstruction of the wound had been done. I believe this is a big reason why this technique is not used more often. The use of second-intent healing must be discussed with the patient, and they must be accepting and have patience in allowing the wound to heal.

This paper outlines a technique that is certainly useful in selected cases. The proper case selection is a skill that has been lost by many younger surgeons in our quest to do the ultimate reconstruction. Certainly, reconstruction is important, but the proper use of second-intent wound healing should be kept in mind. This paper does a good job of reminding us of that.

R.B. Penne, M.D.

7 Pediatric Ophthalmology

Current Issues in Intraocular Lens Implantation in Children

by Leonard B. Nelson, M.D.

Every month there seems to be another article related to the use of intraocular lens (IOL) implantation in the treatment of childhood cataracts. These studies have demonstrated that IOL implantation to correct pediatric aphakia is a safe and effective method to provide both a clear visual axis and optical correction. Although the anatomical results are encouraging, amblyopia remains the major obstacle to a good functional result even with the use of an IOL. Although an IOL provides a considerable convenience not afforded by the use of a contact lens, there are no studies showing that an IOL will provide a better visual outcome.

While the techniques to implant an IOL in children has improved considerably, there are still a number of factors which are of concern. First, the changing refractive status of the developing eye poses a dilemma when one considers IOL implantation. The earlier in life that an IOL is implanted in a child, the greater the refractive change. While the long-term safety of IOLs has been well documented in adults, those findings do not currently span the many years that a lens may be inside the eye of a child.

The data about the long-term safety of IOLs have been, for the most part, obtained in an older, less active patient population. These patients are probably less likely to sustain a traumatic injury that could result in lens movement or wound dehiscence.

At the present time, contact lenses remain an excellent option to correct pediatric aphakia. Until the long-term safety of IOLs in children can be demonstrated, and until it can be proved that IOLs provide better visual outcome than contact lenses, IOL implantation cannot be considered the standard of care in treating childhood cataracts.

Effect of Ongoing Treatment of Amblyopia on Surgical Outcome in Esotropia

Weakley DR Jr, Holland DR (Univ of Texas, Dallas; Children's Med Ctr, Dallas)
J Pediatr Ophthalmol Strabismus 34:275–278, 1997 7–1

Objective.—Although studies have suggested that performing surgery for correcting esotropia (ET) before completion of amblyopia therapy does not adversely affect motor or sensory output, provided amblyopia therapy is continued postoperatively, no definitive studies have been conducted to assess outcome. The effect of such ongoing amblyopia therapy on the surgical success rate in various types of ET were assessed retrospectively.

Methods.—In 1994, 102 patients with amblyopia underwent occlusion therapy for at least 6 weeks before surgery to correct ET and were followed up for at least 1 month. Degree of amblyopia before therapy was compared with degree of amblyopia at the time of therapy. Surgical success rates were based on those with moderate amblyopia who improved to mild amblyopia before surgery. Patients were assessed 4–6 weeks after surgery.

Results.—The surgical success rate in patients with moderate amblyopia was significantly lower than for patients with mild amblyopia (Table 2). Patients with moderate amblyopia were significantly older than those with mild or no amblyopia. When the ages of children with infantile ET who had successful surgery were compared with the ages of similar children who did not have successful surgery, there were no significant differences between age groups. Surgical success rates were similar for all patients with acquired, partially accommodative ET regardless of degree of amblyopia. Patients with acquired, nonaccommodative ET had similar surgical success rates regardless of degree of amblyopia. Surgeons may want to operate in the presence of amblyopia or in acquired ET with amblyopia before deviations become permanent. Whereas surgical success does not appear to be influenced by degree of amblyopia in acquired ET or in infantile ET with mild amblyopia, patients with infantile ET and moderate amblyopia have a significantly lower surgical success rate. These patients had a tendency toward overcorrection, whereas patients with mild amblyopia did as well as patients with no amblyopia.

Conclusions.—Patients with infantile ET and moderate amblyopia have poorer surgical success rates than similar patients with mild or no ambly-

TABLE 2.—Surgical Success Rates for All Patients

Degree of amblyopia	All patients (n=102)	Infantile ET (n=62)	Acquired, partially accommodative ET (n=26)	Acquired, non-accommodative ET (n=14)
None	84.3% (43/51)	77.1% (27/35)	100% (9/9)	100% (7/7)
Mild	81.6% (31/35)	81.0% (17/21)	91.7% (11/12)	60% (3/5)
Moderate	61.5% (8/13)	16.7% (1/6)	100% (5/5)	100% (2/2)

Abbreviation: ET, esotropia.
(Courtesy of Weakley DR Jr, Holland DR: Effect of ongoing treatment of amblyopia on surgical outcome in esotropia. *J Pediatr Ophthalmol Strabismus* 34:275–278, 1997.)

opia. There is no significant effect of surgery on patients with acquired ET regardless of the degree of amblyopia.

▶ It was not too many years ago that it would have been unthinkable to propose to operate on a patient with esotropia before the associated amblyopia was improved. Amblyopia was considered a significant obstacle to long-term successful alignment and needed to be corrected before strabismus surgery. The authors have confirmed the findings of others that for certain types of esotropia, it is reasonable to proceed with surgery even if amblyopia persists. Especially in acquired esotropia, the possible surgical success does not appear to be influenced by the severity of amblyopia. It is these kind of studies that question the "old doctrine," which can have a profound effect on the way we practice pediatric ophthalmology.

L.B. Nelson, M.D.

Perioperative Care of the Strabismus Patient

Olitsky SE, Awner S, Reynolds JD (State Univ of New York at Buffalo)

J Pediatr Ophthalmol Strabismus 34:126–128, 1997 7–2

Objective.—Keys to success in strabismus surgery are good preoperative measurements and avoidance of or proper handling of inadvertent scleral perforations, postoperative retinal detachment or infection, and lost or slipped muscles. The practice patterns followed to meet these goals vary, often without scientific rationale. This study documented surgeon variability in the management of surgical strabismus.

Findings.—The findings were based on a survey of 430 members of the American Association for Pediatric Ophthalmology and Strabismus. The response rate was 82%. The results showed wide variation in practice. Most respondents scheduled surgery after 1 measurement, as long as no complicating factors were present. The rest used 2 visits or more to confirm angle size stability or to establish better rapport. Few surgeons used preoperative antibiotics, but nearly three fourths used topical postoperative antibiotics, usually with a topical steroid. Most respondents said they would not alter their surgical routine for a known or suspected suprachoroidal needle pass. Although most surgeons scheduled the first postoperative visit between 1 and 4 days after surgery, the responses indicated substantial variability with no apparent rationale.

Conclusion.—Surgeons vary considerably in their preoperative and postoperative routines for strabismus correction. On most points examined, there is no consensus. There is near universal agreement, however, regarding the futility of prescribing routine postoperative oral antibiotics and the desire to evaluate postoperative patients within the first week.

▶ The authors attempted to document the trends in managing surgical strabismus patients by a physician survey. The variability in practice patterns was dramatic. However, there were several trends that were noteworthy.

Surgery was scheduled for an appropriate patient after 1 or 2 visits when no mitigating factors, such as amblyopia, were present. A majority of physicians were satisfied with 1 measurement. Very few surgeons use outpatient preoperative antibiotics. Certainly, the low incidence of postoperative infection in strabismus surgery does not warrant this type of treatment. However, the use of chemical prophylaxis of the conjunctiva just before or after surgery was common. The literature does support this practice in decreasing conjunctival flora considerably.

It was interesting that nearly three quarters of the respondents used topical postoperative antibiotics, even without evidence in the literature that it is necessary. Several physicians used postoperative oral antibiotics. Again, the scientific rationale for this is lacking. The timing of the first postoperative examination varied considerably among surgeons. There does not seem to be perfect postoperative timing for recognizing any serious complications.

L.B. Nelson, M.D.

Effects of Strabismus Surgery on Corneal Topography

Nardi M, Rizzo S, Pellegrini G, et al (Univ of Pisa, Italy)

J Pediatr Ophthalmol Strabismus 34:244–246, 1997 7–3

Background.—Extraocular muscle surgery is associated with changes in refraction. A computer-assisted topographic analysis system was utilized to evaluate variation in corneal topography after medial or lateral rectus muscle recessions for strabismus.

Methods.—The study group consisted of the 52 eyes of 36 patients undergoing initial surgery for 4- to 7-mm medial or lateral rectus muscle recessions. The surgery was performed at the University of Pisa between March and September 1992. Corneal topography was performed before surgery and 1, 15, and 30 days after surgery using the Corneal Modeling System. Repeat corneal topographic measurements were performed on healthy controls to validate the measurement technique.

Results.—One day after surgery, a significant change in astigmatic power was observed in the meridian of the recessed muscle, indicating a localized corneal flattening. This induced astigmatism decreased over time. At 30 days after surgery, only 6% of patients had a residual astigmatism higher than 1 D and only 12% had residual astigmatism higher than 0.5 D. This increase was higher for medial rectus recession than for lateral rectus recession.

Conclusions.—These results indicate that recessions of extraocular muscles cause changes in corneal topography, which decrease over time. These changes are mostly located in the meridian of the recessed muscle and in the optical zone. In 6% of patients, these changes remain, at less than 1 D, even after 30 days.

▶ Sometimes after strabismus surgery patients will notice that their vision in the surgically treated eye is decreased. This change in vision usually lasts for a short time, perhaps several weeks. The study has confirmed the results of other investigators that horizontal rectus muscle surgery causes a temporary change in the astigmatic power of the cornea. In 6% of patients, less than 1 D of astigmatism may persist. This could result in amblyopia and should be identified during the postoperative period.

L.B. Nelson, M.D.

Psychosocial Implications of Strabismus Surgery in Adults

Burke JP, Leach CM, Davis H (Univ of Sheffield, England)

J Pediatr Ophthalmol Strabismus 34:159–164, 1997 7–4

Objective.—Little research has been conducted into the psychological problems caused by strabismus. The psychosocial effects of noticeable strabismus in adults and its surgical correction were assessed.

Methods.—A self-reporting repertory grid assessing psychosocial consequences of surgery was completed by 31 adults (15 men), aged 18–68 years, who underwent correction of longstanding poor horizontal alignment. Fifteen personality traits were evaluated. Responses were compared statistically.

Results.—There were 11 men and 9 women with exotropias (XTs), 10 primary and 10 secondary, and 4 men and 7 women with esotropias (ETs), all primary. Of the 15 grids returned, 7 were from men (6 XTs 1 ET) and 8 were from women (5 XTs, 3 ETs). The sample of patients who returned the grids was similar to the sample who did not return the grids. Postsurgery scores were significantly higher than presurgery scores, indicating that ocular realignment improves psychosocial functioning. Respondents believed, before and after surgery, that others would rate them lower than they rated themselves, indicating a lack of self-confidence and self-esteem, even after surgery. Respondents also believed that others would expect them to behave significantly more positively after surgery. Although the costs of treatments for older individuals are sometimes more carefully scrutinized than for younger individuals, study results indicate that strabismus correction is equally important to both groups. Women believed, significantly more than men, that correction would have a more positive effect, and ET patients were significantly more positive than XT patients regarding the effects of correction. Most patients improved from "poor" ocular alignment before surgery to "excellent" alignment afterward.

Conclusion.—Psychosocial implications of corrective surgery for strabismus are not usually considered because of the difficulty in assessing people's perceptions. These considerations should be entered into the health care equation to assess the true value of correction when evaluating the effect of treatment.

► The psychological implications of strabismus on an individual's life have not gained adequate attention in the medical, psychological, or scientific literature. Patients with strabismus, however, have difficulty with self-image, interpersonal relationships, and securing employment. Problems encountered by patients with strabismus do not go away after childhood. The psychological problems encountered by these individuals intensify in the teenage and adult years.

Burke and associates show that adults with strabismus experience various psychosocial difficulties as a result of their ocular motor disorder. When these patients had their alignment corrected, psychosocial functioning improved significantly. Therefore, the benefits of strabismus surgery are multiple and should be readily available to all patients.

L.B. Nelson, M.D.

Ocular and Orbital Trauma From Water Balloon Slingshots: A Clinical, Epidemiologic, and Experimental Study

Bullock JD, Ballal DR, Johnson DA, et al (Wright State Univ, Dayton, Ohio; Univ of Dayton, Ohio; Eye Clinic of Wichita, Kan)

Ophthalmology 104:878–887, 1997 7–5

Introduction.—Water balloons can cause severe ocular and orbital injuries when launched with an elastic slingshot. Since 1988, several dozen such injuries have been reported to the Consumer Product Safety Commission. Eleven previously reported cases and 6 additional cases are presented here, together with an experimental and theoretical study of the kinetic energies involved in slingshot-launched water balloons.

Patients and Methods.—The 6 new cases were 2 males and 4 females who ranged in age from 9 to 28 years. A variety of injuries were sustained (Table 1), including periorbital edema and ecchymoses, traumatic iritis, eyelid lacerations, traumatic cataract, left orbital floor fracture, macular hole formation, and optic atrophy. Among the 11 previously reported cases were 2 female and 8 male patients age 9–34 years. Data on these patients indicated eye injuries that were "severe," "serious," or "permanent" in 4 cases; 1 patient was described as legally blind. Velocity and kinetic energy determinations were obtained by field trials and calculations.

Results.—Epidemiologic analysis showed that most of those injured were children and young adults. Males were involved more often than females, and most injuries occurred during warm weather months. Maximum water balloon velocities ranged from 85 to 92 mph in field trials. Kinetic energies ranged from 176 to 245 J. A calculation of velocities and kinetic energies based on the experimental determination of the ranges traversed by the balloons indicated a range of 39–102 yards, velocities of 43–85 mph, and kinetic energies of 42–245 J.

Discussion.—Serious ocular injuries can result from a water balloon slingshot, marketed on television as a "toy." The energies produced are far in excess of those required to perforate a cornea, rupture a globe, or fracture the bony orbit. In a field demonstration, a 300-gallon water

TABLE 1.—Ocular and Orbital Injuries From Slingshot-launched Water Balloons

Patient No.	Age (yrs)/ Gender	Water Balloon Struck	Injuries	Subsequent Ophthalmic Procedure(s)	Outcome
1	12/M	Right side of face	Hyphema, subconjunctival hemorrhage periorbital edema/ecchymoses	None	20/20
2	16/F	Right periorbital area	Periorbital edema/ecchymoses, subconjunctival hemorrhage, traumatic iritis	None	20/20 OU
3	9/F	Face	Bilateral hyphema, periorbital edema/ ecchymoses, subconjunctival hemorrhages unilateral vitreous hemorrhage, eyelid laceration, medial orbital wall fracture	None	20/20 OU
4	13/M	Face	Bilateral hyphema, periorbital edema/ ecchymoses, maxillary sinus hematomas; unilateral corneal abrasion, traumatic cataract, iris atrophy, sphincter rupture posterior synechiae	Left lensectomy anterior vitrectomy, placement posterior chamber IOL	RE 20/20 LE 20/30
5	28/F	Left periorbital area	Periorbital edema/ecchymoses, subconjunctival hemorrhage, traumatic iritis, facial hypesthesia, retinal hemorrhages, orbital hematoma; bilateral maxillary sinus hematomas	None	RE 20/20 LE 20/25
6	21/F	Face	Left orbital floor fracture, periorbital edema/ ecchymoses, subconjunctival hemorrhage, eyelid laceration, maxillary sinus hematoma; right retinal hemorrhages, hyphema, iris sphincter rupture	Repair left blow-out fracture	Mild left orbital deformity 20/20 OU

Abbreviations: M, male; *F*, female; *IOL*, intraocular lens; *OU*, both eyes; *RE*, right eye; *LE*, left eye.

(Courtesy of Bullock JD, Ballal DR, Johnson DA, et al: Ocular and orbital trauma from water balloon slingshots: A clinical, epidemiologic, and experimental study. *Ophthalmology* 104:878–887, 1997. Published courtesy of *Ophthalmology*.)

balloon launched horizontally from a distance of 20 feet exploded a 12kg watermelon with a mean rind thickness of 12.5 mm.

► Eye injuries are a significant cause of visual impairment and blindness. In this study, the authors highlight the importance of water balloon slingshots as a potential cause of ocular injury. The water balloon slingshot has been advertised as a toy, yet it has the potential to inflict serious ocular injury. The authors have shown that the water balloons can achieve an extremely high kinetic energy, sufficient to cause severe ocular injuries, including permanent blindness. Therefore, the general public needs to become aware of the danger inflicted by the use of this device.

L.B. Nelson, M.D.

Sports-related Ocular Injuries: A Three-Year Follow-up Study

Filipe JAC, Barros H, Castro-Correia J (S João Hosp, Porto, Portugal)

Ophthalmology 104:313–318, 1997 7–6

Background.—Ocular trauma is a major cause of visual morbidity. There are few data of use in preventing sports-related eye injuries and little long-term follow-up information on injured patients. Patients with sports-related ocular injuries were studied, with long-term follow-up.

Patients.—Over a 3-year period, 84 consecutive patients with sports-related eye injuries were prospectively studied. All patients were treated at a Portuguese hospital department of ophthalmology. One patient had injuries to both eyes. The patients were 78 males and 6 females (mean age, 25 years). About one fourth of the patients were less than 18 years of age; 83% were less than 35 years of age. The peak incidence of injuries occurred in March and May. Outdoor and indoor soccer accounted for 38% and 34.5% of the injuries, respectively. The next most commonly implicated sports—involved in 6% or less of cases—were handball, basketball, volleyball, and tennis. The soccer-related injuries were most often incurred by defensive players and forwards most often near the goal post. Sixty-four percent of the soccer injuries occurred when the player was hit with the ball; 16% resulted from fist trauma. None of the patients was wearing protective eyewear at the time of the injury.

Findings.—The patients' visual acuity at presentation was 20/40 or better in 69% of cases and 20/50 or worse in 31%. Six percent of patients were left with visual acuity of 20/300 or worse at final follow-up. The causes of permanent visual loss in these cases were corneoscleral laceration with retinal detachment and proliferative vitreoretinopathy caused by a fingernail scratch, retinal detachment with glaucoma caused by an eyeglass frame lesion, retinal detachment caused by a soccer ball, contusion maculopathy with choroidal rupture caused by a punch, and contusion maculopathy caused by a basketball. Patients who had good visual acuity at presentation usually had good visual acuity at follow-up.

Conclusion.—Sports-related ocular injuries are potentially serious. Many injuries occur in soccer players, especially near the goal post. These injuries warrant special care. Special preventive measures should be followed by 1-eyed athletes, those with pre-existing eye conditions, and athletes in high-risk sports. The severity of injury to the anterior segment in sports-related ocular trauma cannot predict the extent of damage to the posterior segment. All patients with blunt trauma should have regular gonioscopy and peripheral retinal examination to prevent delayed consequences of their eye injuries.

► As soccer has become more popular in the United States, more ocular injuries have been noted. Most of the literature on sports-related eye injuries in the United States reports baseball as the most common sport in which ocular injuries have occurred. In this study from Portugal, the mechanism of ocular injury in soccer was usually direct ball trauma occurring near the goal post. This often resulted in globe contusion. The number of monocular patients injured corroborates the concept that functionally 1-eyed athletes should not participate in sports in which adequate eye protection is not available. I agree with the authors that there is an educational role for eye injury preventive measures, especially in 1-eyed athletes, those with ocular disorders that can predispose them to injury, and athletes involved in high-risk sports.

L.B. Nelson, M.D.

Myopic Shift After Cataract Removal in Childhood

McClatchey SK, Parks MM (Naval Med Ctr, San Diego, Calif; Children's Natl Med Ctr, Washington, DC)

J Pediatr Ophthalmol Strabismus 34:88–95, 1997 7–7

Introduction.—In children who have cataracts removed, correction of the resultant hyperopia is needed. This used to be done with glasses or contact lenses, but now intraocular lens implants are sometimes used. Many surgeons avoid this, however, because of the need to change correction when the eye grows. To select the proper intraocular lens for children undergoing cataract removal, it is necessary to know the natural history of aphakic refractive change and the pattern of myopic shift. Hyperopia in aphakic eyes may decline rapidly in early childhood and less rapidly later on. A link between myopic shift and age was sought in a large group of aphakic children with long-term follow-up. The possible effects of age, cataract type, glaucoma, and other factors on the rate of myopic shift were evaluated as well.

Methods.—The study included 156 aphakic eyes of children who underwent cataract surgery before 10 years of age and had documented refractions for more than 3 years. Each child's refractive correction was achieved with contact lenses and glasses. Glaucoma was treated as indicated. Differences in the rate of myopic shift among different subgroups of children were assessed by stepwise multiple regression.

Results.—Analysis showed that aphakic refraction tended to follow a logarithmic curve. For all eyes, the rate of myopic shift—i.e., the slope of aphakic refraction vs. log of age—was −5.5 Diopters, with a standard deviation of 3.8. The only factor with even a small effect on the rate of myopic shift was age at surgery. The rate of shift tended to be less in very young children than in older children. The rate was slightly but not significantly greater in eyes with unilateral cataract. In 86 eyes with cataracts removed after 6 months of age, age at surgery played a less important role. The rate of myopic shift was greater in patients with unilateral cataract than in those with bilateral cataracts.

Conclusion.—In aphakic children, cataract type and glaucoma have no effect on myopic shift. Rather, the only factors significantly related to the rate of shift are age at surgery and unilateral vs. bilateral cataract. Even so, the effect of these 2 factors is less than the standard deviation of the rate of shift. Eyes treated in a very young patient tend to have a large amount of myopic shift and a high rate of glaucoma. The myopic shift observed in aphakic eyes appears to be caused largely by normal eye growth. Hyperopia in aphakic children follows a logarithmic curve, tending to decline with age.

► Intraocular lens implants have become a more common method of correcting pediatric aphakia. Intraocular lens implants result in a permanent correction of the hyperopia at a fixed power. However, with growth of a child's eye, there is a change in the refractive error. Hyperopia tends to decline with age, although there is a wide variation in the rate of the myopic shift. This shift is determined partly by age at surgery and whether the cataract was unilateral or bilateral. The rate of myopic shift is not determined by cataract type, glaucoma, sex, or best corrected visual acuity. Because of the variability of myopic shift, many ophthalmologists remain reluctant to implant intraocular lenses in young children.

L.B. Nelson, M.D.

Head Turn in 1-Eyed and Normally Sighted Individuals During Monocular Viewing

Goltz HC, Steinbach MJ, Gallie BL (York Univ, Toronto; Eye Research Inst of Canada, Toronto; The Hosp for Sick Children, Toronto)

Arch Ophthalmol 115:748–750, 1997 7–8

Introduction.—A study of 5 children who were enucleated between the ages of 2 weeks and 6 months reported increased head turn in the direction of the remaining eye. The authors' experience, however, was that head turning after unilateral enucleation was usually toward the missing eye. The nature of head turn during monocular viewing was studied in normally sighted and unilaterally enucleated individuals.

Methods.—The enucleated group included 52 children and adults (median age, 10 years) who lost sight in 1 eye because of retinoblastoma. Median age at enucleation was 18 months. None showed evidence of nystagmus. The controls, 28 normally sighted children and adults (median age 9 years), were tested with a patch covering 1 eye. Both groups were videotaped as they walked toward the camera down a 15 m hallway that was illuminated with normal fluorescent lighting. Enucleated individuals were tested with fixation relaxed (looking at the camera) and with fixation forced (trying to identify a small fixation target on the camera); controls were tested in the fixation-forced condition only. Two independent observers rated the incidence and magnitude of head turn.

Results.—Obvious head turn during the fixation-relaxed condition was reported for 17% of enucleated individuals; 58% exhibited no head turn, and 25% showed only a small (5–10 degree) head turn. In the fixation-forced condition, 42% had no head turn, and 30% demonstrated an obvious head turn. When head turn occurred in enucleated individuals, it was most commonly toward the enucleated eye. Neither age at enucleation nor years since eye removal had any significant effect on the incidence and magnitude of head turn in the fixation forced condition. There were no consistent head turn findings in monocularly patched controls.

Conclusion.—Approximately 30% of enucleated individuals showed obvious head turn, usually in the direction of the missing eye. Head turn appears to be an adaptive strategy developed in response to visual field loss and is unrelated to nystagmus.

▶ One-eyed children frequently exhibit a head turn toward the missing eye. This occurs even in the absence of nystagmus. I agree with the author's suggestion that the direction of the head turn moves the remaining eye toward the midline and reduces the occulusion by the nose in the lower contralateral field. In evaluating the degree of head turn, it is imperative that the observer force the subject to fixate on visual targets that are small enough to elicit this adaptive method of viewing.

L.B. Nelson, M.D.

Resolution of Astigmatism After Surgical Resection of Capillary Hemangiomas in Infants

Plager DA, Snyder SK (Indiana Univ, Indianapolis)

Ophthalmology 104:1102–1106, 1997 7–9

Background.—Capillary hemangioma is one of the most common orbital and eyelid tumors of infants. These tumors often spontaneously regress, but may cause significant visual sequelae. The most frequent treatment is intralesional injection of corticosteroids. In 3 cases, complete surgical excision of visually significant astigmatism-inducing hemangiomas in children younger than 1 year was successful.

Methods.—Complete surgical excision of astigmatism-inducing hemangiomas was performed in 3 children, aged 4 months, 6 months, and 9 months. Cosmetic results and refractive change in the surgically treated eye were assessed.

Results.—In all 3 cases, complete surgical excision of the hemangioma resulted in nearly complete resolution of anisometropia and excellent cosmetic results.

Conclusions.—Surgical resection of adnexal hemangiomas in carefully selected infants can lead to excellent cosmetic and visual results. Appropriate patient selection is very important. The ideal patient has a firm, discrete lesion that does not include the skin surface and is anterior to the orbital septum. Removing the compressive force of the hemangioma from the infant sclera permits the eye to assume a more normal shape, which may be necessary to prevent permanent anisometropia. No other therapy for these hemangiomas has this effect.

▶ Intralesional steroid injection is probably the most commonly used method to treat amblyogenic eyelid hemangiomas. Treatment complications with this technique are uncommon but can be severe. The surgical treatment for hemangiomas has been reserved for cosmetic improvement of residual tumor and lid abnormalities left after the mass has resolved. Ophthalmologists have been reluctant to operate on active lesions in infants because of the potential blood loss and poor results such as scarring and inadequate tumor removal. The authors have demonstrated excellent results with surgical resection of selected hemangiomas. They outline specific criteria including relatively firm, discrete lesions, which do not extend to include the skin surface and which are anterior to the orbital septum.

L.B. Nelson, M.D.

8 Neuro-ophthalmology

Graves' Ophthalmopathy: What Should We Do Now?

by Robert C. Sergott, M.D.

During the last year, the lead article in one issue of *The New England Journal of Medicine* attempted to define the relationship between the therapy for hyperthyroidism and the course of Graves' ophthalmopathy.[1] This study followed earlier work advocating the use of systemic corticosteroids for many patients who received radioactive iodine in an attempt to lessen the chances of serious orbital complications.[2]

While both these studies were published in one of the world's most prestigious medical journals, the results are far from conclusive, as was correctly described in an accompanying editorial in the same January 1998 issue of *The New England Journal of Medicine*.[3] However, practicing clinical ophthalmologists now have a new maze of data to weave through in advising their patients about the proper treatment of thyroid eye disease.

This debate and uncertainty are by no means new, dating back almost to the early 19th century when Robert Graves first described the association of hyperthyroidism and proptosis. For over 200 years, patients, endocrinologists, and ophthalmologists have struggled to understand how a gland in the neck could exert such a potentially devastating effect upon the extraocular muscles, orbital fat, and optic nerve.

Clinicians must be acutely aware of one pivotal fact: some patients with Graves' hyperthyroidism will develop vision threatening and cosmetically debilitating orbital disease. And unfortunately in our current medicolegal community, some legal "scholars" will litigate the situation retrospectively, claiming that the use of corticosteroids would have prevented or lessened the patients' Graves' ophthalmopathy.

The practicing clinician is in a devilish quandary; if the patient receives corticosteroids and develops a corticosteroid-related complication, litigation is also a likely occurrence. At the present time, I believe that ophthalmologists need to read these studies and follow the guidelines set forth by Dr. Wilmar Wiersinga in his editorial. In addition, they should directly address this controversy with their patients and maintain a continuing dialogue. The treatment of Graves' ophthalmopathy requires continued patient education.

The following practical clinical messages evolve from Dr. Wiersinga's editorial and should form the basis of our current treatment regimen:

1. The existing studies do not prove that radioactive iodine causes a higher frequency of new or worsening ophthalmopathy.
2. Not all patients should receive corticosteroids after radioactive ablation of their thyroid. Instead, the patients need to be informed of the clinical dilemma of this disease and monitored for any signs of significant deterioration. I define *significant worsening* as the new limitation of restrictive ocular motility, an increase of 2 mm of proptosis, the loss of two or more lines of visual acuity, or the worsening of a scotoma with visual field testing.
3. If such clinical worsening occurs, then the patients should be considered for systemic corticosteroid therapy, provided no general medical reasons contraindicate the use of significant doses of oral prednisone.
4. If patients have severe ophthalmlopathy, it may be reasonable to advise endocrinologists to treat the hyperthyroidism for as long as possible with antithyroid medications before recommending radioactive ablation therapy.

As Dr. Wiersinga points out, there are several other clinical findings that may enable clinicians to decide who needs to be carefully monitored for severe worsening of Graves' ophthalmopathy. The following factors should be considered:

1. Patients who smoke tobacco products.
2. Severe preexisiting ophthalmopathy.
3. High pretreatment triiodothyronine concentrations.
4. High serum concentrations of thyrotropin-receptor antibodies and thyrotropin after treatment.

Clinicians must remain more vigilant in their follow-up assessment and care of patients with Graves' ophthalmopathy. They need to employ corticosteroids when significant worsening occurs following the administration of radioactive iodine. All patients who smoke tobacco must be vigorously counseled to stop smoking and must be warned that failure to stop may result in permanent visual and cosmetic deficits. All patients who receive radioactive iodine should not be treated with corticosteroids. Clinicians must remember that there are no absolutes in the care of Graves' ophthalmopathy except for careful, meticulous, continued care of the patient by specialists with experience and expertise in orbital disease and neuroophthalmology.

References

1. Bartalena L, Marcocci C, Bogazzi F, et al: Relation between therapy for hyperthyroidism and the course of Graves' ophthalmopathy. *N Engl J Med* 338:73–78, 1998.

2. Bartalena L, Marcoccci C, Bogazzi F, et al: Use of corticosteroids to prevent progression of Graves' ophthalmopathy after radioactive iodine therapy for hyperthyroidism. *N Engl J Med* 321:1349–1352, 1989.
3. Wiersinga WM: Preventing Graves' ophthalmopathy. *N Engl J Med* 338:121–122, 1998.

Giant Cell Arteritis: Validity and Reliability of Various Diagnostic Criteria

Hayreh SS, Podhajsky PA, Raman R, et al (Univ of Iowa, Iowa City)
Am J Ophthalmol 123:285–296, 1997 8–1

Introduction.—Giant cell arteritis carries a high risk of severe visual loss if not promptly recognized and treated. Early diagnosis may be difficult, however, because the range of symptoms is quite wide. A prospective study assessed the validity, reliability, sensitivity, and specificity of various signs and symptoms of and diagnostic tests for giant cell arteritis.

Patients and Methods.—Data for the study came from 363 patients referred for temporal artery biopsy from 1973 to 1994. The patients, 123 men and 240 women with a mean age of 72 years, were seen at the ophthalmology department of the University of Iowa Hospitals and Clinics. Many had been referred from other departments because of systemic signs and symptoms suggestive of giant cell arteritis. At least 1 inch of the temporal artery was removed at biopsy. A second biopsy was performed on the other side if results were negative or equivocal, but suspicion was high for giant cell arteritis. All patients underwent detailed clinical evaluation and determination of erythrocyte sedimentation rates. C-reactive protein values were estimated in 223 patients evaluated since 1985. Data on these 2 parameters also were obtained in controls with systemic diseases associated with retinal vein occlusion and nonarteritic anterior ischemic optic neuropathy. The following 3 groups were identified for statistical analysis: 106 patients with positive temporal artery biopsy for giant cell arteritis, 257 patients negative biopsy, and 749 controls.

Results.—Signs and symptoms recorded were headache, fever, anorexia and weight loss, jaw claudication, malaise, myalgia, abnormal temporal artery, scalp tenderness, neck pain, and anemia. The odds of a positive biopsy for giant cell arteritis were 9 times greater with jaw claudication, 3.4 times greater with neck pain, and 2 times greater for age 75 years or older. The odds of a positive biopsy were increased 2 times with an erythrocyte sedimentation rate of 47–107 mm/hr and 3.2 times with C-reactive protein greater than 2.45 mg/dL.

Discussion.—Early diagnosis is crucial to the prevention of blindness in patients with giant cell arteritis. In this series of patients, the clinical criteria most strongly associated with a positive diagnosis were jaw claudication, C-reactive protein greater than 2.45 mg/dL, neck pain, and an erythrocyte sedimentation rate of at least 47 mm/hr. The C-reactive protein level was the most sensitive parameter (100%). A combination of C-reactive protein with erythrocyte sedimentation rate yielded a specificity of 97%.

► All clinicians are hoping that someday there may be a simple way to diagnose giant cell arteritis. Although C-reactive protein may be another weapon in our diagnostic armamentarium, it is not specific. This disease remains of paramount importance for prompt diagnosis since prevention of visual loss is critical. Once visual loss has ensued, no therapy has proven to be effective. Therefore, C-reactive protein may be somewhat helpful, but nothing replaces the clinician's high index of suspicion for this entity. Since the publication of this paper, we have had 3 patients with biopsy-proven giant cell arteritis who have had normal C-reactive proteins. Therefore, C-reactive proteins certainly may be beneficial in some situations, but again, it does not replace good clinical judgment and consideration of the patient's entire situation.

R.C. Sergott, M.D.

Postprandial Transient Visual Loss: A Symptom of Critical Carotid Stenosis

Levin LA, Mootha VV (Univ of Wisconsin, Madison)

Ophthalmology 104:397–401, 1997 8–2

Background.—Severe stenosis of the carotid circulation can cause transient visual loss from retinal or choroidal hypoperfusion. Such visual loss, which lasts from several minutes to hours, can be induced by situations that increase retinal oxygen demand or reduce perfusion pressure. Two patients with severe carotid occlusive disease who experienced visual loss after eating a meal were seen.

Case Report 1.—Woman, 59, had a 6-week history of transient visual loss in the left eye, occurring daily 1 hour after eating lunch, which was her largest meal of the day. The visual loss usually lasted about 3 hours. Frequently, these episodes were accompanied by right arm numbness and weakness. This patient's medical history was significant for insulin-dependent diabetes mellitus of 10 years' duration, essential hypertension, hypercholesterolemia, hypothyroidism, and a 144 pack-year history of smoking. Fundus examination demonstrated flat discs, background diabetic retinopathy in the right eye, and many peripheral blot hemorrhages in the left eye. On angiography, 90% stenosis of the left proximal internal carotid artery and 50% stenosis of the right carotid siphon were seen. Uncomplicated left carotid endarterectomy resulted in complete resolution of the episodes of visual loss and the arm symptoms.

Case Report 2.—Woman, 65, had a 6-month history of transient bilateral visual loss precipitated by eating a meal or standing from a sitting or lying position. She described these episodes as looking like "mud had been thrown over the bathroom walls." The episodes lasted for 2 minutes to 1.5 hours and were often accompanied by feeling faint. This patient was hypertensive and a heavy smoker. Carotid endarterectomy was not considered because of the patient's advanced metastatic disease.

Discussion.—Both of these patients had splotchy visual loss precipitated by eating a meal. The nature of the visual loss was very characteristic of that associated with hypoperfusion of the retina and choroid: the scotomas occurred in a blotchy pattern, did not travel across the visual field, and lasted several minutes to hours. These patients' visual loss, provoked by eating a meal, may have been caused by a combination of mesenteric steal, reduced cardiac output, and abnormal vasomotor control in the presence of severe carotid disease, resulting in reduced perfusion of the retinal and choroidal circulations.

▶ The authors describe a very clinically useful symptom of high-grade carotid occlusive disease. As the baby boomer generation moves into the fifth, sixth, and seventh decades of life, carotid occlusive disease is becoming more and more common. In addition, with the results of the highly controlled surgical studies showing benefit of carotid artery surgery, the recognition of this disease is critical. Carotid artery surgery just 7–10 years ago was felt to be useless, but then the studies were controlled very carefully for the quality of the surgeon and the postoperative care and, indeed, a benefit was shown.

Levin and Mootha describe 2 patients who suffered loss of vision after eating a meal. Both individuals had high-grade carotid occlusive disease. The quality of the patients' visual loss was that of retinal and choroidal ischemia in that a blotchy pattern occurred lasting for several minutes but without spread across the visual field. This short, but extremely well written, paper highlights a very useful clinical symptom that practicing ophthalmologists need to remember.

R.C. Sergott, M.D.

Carotid Endarterectomy Trends in the Patterns and Outcomes of Care at Academic Medical Centers, 1990 Through 1995

Holloway RG Jr, Witter DM Jr, Mushlin AI, et al (Univ of Rochester, NY; Association of American Medical Colleges, Washington, DC; Duke Univ, Durham, NC)

Arch Neurol 55:25–32, 1998 8–3

Purpose.—Recent years have seen widespread diagnostic and management changes for patients undergoing carotid endarterectomy (CEA). However, the impact of these changes remains undefined. As the CEA rate continues to increase, the rate of carotid arteriography has been declining steadily. All of these changes are taking place in the context of ongoing efforts to deliver health services more efficiently. Trends in inpatient care, patient characteristics, and outcomes for patients undergoing CEA during the 1990s were retrospectively analyzed.

Methods.—Administrative data on 7,019 admissions for CEA from 1990 through 1995 were reviewed. The analysis looked at changes in patient demographics and comorbidity over time; changes in CEA frequency, length of stay, and inpatient use of cerebral arteriography; and associated changes in patient outcomes.

Results.—During the study period, the number of CEAs performed per year more than doubled. At the same time, the percentage of admissions for patients aged 65 years or older increased from 65% to 75%. Length of hospital stay was reduced by half, as was the percentage of patients requiring ICU admission and the percentage requiring inpatient cerebral arteriography. Despite all of these changes, there was no apparent impact on patient outcomes.

Conclusions.—In the first half of the 1990s, the number of CEAs performed increased, and the procedure was offered to an increasingly older patient population. There have been many striking changes in inpatient management, including great reductions in postoperative arteriography to confirm arterial patency, with no apparent adverse effects on patient outcome. Any attempt to reduce utilization of medical services—particularly in a delicate procedure such as CEA—should be accompanied by early, rigorous assessment studies like this one.

▶ Carotid endarterectomy generates more controversy than any other operation in the country. In the hands of highly trained surgeons at experienced medical centers, CEA seems to have a place for patients with hemodynamically significant carotid stenosis.

This study demonstrates that cost-effective prompt evaluation and improved intensive care procedures do not adversely impact patient outcome. For example, routine postoperative cerebral angiography is now rarely performed. This type of retrospective study is very valuable so that patients and practitioners know that new management strategies do not compromise the quality of care.

R.C. Sergott, M.D.

The Clinical, Neuroradiographic, and Endocrinologic Profile of Patients With Bilateral Optic Nerve Hypoplasia

Siatkowski RM, Sanchez JC, Andrade R, et al (Univ of Miami, Fla; Universidad Catolica, Guayaquil, Ecuador)

Ophthalmology 104:493–496, 1997 8–4

Background.—About 40 years ago, deMorsier reported a series of patients with optic nerve hypoplasia, poor vision, hypotelorism, and absence of the septum pellucidum. In 1970, Hoyt et al. discovered that hypopituitarism was associated with this syndrome. The clinical, neuroradiographic, and endocrinologic findings in 1 series of patients with bilateral optic nerve hypoplasia (BONH) were reviewed.

Methods.—The records of 35 children with BONH were reviewed. Data on visual acuity, refractive error, and the presence of nystagmus and strabismus were noted. Full endocrinologic assessment and MRI or CT scanning were done in 26 children.

Findings.—Visual acuity was 20/60 or better in 10% of the eyes. Thirty-four percent had no light perception. Eighty-six percent of the eyes had an acuity of less than 20/200. Eighty percent of the patients were legally blind. Eighty-six percent had nystagmus or strabismus, or both. In 46%, the septum pellucidum and corpus callosum were absent on neuroimaging. Endocrinologic abnormalities were present in 27% of the patients, growth hormone deficiency being most common. Eleven and a half percent of the children had panhypopituitarism.

Conclusions.—The visual prognosis of children with BONH is generally poor. However, 10% have excellent acuity. Only one fourth of the patients had endocrine abnormalities, in contrast to previous reports. Only 11.5% had full-blown deMorsier syndrome.

► Bilateral optic nerve hypoplasia is being recognized more and more frequently. It is of critical importance for ophthalmologists to be aware of this syndrome because the diagnosis of BONH in these children has implications not only for how they are cared for visually, but also for the endocrine disturbances they may have, as is reviewed in this article. In addition, BONH may go unrecognized in some of these patients until the time of strabismus surgery. With the stress of general anesthesia, the hypoadrenal state may become evident and actually threaten the patient's life. Therefore, the ophthalmologist in this situation must be aware of not only the visual problems but also the other manifestations of this disease.

R.C. Sergott, M.D.

Pathogenesis of Acute Monocular Blindness From Leaking Anterior Communicating Artery Aneurysms: Report of Six Cases

Chan JW, Hoyt WF, Ellis WG, et al (Univ of California, San Francisco; Univ of California, Davis)

Neurology 48:680–683, 1997 8–5

Background.—Sudden visual loss in 1 eye is an uncommon focal sign of anterior communicating artery aneurysm. Six patients with acute monocular blindness from leaking anterior communicating aneurysms were treated at 1 center during a 37-year period.

Case Reports.—The patients were 4 women and 2 men, aged 26 to 49 years. In 2 patients, the pathogenic mechanism of acute monocular blindness was demonstrated by surgical and pathologic evidence. As the aneurysm enlarged, the down-pointing dome compressed the optic nerve from above and adhered to it. When the aneurysm ruptured through the adherent dome, it bled directly into the optic nerve. Severe headache and monocular blindness resulted. In the remaining patients, an alternative mechanism was suggested. The aneurysm apparently compressed the nerve directly in these patients.

Discussion.—This report is the first to show the probable mechanism of visual loss with pathologic specimens in patients with monocular blindness from bleeding from an aneurysm of the anterior communicating artery aneurysmal bleeding. Autopsy findings in 2 patients showed unusual aneurysms that pointed down toward the optic nerve, large enough to touch the nerve sheath. In 1, the aneurysm had compressed the nerve gradually, resulting in the visual symptoms. The aneurysm adhered to the nerve, possibly through repeated intramural capillary leaks and fibrosis, rupturing in the area of adhesion. This sent a pulsating, needle-like jet of blood into the optic nerve, expanding it and causing blindness. Under arterial pressure, blood dissected up the optic nerve into the chiasm and adjacent brain, eventually breaking into the subarachnoid space.

▶ Anterior communicating artery aneurysms are unusual neuro-ophthalmic problems. However, it is of critical importance for ophthalmologists to recognize this disorder because the management of this problem is obviously so much different from that of inflammatory optic neuropathies. This article emphasizes the acute loss of vision occurring with anterior communicating artery aneurysms and provides clinicopathological correlation so that the entire disease process may be better understood. Ophthalmologists should be aware of this syndrome when patients are seen with painful unilateral visual loss and their headache is not typical of optic neuritis. If there are any meningeal symptoms present at the time of the visual loss, such as nausea, vomiting, or neck stiffness, immediate MRI scanning is indicated.

R.C. Sergott, M.D.

Radiation Optic Neuropathy After Stereotactic Radiosurgery

Girkin CA, Comey CH, Lunsford LD, et al (Univ of Alabama, Birmingham; Univ of Pittsburgh, Pa; Piedmont Hosp, Atlanta, Ga)

Ophthalmology 104:1634–1643, 1997 8–6

Background.—Patients undergoing stereotactic radiosurgery receive a single, high dose of ionizing radiation to a stereotactically localized area within the brain. Some of the lesions treated by this technique are located next to the anterior visual pathways. External beam radiation therapy can cause delayed injury to the anterior visual pathways. Such changes most often occur 8–18 months after treatment, with an acute onset. Four cases of optic neuropathy occurring after stereotactic radiosurgery for perichiasmal tumors were described.

Patients.—The patients were 2 men and 2 women, ages 33–62, undergoing gamma knife therapy for meningioma or pituitary adenoma. About 7–30 months after treatment, the patients had optic neuropathy, signaled by an abrupt change in visual function. On gadolinium-enhanced MRI scans performed in 3 patients, swelling and enhancement of the affected part of the visual apparatus was seen. All patients received systemic corticosteroids; 1 showed partial recovery.

Conclusions.—Optic neuropathy is a rare complication of stereotactic radiosurgery for lesions located near the visual pathways. The clinical course is similar to that occurring after conventional radiotherapy. The best way to prevent this complication is careful, MRI-guided dose planning, with a maximal radiation dose to the visual pathways of less than 8 Gy.

▶ Although stereotactic radiosurgery ("gamma knife") has clear and compelling advantages in some cases over conventional radiation therapy, radiation necrosis of the afferent visual system may still occur. Clinicians must exercise extreme caution in advocating any type of radiation when the lesion is in close proximity to the optic nerves and chiasm.

As this study reiterates, treatment of radiation necroses is not currently possible. Therefore, even the prompt institution of corticosteroids and/or hyperbaric oxygen is not helpful. Some other recent studies have advocated anticoagulation for radiation necrosis because the basic pathology is a radiation vasculitis. No definitive studies exist about radiation necrosis and anticoagulation, but it remains as another desperation therapeutic option.

R.C. Sergott, M.D.

Bilateral Superior Ophthalmic Vein Enlargement Associated With Diffuse Cerebral Swelling: Report of 11 Cases

Khanna RK, Pham CJ, Malik GM, et al (Henry Ford Hosp, Detroit)
J Neurosurg 86:893–897, 1997 8–7

Background.—Patients with carotid-cavernous fistulas, intraorbital abnormalities, and parasellar tumors may be found to have unilateral superior ophthalmic vein (SOV) enlargement. This syndrome is characterized by increased retrograde SOV flow, SOV obstruction, or cavernous sinus compression. With some exceptions, SOV enlargement is almost always unilateral. One group of patients with bilateral SOV enlargement associated with cerebral edema that resolved with treatment was reported.

Methods and Findings.—Eleven patients with bilateral SOV enlargement associated with cerebral swelling on CT were studied. Patient age ranged from 15 to 59 years. Cerebral swelling and increased intracranial pressure resolved after various surgical procedures. After treatment, the bilaterally enlarged SOVs returned to a normal size (Fig 1).

Conclusions.—Bilateral enlargement of the SOVs probably occurs more often in patients with cerebral edema than is currently appreciated. After

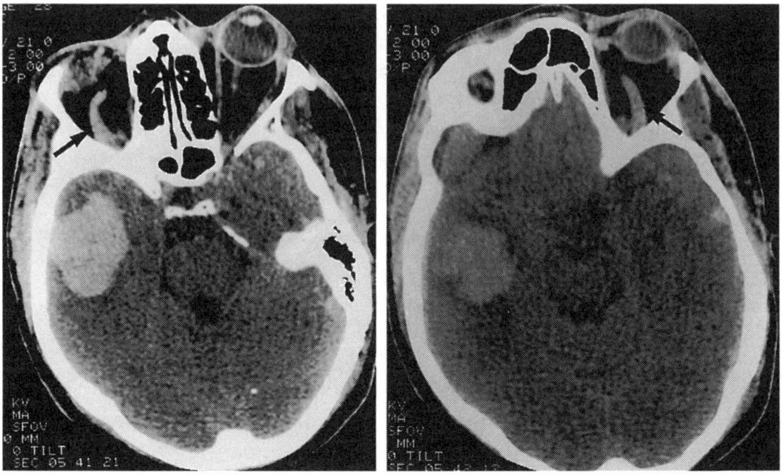

FIGURE 1.—Initial CT scans in a patient with bilateral SOV enlargement. **Left**, note the enlarged right superior ophthalmic vein (*arrow*) as well as the right temporal hemorrhage. The ethnoid air cells, sphenoid sinus, and mastoid air cells are clear. **Right**, the left superior ophthalmic vein is also enlarged (*arrow*). (Courtesy of Khanna RK, Pham CJ, Malik GM, et al: Bilateral superior ophthalmic vein enlargement associated with diffuse cerebral swelling: Report of 11 cases. *J Neurosurg* 86:893–897, 1997.)

corroboration by other clinical criteria and CT scanning for increased ICP, this finding usually reflects significant intracranial hypertension, and early aggressive treatment may be needed. A prospective study with MRI and venography should ultimately provide a better understanding of the mechanism(s) involved in SOV enlargement.

► The authors report a clinically useful observation of enlarged SOVs in patients with cerebral edema. These patients need to be distinguished from other individuals with carotid-cavernous fistulas and septic cavernous sinus thrombosis.

The authors' observation appears valid given the prompt resolution of the enlarged SOVs with reduction of the cerebral edema. Although not described in this study, we have observed a similar patient who came to neuroophthalmologic attention because of a unilateral cavernous sinus syndrome. CT scanning revealed an enlarged SOV and with resolution of the cerebral edema, both the patients' clinical and neuroradiologic findings improved. Therefore, this report does have clinical application.

R.C. Sergott, M.D.

A Double-blind Controlled Study of Gabapentin and Baclofen as Treatment for Acquired Nystagmus

Averbuch-Heller L, Tusa RJ, Fuhry L, et al (Case Western Reserve Univ, Cleveland, Ohio; Bascom Palmer Eye Inst, Miami, Fla; Ludwig-Maximilians Univ, Munich; et al)

Ann Neurol 41:818–825, 1997 8–8

Introduction.—The symptoms of acquired nystagmus may be alleviated if the ocular oscillations are reduced or abolished, but few reliable clinical therapies are available. A double-blind, crossover trial compared gabapentin to baclofen as therapy for acquired nystagmus.

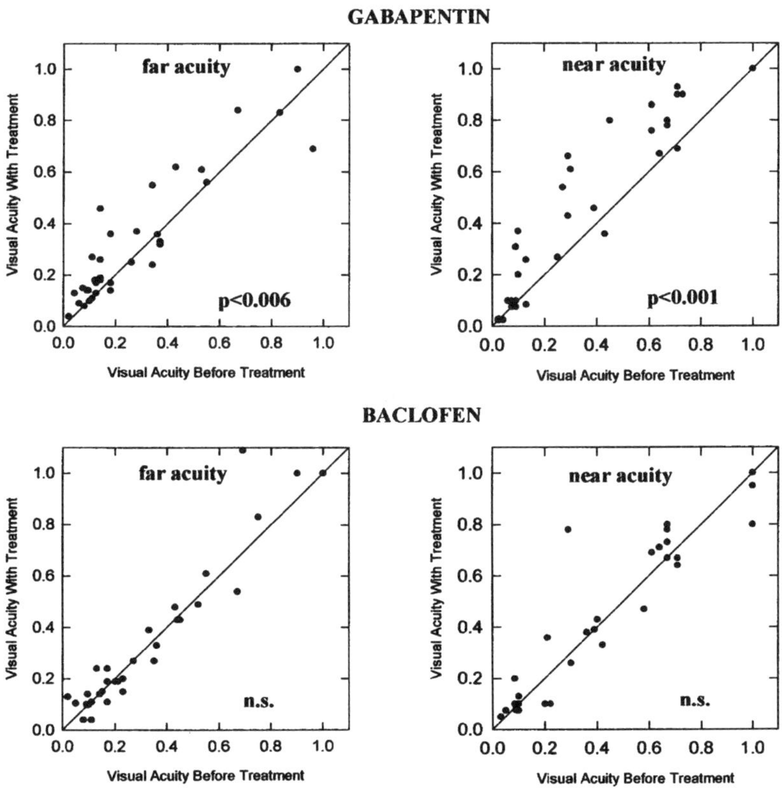

FIGURE 2.—Comparison of visual acuity, expressed as a decimal, before and at the end of the treatment phase with gabapentin or baclofen in the patients with acquired pendular nystagmus (patients 1–15). Each *data point* compares corresponding measurements while the right, the left, or both eyes view either the chart at distance (*far acuity*) or a near card (*near acuity*). The *solid line* at 45 degrees represents no change between pretreatment and treatment values. *Data points above the line* represent improvement in visual acuity with treatment, and those *below* represent deterioration with treatment. Gabapentin produced statistically significant improvements in both far and near visual acuity (indicated by *P* values), whereas the changes produced by baclofen were not significant (*n.s.*). (Reprinted from *Annals of Neurology*, courtesy of Averbuch-Heller L, Tusa RJ, Fuhry L, et al: A double-blind controlled study of gabapentin and baclofen as treatment for acquired nystagmus. *Ann Neurol* 41:818–825, 1997.)

Methods.—Fifteen patients had acquired pendular nystagmus (APN) and 6 had jerk nystagmus that was either downbeat or torsional downbeat. Several had tried a variety of medications with only minor or temporary relief. Treatment consisted of gabapentin (up to 900 mg/day) and baclofen (up to 30 mg/day). Experimental studies suggest that γ-aminobutyric acid (GABA) plays an important role in the mechanism by which gaze is held steady during visual fixation, and both gabapentin and baclofen involve GABAergic mechanisms. Visual acuity and nystagmus were measured before and after 2 weeks of administration of each agent.

Results.—Twenty patients completed both 2-week test periods. Only gabapentin significantly improved visual acuity in patients with APN; median eye speed was significantly reduced in all 3 planes with gabapentin, but baclofen affected only the vertical plane (Fig 2). Eight patients with APN elected to continue gabapentin treatment. With both therapies, patients with downbeat or torsional downbeat nystagmus had less consistent changes in median slow-phase eye speed. Only 1 of 6 patients had consistent reduction in median eye speed, and the 2 drugs were similarly effective in this case.

Conclusion.—Gabapentin proved to be an effective therapy for most patients with APN. Visual acuity was improved and all components of the nystagmus were reduced. Ataxia may be worsened, however, and care should be taken to avoid falls. Both gabapentin and baclofen may benefit some patients with downbeat nystagmus.

► For decades, nystagmus has been like most neuro-ophthalmologic disorders: diagnosable but untreatable. Now, basic science research is beginning to return clinical dividends. This study demonstrates clearly that gabapentin (300 mg by mouth, 3 times a day) improved visual acuity and nystagmus parameters in patients with APN. Some patients with downbeat nystagmus seemed to improve with gabapentin or baclofen (10 mg by mouth, 3 times a day). Both medications were well tolerated; however, gabapentin did increase ataxia and imbalance in some patients. Therefore, patients need to be cautioned about the potential dangers of falling.

R.C. Sergott, M.D.

Axonal Transection in the Lesions of Multiple Sclerosis

Trapp BD, Peterson J, Ransohoff RM, et al (Cleveland Clinic Found, Ohio; Haukeland Hosp, Bergen, Norway)

N Engl J Med 338:278–285, 1998 8–9

Objective.—The cause of multiple sclerosis is unknown, although environmental and genetic factors play a role in susceptibility. At the onset of multiple sclerosis, MRI scans may show breakdown of the blood-brain barrier. Even with anti-inflammatory or immunosuppressive therapy, progressive neurologic deterioration—perhaps reflecting axonal loss—occurs

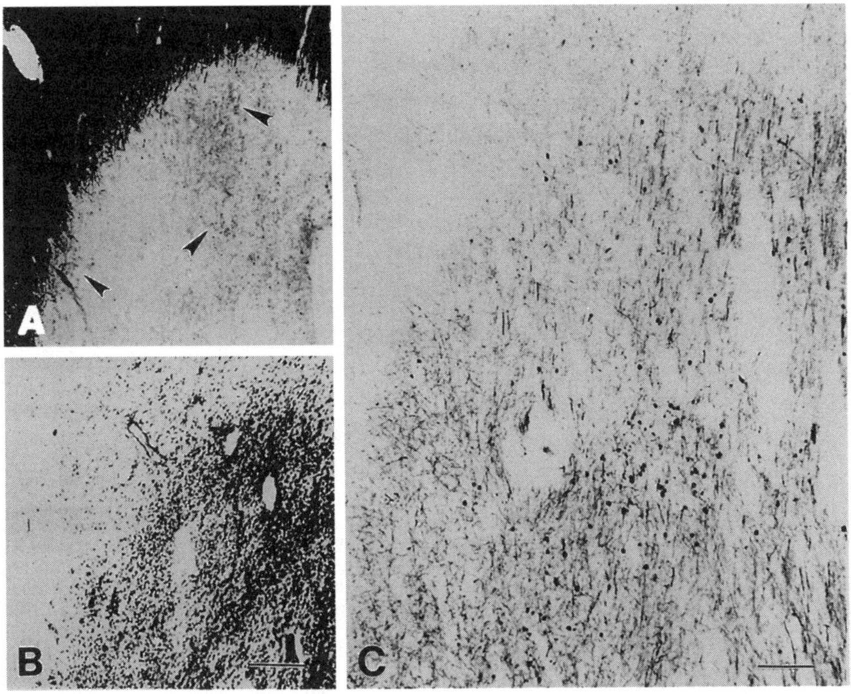

FIGURE 1.—Serial sections of multiple sclerosis lesions immunostained for myelin (**panel A**), major histocompatibility complex (MHC) class II (**panel B**), and nonphosphorylated neurofilaments (**panel C**). This figure shows an active multiple sclerosis lesion characterized by loss of myelin (**panel A**), myelin debris within the demyelinated area (**panel A, arrowheads**), even distribution of numerous MHC class II–positive cells throughout the demyelinated area (**panel B**), and abundant expression of nonphosphorylated neurofilaments within the lesion (**panel C**). The *scale bars* in **panels A** and **B** represent 400 μm; the *scale bar* in **panel C** represents 235 μm. (Reprinted by permission of *The New England Journal of Medicine*, from Trapp BD, Peterson J, Ransohoff RM, et al: Axonal transection in the lesions of multiple sclerosis. *N Engl J Med* 338:278–285. Copyright 1998, Massachusetts Medical Society. All rights reserved.)

in most patients with this condition. One report suggested axonal accumulation of the amyloid precursor protein in multiple sclerosis lesions, possibly related to irreversible axonal damage. The pathologic changes of the axons in multiple sclerosis were analyzed by 3-dimensional imaging of brain sections.

Methods.—Autopsy specimens of brain from 11 patients with multiple sclerosis and 4 subjects without brain disease were studied. A total of 14 active multiple sclerosis lesions (Fig 1) and 33 chronic active lesions (Fig 2) were examined for demyelination and other abnormalities, along with samples of normal-appearing white matter. The finding of terminal axonal ovoids was used as an indicator of axonal transection.

Results.—Multiple sclerosis lesions were consistently associated with transected axons. The more severe the inflammation within the lesions, the greater the frequency of transected axons.

Conclusions.—Axonal transection consistently follows demyelination in multiple sclerosis lesions in the brain. The axons appear to be a major

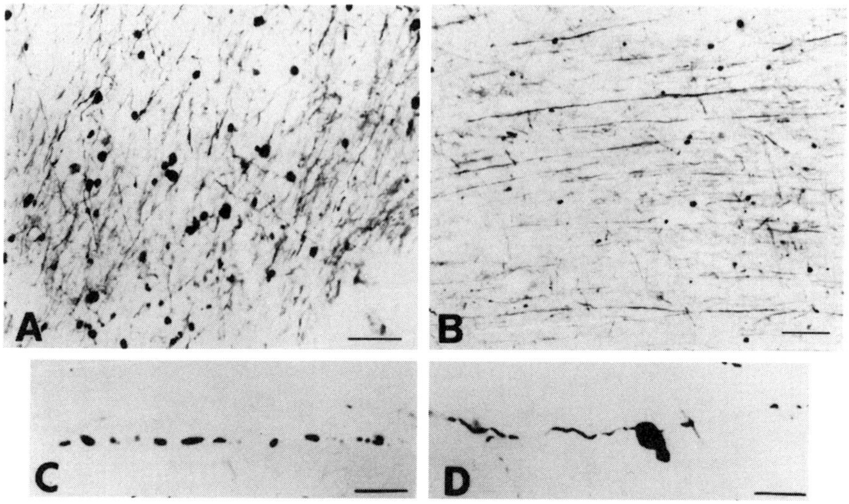

FIGURE 2.—Patterns of axonal pathologic changes in multiple sclerosis lesions. In active lesions (**panel A**), SMI-32–positive ovoids and axons are abundant. At the edges of chronic active lesions (**panel B**), nonphosphorylated-neurofilament-positive axons and ovoids are less abundant and the ovoids are smaller. Most nonphosphorylated-neurofilament-positive axons in multiple sclerosis have a normal appearance (**panels A** and **B**). Some have discontinuous staining for nonphosphorylated neurofilaments (**panel C**), which is characteristic of axonal degeneration. Other axons have constrictions, dilatations, or large swellings (**panel D**). The *scale bars* in **panels A** and **B** represent 60 μm; the *scale bars* in **panels C** and **D** represent 52 μm. (Reprinted by permission of *The New England Journal of Medicine*, from Trapp BD, Peterson J, Ransohoff RM, et al: Axonal transection in the lesions of multiple sclerosis. *N Engl J Med* 338:278–285. Copyright 1998, Massachusetts Medical Society. All rights reserved.)

target of disease in multiple sclerosis. The findings strengthen the rationale for early anti-inflammatory treatment in multiple sclerosis, because axonal transection is most frequent in inflamed areas. The ramifications of reduced N-acetyl aspartate in multiple sclerosis lesions need to be clarified, and new approaches to monitoring and treating the axonal pathologic changes are needed.

► Trapp and colleagues have published a paper of potential landmark significance. While the basic injury in multiple sclerosis is an attack upon the CNS myelin and/or oligodendrocytes, this study established axonal damage as an important part of these lesions. Although other investigators have suggested that axons may be involved, traditional neuropathologic dogma discounted this hypothesis.

This study provides theoretical evidence for the more aggressive treatment of recent multiple sclerosis lesions with anti-inflammatory medication in an effort to protect axons from secondary bystander injury. Future strategies designed to restore neurologic function must include not only stimulators for remyelination but also promoters of axonal regeneration.

R.C. Sergott, M.D.

9 Imaging

Telemedicine: A Trojan Horse

by Robert I. Grossman, M.D.

As a neuroradiologist, I appreciate that image is everything—well, almost everything. Most non-radiologists are either envious or critical of a specialty that has a primarily consultative role in patient care. The combination of these two aspects of my specialty make it particularly attractive for telemedicine. In fact, it is probably more advanced in this respect to most other medical disciplines. Having participated in this process for the past few years, I offer a few observations that may be pertinent to other areas of medicine, such as ophthalmology, in which image is perhaps just as important as in radiology.

Telemedicine is clearly a "hands-off" practice. You have no patient contact and are dependent on those at the other end of the camera. The way your consultation is conveyed to the requesting physician is most important. In radiology most of the consultations are written reports; however, in certain instances, only verbal reports are requested. The modulation transfer function of the consultation is thus suboptimal. As you might expect, thorny legal issues rear their ugly faces constantly as you provide opinions and guidelines for therapy to physicians that you probably don't know and patients with whom you have no relationship. I do not wish to dwell on the legal aspects of telemedicine, but I suggest the reader consider these items:

1. Licensure when performing such consultations across state lines.
2. Associated malpractice coverage for these consultations.
3. Breaching of patient confidentiality,
4. Venue of laws and litigation.

Paper trails are poor, and looking at a picture on a monitor is very different than examining a patient up close and personal.

I find film reading to be much faster for MR than reading from a workstation. CT of the brain, however, is just the opposite. One of the reasons for this is the number of images. MR has so many more images than CT that it requires a number of different screen changes. With film on an alternator, one rapidly assesses the myriad of images without mouse clicks and screen changes. The computer cannot match the alternator in terms of speed. It is analagous to reading a novel on a computer. It is yet to be determined which format is more accurate. The workstation enables the reader to view multiple window settings. Subtle abnormalities can be detected, but any such diversions are time-consuming and may not be cost-effective. For ophthalmologists, there will be fewer images. Windowing, however, is critical. One needs high resolution for monitors to detect minimal abnormalities. With suboptimal windowing or equipment these lesions may be occult.

One particularly annoying problem is reading cases that are at a lower standard than your own. Obviously, the physician is a small cog in the economics wheel, but it is incredibly frustrating to be asked to read an MR of the cervical spine in which the axial sections are too thick or the images are of significantly lower resolution to potentially preclude seeing important pathology. Agreement on imaging protocols is essential for successful relationships. Quality must be assured at all levels of this business. Presently, there are only non-binding standards in radiology, and the financial aspects of this modality may govern quality of care issues.

There are many rationalizations regarding telemedicine as a methodology that will provide expertise to those regions that lack, for whatever reason, that depth of knowledge. The military forces benefit by rapid consultations and triage under battlefield conditions. Yet, in my opinion, telemedicine is presently an economic exercise. The end game is potentially devastating to our fundamental medical practice. Imagine every case, be it ophthalmology, radiology, dermatology, etc., being put out to bid on the "medical internet." The local entrepreneur from Oppolusis, LA is underbid by the Harvard-trained ophthalmologist practicing in Bangladesh. Any specialty or diagnosis where "image is everything" is susceptible to this scenario. Happy New Year.

Effect of Mandatory Radiology Consultation on Inpatient Imaging Use: A Randomized Controlled Trial

Bree RL, Kazerooni EA, Katz SJ (Univ of Michigan, Ann Arbor)

JAMA 276:1595–1598, 1996 9–1

Background.—Utilization review for diagnostic imaging has been widely adopted because of the belief that these tests are used excessively, but there is no consensus on the best technique for control utilization. A randomized, controlled trial examined the effect of mandatory consultation service on radiology resource use in inpatient internal medicine services. The authors hypothesized that radiology resource use would be lowered by at least 20% through the mechanism of request denials or changes.

Methods.—The study setting was 4 internal medicine services at a university hospital. Six radiologists performed the intervention on 2 of the services over a 12-month period; the other 2 services were controls. A total of 1,022 patients were admitted to intervention services, and 1,178 were admitted to control services. All radiology studies except emergencies required approval by the attending radiologist. Consultants were urged to substitute lower cost, but equally effective, tests for higher cost tests. The following 4 classes of radiology tests were examined: X ray, MRI, CT, and US.

Results.—Outcome was determined on the basis of relative resource costs, number of examinations per patient, proportion of patients who underwent 1 or more tests, and mean length of stay (LOS). Relative resource costs were measured in relative value units (RVUs). The intervention and control groups were similar in age, sex, and distribution of diagnosis-related groups (DRGs). Mean RVUs did not differ significantly for intervention (356.1) and control groups (336.0), even after adjustment for differences in DRGs. The mean quantity of examinations per admission, percentage of patients undergoing radiologic examinations, and LOS were all similar or identical for the mandatory consultation and control services.

Discussion.—Radiology resource use was not reduced in these internal medicine services by the implementation of a mandatory precertification program for inpatients. The consultation was time-consuming, and only a few requests were denied. However, managed care organizations might achieve cost savings, if outpatient radiology resource use were targeted.

▶ I chose this article because of its implications not only in radiology but also throughout medicine. The investigators prospectively studied the use of mandatory radiology consultation on the academic inpatient practice as a means of decreasing utilization of radiology resources. Such resource management is certainly coming in the near future as an approach to ordering of studies and procedures.

In this particular study, each radiologic examination required approval by the attending radiologist before it was performed. The cost of providing this consultation over the duration of the study was estimated to be approximately $20,000. The results of the study, which demonstrated that the mean RVUs and the mean LOS of patients were statistically similar between the intervention group and the control group, were not anticipated.

There were several factors that probably contributed to this lack of efficacy in controlling the studies requested. The reasons listed by the authors include the following: (1) Physicians were not sufficiently influenced by the intervention, which contradicts the belief that physicians respond to the threat of review by performing fewer procedures or ordering fewer studies. (2) There may have been failure of the radiology consultants because of a reluctance on their part to perform precertification. This also suggested that radiologists may not be properly trained to judge the appropriateness of particular studies.

The authors of an editorial associated with this publication[1] suggest other reasons, including the following: (1) substitution of other examinations; (2) added value by the interactive radiologic consultant by communication and education; (3) no incentive for the consulting radiologist to reduce utilization.; (4) gatekeepers have no authority; (5) a lack of guidelines for appropriateness; and (6) a bias in the environment in which these consultants were operating.

As a radiologist involved in a busy academic practice, I see many cases in which appropriateness criteria would aid in providing cost-effectiveness examinations. In this era in which radiologic examination is being viewed as a cost center, it is important for the radiologist to be a consultant as well as a diagnostician. From the perspective of the ophthalmologist, it makes perfect sense to speak with your radiologist before ordering a particular examination. Indeed, appropriateness criteria must be developed along organ-oriented lines. Thus, if one is looking for a retrobulbar lesion, the most appropriate study would be an MRI. Whereas, if the ophthalmologist is concerned about a young patient who may have retinoblastoma, the most efficient approach to look for calcification would be CT, which is better than MRI. The issue is that once appropriateness guidelines are agreed on, cost-efficiency is optimized. This has positive implications for everyone.

What this study emphasizes is that consultation precertification alone does not go far enough in decreasing cost. I applaud the authors for undertaking this difficult study, which provided some interesting results. I believe these results may have more general implications throughout medicine.

R.I. Grossman, M.D.

Reference

1. Forman HP, McClennan BL: Meeting of managerial science with medicine: The pace quickens (editorial). *JAMA* 276:1599–1600, 1996.

Visual Function 5 Years After Optic Neuritis: Experience of the Optic Neuritis Treatment Trial

Beck RW, for the Optic Neuritis Study Group (Univ of Arkansas, Little Rock; et al)

Arch Ophthalmol 115:1545–1552, 1997 9–2

Introduction.—The efficacy of corticosteroids in the treatment of acute optic neuritis was assessed in the Optic Neuritis Treatment Trial. Visual recovery was accelerated with treatment with high-dose intravenous followed by oral corticosteroids, but no long-term benefit to vision was provided by this treatment. A short-term reduction in the rate of development of clinically definite multiple sclerosis was produced by this treatment as well. A long-term view of the clinical course of optic neuritis was possible with a 5-year follow-up of this group, in which the visual changes and frequency of recurrent optic neuritis were reported.

Methods.—There were 397 patients who had 5-year follow-up vision testing, which included measures of contrast sensitivity, visual acuity, visual field, and color vision.

Results.—In most patients, after 5 years, visual function test results in the eyes with optic neuritis were normal or only slightly abnormal. In 87%

of patients, the visual acuity in the affected eyes was 20/25 or better. In 7% of patients, the visual acuity was 20/25 to 20/40. In 3%, it was 20/50 to 20/190. In 3%, it was 20/200 or worse. In 28% of patients, optic neuritis recurred and was more frequent in patients with prednisone or with multiple sclerosis. Normal or almost normal visual function was retained in most eyes in which optic neuritis recurred.

Conclusions.—In the 5 years after an attack of optic neuritis, most patients retained good-to-excellent vision, even if the optic neuritis recurred. In patients with multiple sclerosis and those treated with oral prednisone alone, recurrences were more frequent. Management recommendations were not altered after the completion of the 5-year follow-up treatment trial. The only factors associated with an increased 5-year risk of clinically definite multiple sclerosis were a history of prior nonspecific neurologic symptoms and prior optic neuritis among patients with brain MRI lesions. However, a normal brain scan should not be taken to signify that multiple sclerosis will not develop, because the percentage of patients with no MRI lesions in whom clinically definite multiple sclerosis developed (16%) was sufficiently high.

► This study of 397 patients followed up over a 5-year course presents some most interesting results. The vast majority of patients retained excellent visual acuity. The rate of recurrence of optic neuritis was more frequent in patients with multiple sclerosis (MS) and in those patients treated with oral prednisone. The adverse effect of prednisone occurred predominantly in patients who did not have clinical or MRI evidence of MS. Why this occurred is quite puzzling and perhaps merits further investigation.

The investigators again underscore the utility of MRI in predicting the development of clinically definite MS in patients that have optic neuritis. The cumulative probability of clinically definite MS was 16% in patients with no brain MRI lesions, 37% in patients with 1 or 2 lesions, and 51% in patients with 3 or more lesions.

I personally have never liked these criteria because they are dependent on many technical parameters as well as the sensitivity/specificity of the particular readers. There are now better, more sensitive indicators of lesions in these patients including magnetic resonance spectroscopy and magnetization transfer measurements.

Clinical features associated with the low risk of clinically definite MS included lack of pain, presence of optic disc edema, and mild visual loss.

This is an excellent study with a rather unsuspected result—the possible deleterious affect of oral prednisone in the dosages prescribed. It also points out the prognostic power of MRI, which will be used in the future to be the arbiter of drug efficacy in lesions that affect the CNS.

R.I. Grossman, M.D.

Optic Nerve Contact and Compression by the Carotid Artery in Asymptomatic Patients

Jacobson DM, Warner JJ, Broste SK (Marshfield Clinic, Wis; Marshfield Med Research and Education Found, Wis)

Am J Ophthalmol 123:677–683, 1997 9–3

Objective.—Magnetic resonance imaging studies have identified a group of patients with progressive retrobulbar optic neuropathies as a result of optic nerve compression by the supraclinoid carotid artery. The frequency of carotid artery compression of the optic nerve in asymptomatic patients and the significance of this finding in patients with unexplained progressive retrobulbar optic neuropathy were examined in an MRI study.

Methods.—Magnetic resonance studies, including T1-weighted coronal images, were performed on 100 asymptomatic patients (47 males; average, age 51 years) for reasons other than vision, optic neuropathy, or carotid artery disorders. Using the MR image, investigators graded the relation

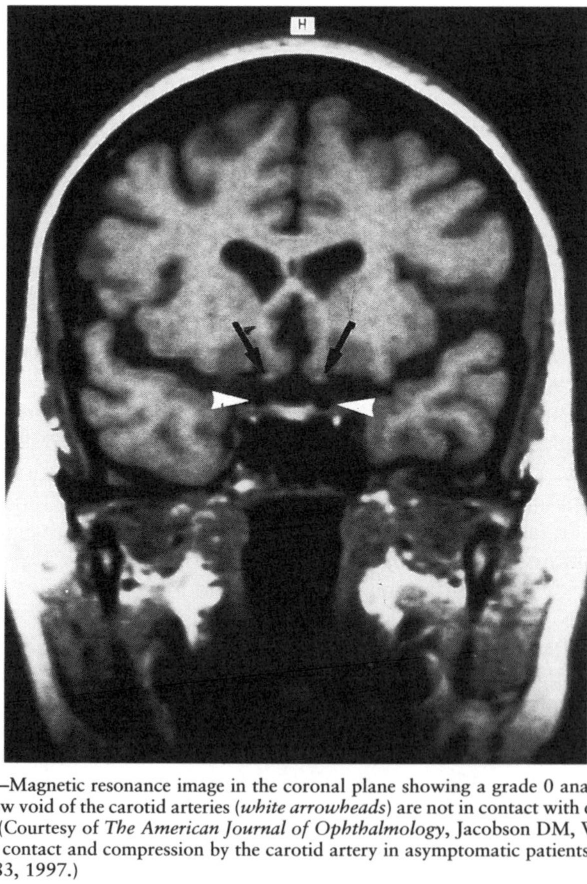

FIGURE 1.—Magnetic resonance image in the coronal plane showing a grade 0 anatomical relation. Note that the flow void of the carotid arteries (*white arrowheads*) are not in contact with either optic nerve (*black arrows*). (Courtesy of *The American Journal of Ophthalmology*, Jacobson DM, Warner JJ, Broste SK: Optic nerve contact and compression by the carotid artery in asymptomatic patients. *Am J Ophthalmol* 123:677–683, 1997.)

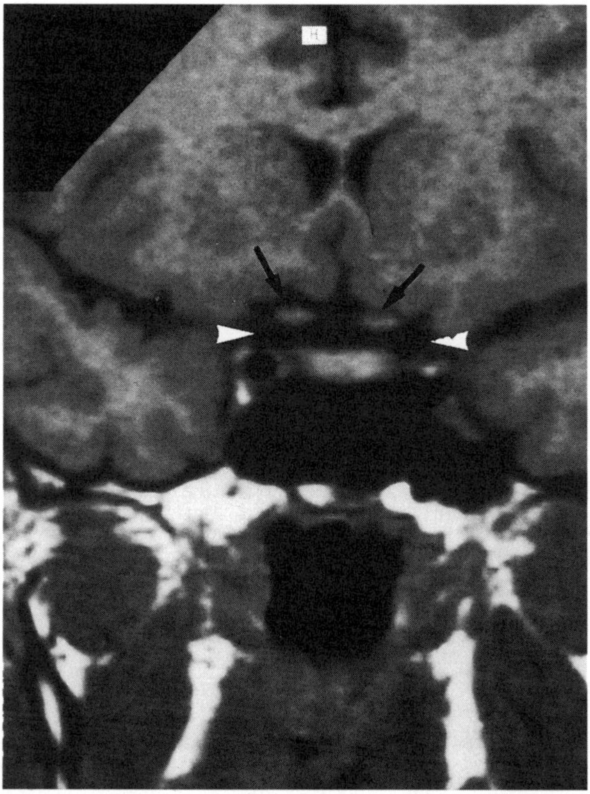

FIGURE 2.—Magnetic resonance image in the coronal plane showing a grade 1 anatomical relation. Note that the flow void of both carotid arteries (*white arrowheads*) are in contact with the optic nerves (*black arrows*) but do not distort their normal oval contour and horizontal orientation. (Courtesy of *The American Journal of Ophthalmology*, Jacobson DM, Warner JJ, Broste SK: Optic nerve contact and compression by the carotid artery in asymptomatic patients. *Am J Ophthalmol* 123:677–683, 1997.)

between the carotid artery and the optic nerve on a 0–2-scale (Figs 1, 2, and 3). Final grades were established by consensus between 2 independent reviewers. The variables were analyzed by multiple regression analysis.

Results.—The reviewers disagreed in only 10 observations, which yielded for an overall agreement of 87.5%. There was no contact or compression in 13 patients, unilateral contact in 33, bilateral contact in 24, compression on 1 side but no contact or compression on the other side in 5, compression on 1 side and contact on the other side in 13, and compression on both sides in 12. The risk of compression increased significantly with increasing diameter of the carotid artery. Age was a significant predictor of carotid artery diameter.

Conclusion.—The risk of compression of the optic nerve by the carotid artery increases significantly with the diameter of the artery. Age is significantly related to carotid artery diameter. Although there was a high frequency of contact between the carotid artery and the optic nerve, the

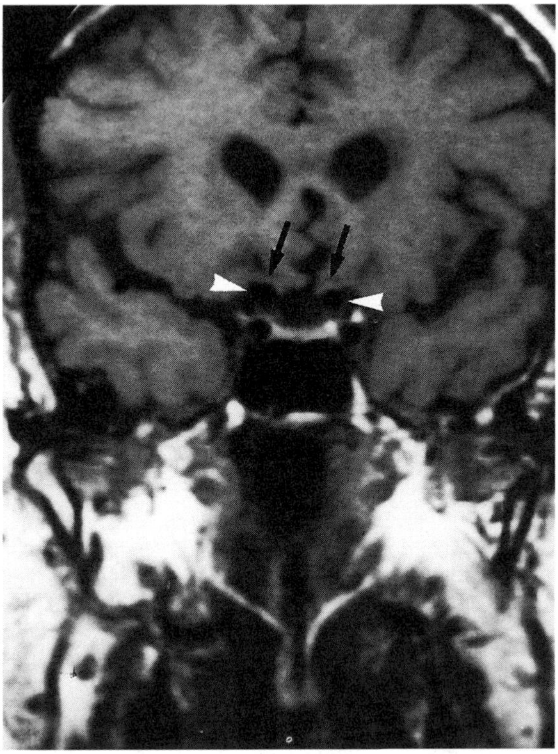

FIGURE 3.—Magnetic resonance image in the coronal plane showing a grade 2 anatomical relation. Note that the flow void of both carotid arteries (*white arrowheads*) not only is in contact with the optic nerves (*black arrows*) but also is displacing them upward and slightly medially, distorting their normal oval contour and causing them to appear draped over the top of the arteries. (Courtesy of *The American Journal of Ophthalmology*, Jacobson DM, Warner JJ, Broste SK: Optic nerve contact and compression by the carotid artery in asymptomatic patients. *Am J Ophthalmol* 123:677–683, 1997.)

frequency of compression was low. Anatomical variations that could have affected the proximity of the carotid artery and the optic nerve could not be determined because of the retrospective nature of this study. Additional studies with larger numbers of patients should be conducted.

► There is renewed interest in the evaluation of vascular compression of the optic nerve in patients with unexplained optic neuropathy and normal tension glaucoma.[1] This study sought to evaluate the relationship between the optic nerve and carotid artery as seen on coronal T1-weighted images. What they did not study was the relationship between this compression and visual symptoms.

In terms of the methodology, the investigators looked at the prechiasmatic intracranial optic nerves in 1 particular location. I would, perhaps, have studied several different slices in this region, particularly the optic nerve, as it immediately emerges from the optic canal. Their choice for the image location was necessitated by difficulty in analyzing the relationship of the

NO POSTAGE NECESSARY IF MAILED IN THE UNITED STATES

BUSINESS REPLY MAIL

FIRST-CLASS MAIL PERMIT NO 135 ST LOUIS MO

POSTAGE WILL BE PAID BY ADDRESSEE

SUBSCRIPTION SERVICES
MOSBY–YEAR BOOK, INC.
11830 WESTLINE INDUSTRIAL DRIVE
ST. LOUIS MO 63146-9988

NO POSTAGE NECESSARY IF MAILED IN THE UNITED STATES

BUSINESS REPLY MAIL

FIRST-CLASS MAIL PERMIT NO 135 ST LOUIS MO

POSTAGE WILL BE PAID BY ADDRESSEE

Mosby

PAT NEWMAN
11830 WESTLINE INDUSTRIAL DRIVE
PO BOX 46908
ST. LOUIS MO 63146-9934

Want to speed up the process?

To order the *Year Book*, you also may call 1-800-426-4545

To subscribe to the journal today, call toll-free in the U.S.: 1-800-453-4351 or fax 314-432-1158 Outside the U.S., call: 314-453-4351

Visit us at:
www.mosby.com/Mosby/Periodicals

Mosby–Year Book, Inc.
Subscription Services
11830 Westline Industrial Drive
St. Louis, MO 63146 U.S.A.

Mosby

carotid artery and any portion of the intracanalicular optic nerve. What potentially is missed is the portion of the optic nerve that ascends vertically to the point where it was evaluated in this study (just in front of the chiasm). Their approach to the observations regarding optic nerve compression was appropriate, and Kappa statistics confirmed a high degree of interreader agreement regarding this finding.

The results of this investigation indicate that there appears to be significant asymptomatic compression of the intracranial optic nerve. The conclusion of the research—to exclude all other potential sources of the pathologic condition before attributing any optic nerve findings to vascular compression—is important. I would also argue that many of the vascular compression syndromes may be less clear cut than we acknowledge. Further research is warranted to understand the significance of such normal/asymptomatic anatomical variations.

R.I. Grossman, M.D.

Reference

1. Golinick KC, Hund PW, Stroman GA, et al: Magnetic resonance imaging in patients with unexplained optic neuropathy. *Ophthalmology* 103:515–520, 1996.

Orbital Venous Anomalies

Wright JE, Sullivan TJ, Garner A, et al (Moorfields Eye Hosp, London; Inst of Ophthalmology, London)

Ophthalmology 104:905–913, 1997 9–4

Objective.—Vascular masses with venous anomalies are common orbital lesions seen at the Orbital Clinic, Moorfields Eye Hospital, London. These anomalies are divided into those with a venous connection (varices) and those without (lymphangiomas). The natural history, likely nature, behavior, and optimal treatment of these lesions were investigated.

Methods.—Between 1968 and 1992, 158 patients (62 males), with primary orbital venous anomalies or lymphangiomas, were treated at the Orbital Clinic. Patients were followed up for 1 month to 25 years. Pathologic examinations were conducted on 57 surgical specimens.

Results.—Clinical symptoms at the initial visit included swelling or a mass on the eyelids, spontaneous hemorrhaging, and pain. There were extraorbital vascular lesions in 29 patients, restricted gaze in 44, and a reduction of 2 or more Snellen lines in 52. The lesions were located in the anterior part of the orbit in 125 patients. There was a dark blue mass or fullness of the eyelid in 104 and conjunctival and episcleral involvement in 68. Proptosis, present at rest, in 96 patients and developing later in 13, worsened with the Valsalva maneuver. Orbital hemorrhaging occurred in 88 patients. Lesions increased in size in 102 patients either at intervals or progressively. Radiographic examinations showed no demonstrable arte-

TABLE 3.—Radiographic Investigations

Investigation	No.	(%)
Plain skull radiographs (78)		
Normal	26	(33)
Abnormal	52	(67)
Orbital enlargement	43	(55)
Phleboliths	20	(26)
Enlarged superior orbital fissure	5	(6)
CT scans (91)		
Normal	1	
Abnormal	90	
Orbital mass	90	(98)
Orbital enlargement	67	(74)
Phleboliths	41	(45)
Orbital venograms (42)		
Normal	2	
Abnormal	40	
Abnormal ophthalmic vein	27	(64)
Mass filling from adajacent vein	13	(31)

(Published courtesy of *Ophthalmology*, from Wright JE, Sullivan TJ, Garner A, et al: Orbital venous anomalies. *Ophthalmology* 104:905–913, 1997.)

rial supply (Table 3). Venous anomalies gave MRI signals of low intensity for vascular channels and signals of high intensity for areas of thrombosis or hemorrhaging. There were 67 patients who did not want surgery despite the fact that 33 had had 1 or more hemorrhages. Of the 91 patients who had surgery, 11 required anterior orbitotomies for suddenly enlarged lesions. Histopathologic examinations were performed on 45 orbital, 4 preseptal, and 8 orbital and preseptal lesions. Sixteen specimens showed thrombotic vascular occlusions with calcified phleboliths in 3 and intravascular papillary endothelial cell hyperplasia in 4. Most of these lesions appeared in childhood; 43% of patients in this study were younger than 6 years. Growth of the lesions probably result from bleeding into the network of vessels rather than a proliferation of new vessels.

Conclusion.—Results of this study indicate that this orbital lesion is an abnormality of the orbital venous system. Investigators recommend discarding the term lymphangioma and using instead "orbital venous anomaly." Indications for surgery include a well-defined lesion causing a cosmetic problem or significant proptosis, hemorrhaging causing proptosis, or pressure on the optic nerve and pain.

► This paper is a beautiful review of an extremely large series (158 patients) with what has been previously described as lymphangiomas or orbital varicies. Of the 158 patients, histologic specimens were available in 57 patients. The controversy that this report attempts to resolve revolves around whether 2 distinct categories of vascular abnormalities exist. These vascular abnormalities would be orbital varices, in which a definite venous connection is seen, and lymphangiomas, in which there is no venous connection. Previous investigators believe that hemorrhaging is more frequent in lymphangiomas than in orbital varices.[1] In this series, 61% of patients had proptosis that, in many cases, was increased by the Valsalva maneuver. Fifty-five percent of the patients had orbital hemorrhaging and this hemorrhaging represented a major factor in lesion enlargement.

Unfortunately, radiographic investigations in this report were significantly limited (Table 3), and only 3 patients underwent MRI. In these 3 patients, there was a variable signal in the lesion with hemorrhaging and flow voids were demonstrated. Phleboliths were present in 45% of the patients.

The paper presents not only a nice history of the pathologic features and pathogenesis of these lesions but also the debate regarding whether these are true lymphangiomas or orbital varices.

In this study, there was no statistically significant difference in the incidence of hemorrhaging between those lesions with a venous connection and those more isolated lesions. Rather, there appeared to be a seamless range of clinical presentations such that it proved impossible to define distinct groups of patients. The investigators thus favor a venous origin primarily because of (1) enlargements in the mass with any rise in venous pressure; (2) phleboliths in patients without any connection with veins; and (3) the fact that the highest percentage of lesions were in the upper inner quadrant, the position of the largest vein. In this case, deep dissection usually failed to identify a normal superior ophthalmic vein, which had been largely replaced by the vascular lesion.

Lastly, the authors note that histopathologic differentiation between lymphatic and venous channels in these patients is extremely difficult. However, vascular elements are invariably encountered. In this series, the lesions were composed of abnormal venous channels. In the preseptal region, although predominantly venous, there were some lymphatic-like vessels. However, no significant lymphatics were ever found in structures located deep in relation to the orbital septum. From the results of this study, one would agree that these lesions represent orbital venous anomalies and the historical term *lymphangioma* should probably be discarded.

The paper also contains some interesting comments regarding the natural history and management of this condition, which the authors believe should generally be conservative. The study is important because it provides necessary data to substantiate the investigators' hypothesis that lymphangiomas are most likely just orbital venous anomalies. The authors should be congratulated for this important work.

R.I. Grossman, M.D.

Reference

1. Harris GJ, Sakol PJ, Bonavolonta G, et al: An analysis of thirty cases of orbital lymphangioma: Pathophysiologic considerations and management recommendation. *Ophthalmology* 97:1583–1592, 1990.

Serial Dynamic Magnetic Resonance Imaging of Orbital Cavernous Hemangioma

Ohtsuka K, Hashimoto M, Akiba H (Sapporo Med Univ, Japan)

Am J Ophthalmol 123:396–398, 1997 9–5

Background.—The MR imaging features of cavernous hemangioma may overlap with those of neurofibroma, hemangiopericytoma, schwannoma, or other mesenchymal tumors. The value of serial dynamic MRI after rapid IV injection of contrast material in diagnosing orbital cavernous hemangioma was determined.

Patients and Findings.—Two patients with orbital cavernous hemangioma underwent MRI, with gadolinium-diethylenetriamine pentaacetic acid (DTPA), 0.1 mmol/kg, injected IV in 10 seconds. About 50 seconds after rapid injection in both patients, 1 small point at the posterior pole of the tumor was enhanced initially. The orbital cavernous hemangiomas displayed a unique enhancement pattern. The initial enhancement point represented the point of connection of the feeding vessels to the tumor (Figs 1 and 2).

Conclusions.—Cavernous hemangiomas on nonenhanced MRI cannot be differentiated from schwannoma, neurofibroma, or other mesenchymal

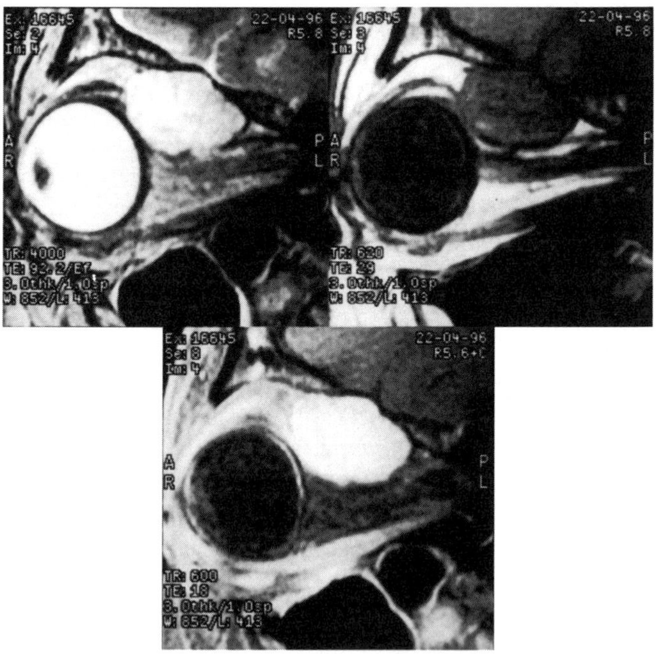

FIGURE 1.—Patient 2. Magnetic resonance imaging of the parasagittal sections of the orbital cavernous hemangioma. **Top left**, T2-weighted image. **Top right**, T1-weighted image. **Bottom**, gadolinium-diethylenetriamine pentaacetic acid–enhanced T1-weighted image with a fat-suppression technique. (From Ohtsuka K, Hashimoto M, Akiba H: Serial dynamic magnetic resonance imaging of orbital cavernous hemangioma. *Am J Ophthalmol* 123:396–398, 1997.)

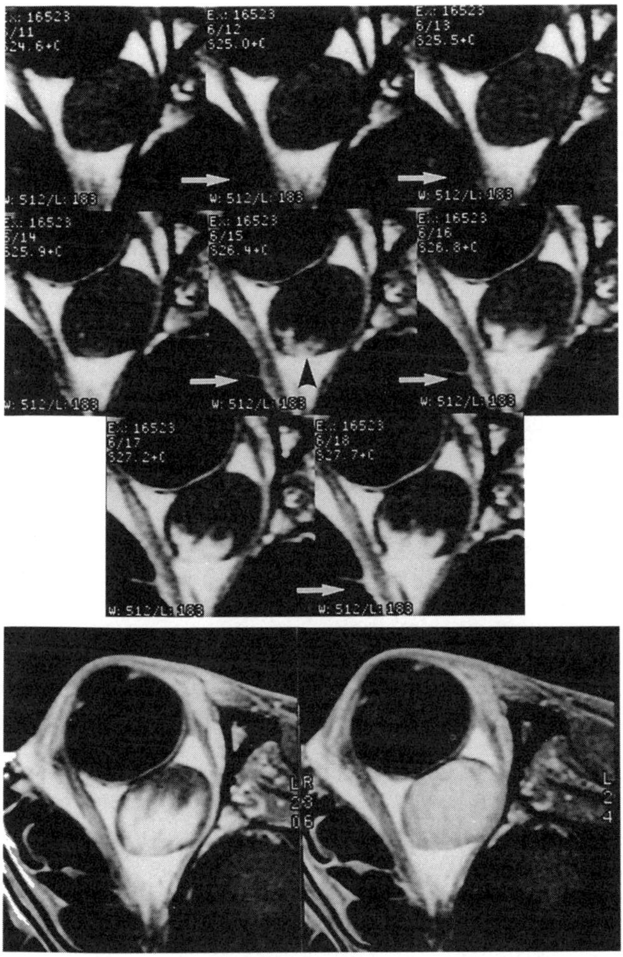

FIGURE 2.—Patient 1. **Top,** an example of early-phase serial dynamic MRI of the orbital cavernous hemangioma. Serial axial images were arranged from upper left (immediately after the rapd IV injection of gadolinium-diethylenetriamine pentaacetic acid to bottom right (70 seconds after the injection) at intervals of 10 seconds (*white arrows*). The *black arrowhead* indicates the initial enhancement point of the tumor. **Bottom,** an example of late-phase serial dynamic resonance imaging. The **left panel** shows axial images of the lesion 17 minutes after the injection. The **right panel** shows the same region 22 minutes after the injection. (From Ohtsuka K, Hashimoto M, Akiba H: Serial dynamic magnetic resonance imaging of orbital cavernous hemangioma. *Am J Ophthalmol* 123:396–398, 1997.)

tumors. Even in the late phase after gadolinium-DTPA administration, schwannoma, neurofibroma, and fibrous histiocytoma show heterogeneous enhancement. Conversely, homogeneous enhancement occurs in capillary hemangioma, orbital varix, hemangiopericytoma, and lymphoproliferative disorders. Thus, serial MRI is useful for the differential diagnosis of cavernous hemangioma.

► In this paper, the authors have employed dynamic MRI after infusion of a bolus of gadolinium. The technique provides very interesting images (Fig 2) of the dynamic changes that this vascular lesion undergoes after contrast injection. In this figure, it is observed that the enhancement begins in one particular region of the lesion and then proceeds to enhance the entire mass. The authors believe this contrast pattern is unique and could be useful to distinguish cavernous hemangiomas of the orbit from schwannoma, neurofibroma, or other mesenchymal lesions that would tend to demonstrate heterogeneous enhancement. They also point out that capillary hemangioma, orbital varix, hemangiopericytoma, and lymphoproliferative disorders show homogeneous enhancement. The enhancement pattern of the cavernous hemangioma can be described as emanating from an initial point in the lesion and subsequently diffusing throughout the entire lesion. That initial area represents the vascular pedicle to the lesion and may have surgical implications.

The proposed technique is useful and may have broader applications in tumors of the brain. One potential problem is that the method represents another pulse sequence to employ. Additionally, most cavernous hemangiomas are rather obvious from their configuration (smoothly marginated), location (intraconal), and clinical presentation.

R.I. Grossman, M.D.

Detection and Localization of Steel Intraocular Foreign Bodies Using Computed Tomography: A Comparison of Helical and Conventional Axial Scanning

Chacko JG, Figueroa RE, Johnson MH, et al (Med College of Georgia, Augusta)

Ophthalmology 104:319–323, 1997 9–6

Background.—Appropriate treatment of ocular trauma relies on the accurate detection and localization of intraocular foreign bodies. The sensitivity and specificity of conventional axial and helical CT were determined in an experimental model.

Methods.—Small steel foreign bodies, ranging from 0.048 to 0.179 mm^3, were placed in intraocular and episcleral locations in eye bank eyes mounted in the orbits of a human skull. The orbits were then scanned using helical and conventional axial methods.

Findings.—Both scanning protocols were able to detect steel foreign bodies as small as 0.048 mm^3. The helical scans appeared to be more sensitive than conventional axial scanning. However, the difference in outcomes was nonsignificant. Sensitivity depended on the size of the foreign body, ranging from 45% to 65% for the smaller ones to 100% for the

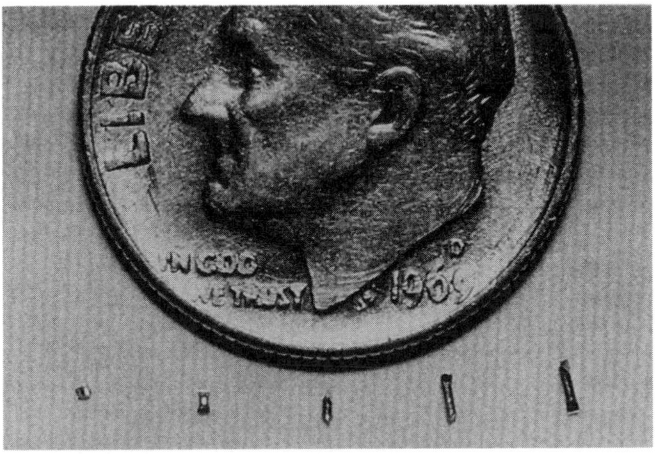

FIGURE 1.—Examples of metallic (steel) foreign bodies used in experiment. The diameter of each is 0.39 mm. The lengths range from 0.4 to 1.5 mm. The corresponding volumes range from 0.048 to 0.179 mm^3. A U.S. dime is shown for size comparison. (Published courtesy of *Ophthalmology*, from Chacko JG, Figueroa RE, Johnson MH, et al: Detection and localization of steel intraocular foreign bodies using computed tomography: A comparison of helical and conventional axial scanning. *Ophthalmology* 104:319–323, 1997.)

larger ones. Multiplanar image reformatting was useful in optimizing accuracy (Figs 1, 2, 4, and 5).

Conclusions.—Helical CT scanning, using 3- or 1-mm thick sections and a 1:1 pitch, provides a fast, very sensitive, specific technique for detecting and localizing small steel intraocular foreign bodies. It may be better than conventional 3-mm axial scanning. The rapid scanning time

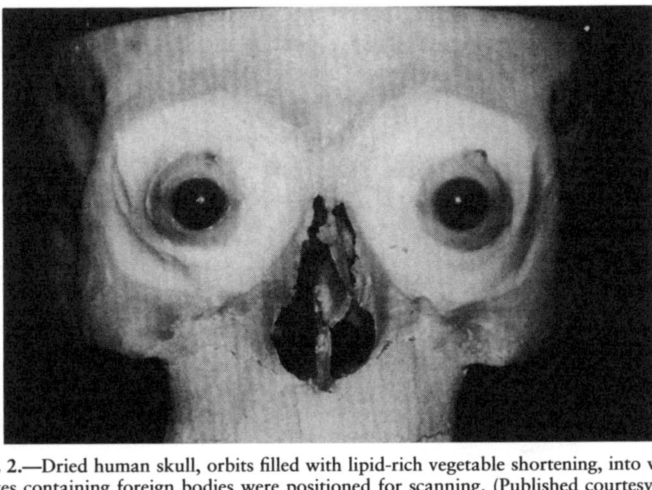

FIGURE 2.—Dried human skull, orbits filled with lipid-rich vegetable shortening, into which human cadaveric eyes containing foreign bodies were positioned for scanning. (Published courtesy of *Ophthalmology*, from Chacko JG, Figueroa RE, Johnson MH, et al: Detection and localization of steel intraocular foreign bodies using computed tomography: A comparison of helical and conventional axial scanning. Ophthalmology 104:319–323, 1997.)

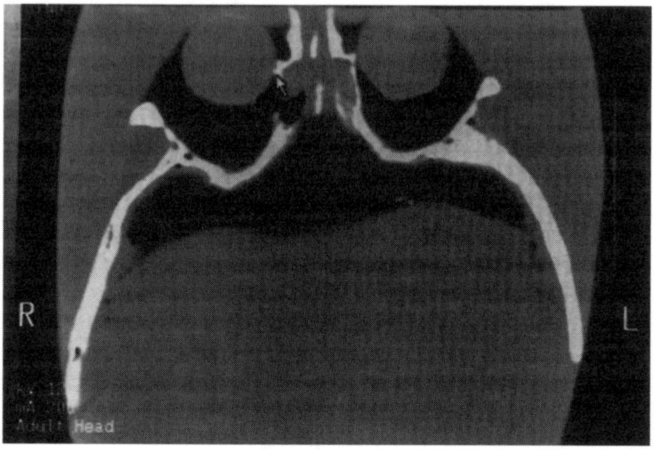

FIGURE 4.—Axial image obtained from a conventional axial scan (3-mm partition, computer reformatted to 1 mm) shows a 0.06 mm^3 extraocular steel foreign body partially obscured by its close proximity to the medial orbital wall bone (*arrowhead*). (Published courtesy of *Ophthalmology*, from Chacko JG, Figueroa RE, Johnson MH, et al: Detection and localization of steel intraocular foreign bodies using computed tomography: A comparison of helical and conventional axial scanning. *Ophthalmology* 104:319–323, 1997.)

and the relatively small value of the eye and orbit make helical CT especially well suited for assessing these structures after trauma.

► This study is a comparison between newer helical and older conventional CT images. The results demonstrate that helical scans appear to provide higher levels of sensitivity compared to conventional axial scanning. However, the data were not statistically significant. The study, although not specifically designed to show the utility of reformatted helical images, does nicely demonstrate its potential. This can be noted from Figure 5. I believe that helical reformatted images are particularly useful to the surgeon who needs precise localization of an intraocular foreign body. One interesting finding was that conventional 3-mm axial and 3-mm helical scans provided similar levels of accuracy. Additionally, 3-mm helical scans compared to 1-mm helical scans required shorter scan time and decreased exposure to ionizing radiation. The real utility of 1-mm helical images is their ability to detect extremely small metallic foreign bodies.

I particularly think the reformatting capability of helical imaging in which regions of interest are sampled in a seamless fashion enables postprocessing of data with decreased slice thickness, and multiplanar reformatting without much loss of resolution. If available, helical CT is the method of choice for imaging metallic intraocular foreign bodies.

R.I. Grossman, M.D.

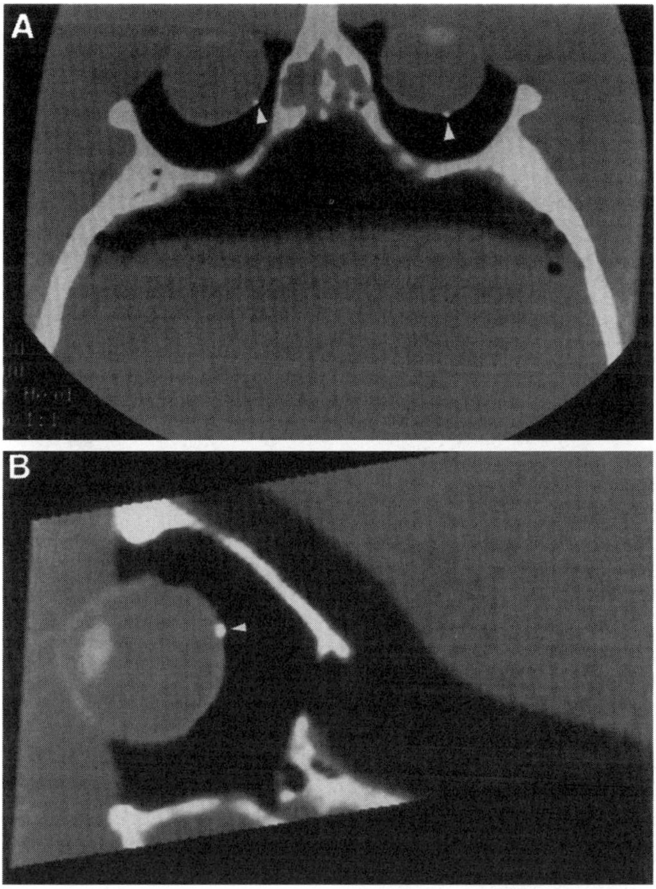

FIGURE 5.—**A**, axial image obtained from helical scan (3-mm partition, 1:1 pitch, computer-reformatted to 1 mm) shows foreign bodies in each globe (*arrowheads*). The size of each foreign body is 0.149 mm^3. **B**, sagittal reconstruction of image data from helical scan in **A** shows extraocular location of foreign body adjacent to left globe (*arrowhead*). (Published courtesy of *Ophthalmology*, from Chacko JG, Figueroa RE, Johnson MH, et al: Detection and localization of steel intraocular foreign bodies using computed tomography: A comparison of helical and conventional axial scanning. *Ophthalmology* 104:319–323, 1997.)

Orbital Involvement in Allergic Fungal Sinusitis

Klapper SR, Lee AG, Patrinely JR, et al (Baylor College of Medicine, Houston; Univ of Texas, Houston)

Ophthalmology 104:2094–2100, 1997 9–7

Introduction.—A form of paranasal sinus mycosis is allergic fungal sinusitis, which occurs in as many as 7% of patients with chronic sinusitis. Reports in the ophthalmic literature are rare of patients experiencing orbital symptoms. A thorough understanding of this condition is essential because the management of allergic fungal sinusitis is profoundly different

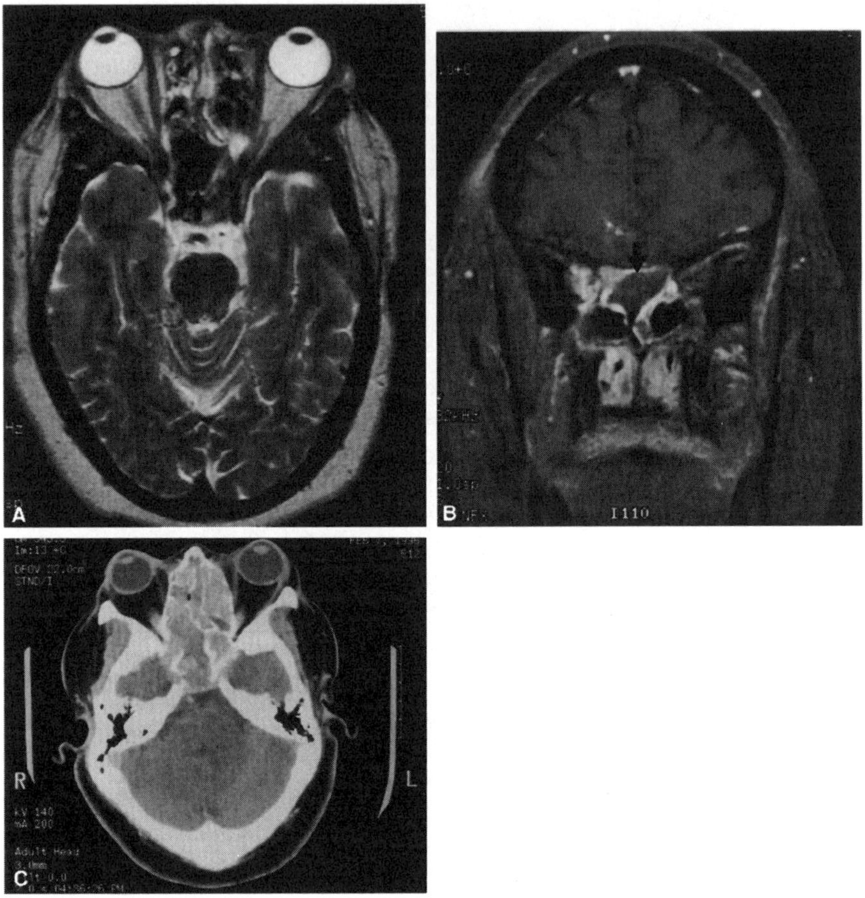

FIGURE 1.—Case 1. **A,** axial T2-weighted MR image shows a decrease in signal intensity within the sphenoid sinus (*arrow*). **B,** coronal T1-weighted image obtained after IV gadolinium contrast administration shows an isointense signal abnormality within the sphenoid sinus (*arrow*), increased signal intensity along the posteromedial aspect of the right orbit, and enhancing soft tissue within the nasal cavity. **C,** axial CT scan after IV contrast administration shows a soft tissue mass within the paranasal sinuses and nasal cavity, with bone destruction in the region of the ethmoid sinuses. (Published courtesy of *Ophthalmology*, from Klapper SR, Lee AG, Patrinely JR, et al: Orbital involvement in allergic fungal sinusitis. *Ophthalmology* 104:2094–2100, 1997.)

from the treatment of invasive fungal sino-orbital disease. Two cases with allergic fungal sinusitis are described.

Case 1.—Woman, 51, had decreased vision in the right eye, and binocular, horizontal diplopia for 2 weeks. Possible enlargement of the pituitary gland, abnormal signal intensity in the right posterior orbit, and pansinusitis were observed on MRI (Fig 1). Fungal sinus disease, sarcoidosis, Wegener granulomatosis, orbital inflammatory syndrome, syphilis, tuberculosis, systemic vasculitis, primary

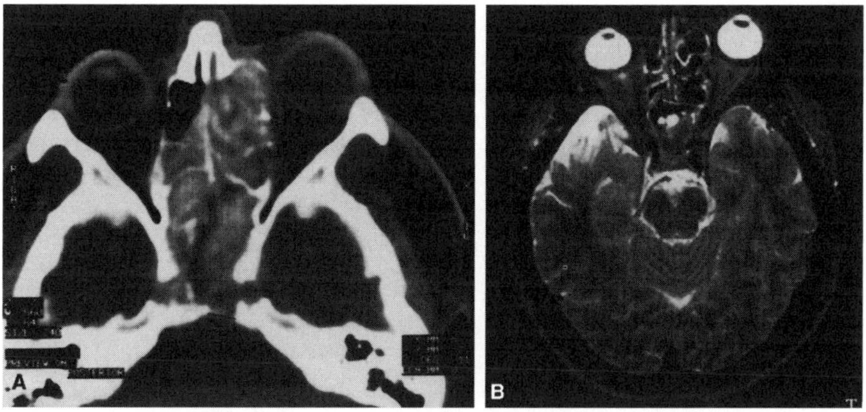

FIGURE 3.—Case 2. **A,** axial CT scan of the orbits shows a soft tissue mass filling the ethmoid and sphenoid sinuses, with extension into the anterior medial left orbit. **B,** axial T2-weighted scan shows increased signal intensity of the ethmoid (*arrow*) and sphenoid sinus mucosa and a marked decrease in signal intensity within the left ethmoid sinus and anterior mucosa and a marked decrease in signal intensity within the left ethmoid sinus and anterior sphenoid sinus. (Published courtesy of *Ophthalmology*, from Klapper SR, Lee AG, Patrinely JR, et al: Orbital involvement in allergic fungal sinusitis. *Ophthalmology* 104:2094–2100, 1997.)

sinus or metastatic carcinoma, and lymphoma were included in the differential diagnosis. *Aspergillus flavus* was isolated. There was complete opacification of the paranasal sinuses, bilateral nasal polyposis and retained secretions, bone destruction in the region of the ethmoid sinuses, and abnormal soft tissue enhancement of the right cavernous sinus and right orbital apex at CT. Sphenoidotomy, total ethmoidectomies, bilateral endoscopic polypectomies, and maxillary antrostomies were performed. Treatment was begun with oral itraconazole and IV methylprednisolone. Symptoms resolved by 3 months after surgery.

Case 2.—Man, 26, had a 3-month history of an epiphora in the left eye and a mass in the left medial canthal region. Diffuse opacification of all the paranasal sinuses except for the right maxillary sinus and right anterior ethmoid air cells, and extension of the left ethmoidal sinus disease in the left posterior orbit were seen on CT (Fig 3), and pansinusitis on MRI. An anterior orbitotomy, left-sided Caldwell-Luc maxillotomy, and external frontoethmoidectomy were performed. *Bipolaris spicifera* was cultured. Further sinus surgery was performed 2 months later; and 1 year after that, symptoms resolved.

Conclusion.—Both patients had distinguishing radiologic and pathologic features. In one patient, *A. flavus* was cultured, and *B. spicifera* was cultured in the other patient. Surgical debridement, aeration of the involved sinuses, and systemic and topical corticosteroids will help to adequately manage allergic fungal sinusitis, unlike invasive forms of mycotic disease. Fungal sinusitis has 4 classifications: acute fulminant, chronic

TABLE 1.—Classification of Fungal Sinusitis

Type	Immune Status	Clinical Course	Role of Fungus	Histopathology	Treatment
Acute fulminant	Immunocompromised	Acute	Pathogen	Angioinvasion, tissue necrosis	Radical surgical debridement, systemic antifungal therapy
Chronic indolent	Immunocompetent, nonatopic*	Chronic	Pathogen	Granulomatous inflammation, tissue invasion	Surgical debridement, systemic antifungal therapy
Fungus ball	Immunocompetent nonatopic	Chronic	Saprophyte	Noninvasive tightly packed fungal hyphae	Surgical debridement
Allergic	Immunocompetent, atopic	Chronic	Allergen	Allergic mucin with noninvasive fungal hyphae	Surgical debridement, systemic/topical corticosteroids

*These patients may have a history of allergy.

(Published courtesy of *Ophthalmology*, from Klapper SR, Lee AG, Patrinely JR, et al: Orbital involvement in allergic fungal sinusitis. *Ophthalmology* 104:2094–2100, 1997.)

TABLE 2.—Clinical, Radiologic, and Pathologic Features of Allergic Fungal Sinusitis

Clinical history	Nasal polyposis, nasal obstruction Chronic, recurrent sinusitis unresponsive to conventional medical therapy
Immune status	Immunocompetent, atopic
Type I hypersensitivity	Peripheral eosinophilia, immediate skin reactivity to fungal antigen(s), serum precipitin (IgG) antibodies against fungal antigen(s), elevated total serum IgE
Radiologic features	
CT	Multiple sinus involvement with marked attenuation on noncontrast views, frequent bone erosion or remodeling
MRI	
T_1 weighted	Isointense or slightly decreased signal intensity of involved sinus cavities; increased signal intensity of inflamed sinus mucosa
T_2 weighted	Markedly decreased signal intensity of involved sinus cavities; increased signal intensity of inflamed sinus mucosa
Pathology	
Gross	Thick (“peanut butter-like”), tenacious, green or brown mucus
Histologic	Allergic mucin: embedded eosinophils, Charcot-Leyden crystals, and extramucosal fungal hyphae
Microbiology	Dematiaceous (darkly pigmented) fungi: Bipolaris, Exserohilum, Curvularia, and Alternaria; Aspergillus species
Treatment	Debridement of fungal debris and aeration of involved sinuses; systemic/topical corticosteroids; role of topical antifungals and immunotherapy not established

Abbreviations: IgG, immunoglobulin G; *IgE*, immunoglobulin E.
(Published courtesy of *Ophthalmology*, from Klapper SR, Lee AG, Patrinely JR, et al: Orbital involvement in allergic fungal sinusitis. *Ophthalmology* 104:2094–2100, 1997.)

indolent, fungus ball, and allergic (Table 1). Clinical history of patients with allergic fungal sinusitis usually includes nasal polyposis, nasal obstruction, and chronic, recurrent sinusitis unresponsive to conventional medical therapy (Table 2).

► This is a nice review of allergic fungal sinusitis, which represents a subset of sino-orbital disease. Table 1 is a classification of fungal sinusitis. Patients presenting with allergic fungal sinusitis have a history of nasal polyposis and nasal obstruction. The MR characteristics demonstrate markedly decreased signal on T2-weighted images, in association with bone erosion and remodeling. There is clearly controversy regarding the infectious component of this allergic disease. For the ophthalmologist these patients can present with visual loss, diplopia, proptosis, and epiphora. What is interesting is that no ideal treatment has been identified. Identification of allergic fungal sinusitis is important because it does not require aggressive surgical treatment or toxic antifungal medication. Rather, this is a fungal allergen producing what appears radiologically to be a chronic sinus infection. The diagnosis is made by biopsy of fungal cultures. This material contains eosinophils, Charcot-Leyden crystals (degradation product of eosinophils), and extramucosal fungal hyphae termed "allergic mucin." The authors have identified a problem that is less well appreciated than most ophthalmologists and radiologists acknowledge. The condition should be considered in the appropriate clinical setting.

R.I. Grossman, M.D.

Evidence of Optic Pathway Gliomas After Previously Negative Neuroimaging

Massry GG, Morgan CF, Chung SM (Saint Louis Univ)

Ophthalmology 104:930–935, 1997 9–8

Objective.—Optic gliomas (pilocytic astrocytomas) are rare, potentially fatal tumors that are possibly associated with neurofibromatosis type 1 (NF1). When the chiasm or adjacent hypothalamus is involved, mortality is significantly increased. Routine CT or MR imaging scans in patients with NF1 is recommended. Whether a negative imaging study means that optic gliomas will not develop in the future depends on whether gliomas are congenital or acquired. Completed tomographic or MRI studies of 360 patients examined at the Neurofibromatosis Clinic at Cardinal Glennon Children's Hospital between 1988 and 1994 were retrospectively reviewed for signs and symptoms of intraorbital or intracranial disease.

> *Case 1.*—A girl, 2½ months, with new onset seizures, no predisposing factors for seizures, and a family history of NF1 was examined. She had 7 café-au-lait spots. An electroencephalogram showed ictal and intraictal right hemisphere discharges. Magnetic resonance imaging revealed hyperintense areas in the right tem-

poral lobe and right cerebellar hemisphere. The child did well on phenytoin (Dilantin) and valproate therapy for 3 years when breakthrough seizures developed. Magnetic resonance imaging revealed a right optic glioma. The family refused treatment. The patient began to decline 6 months later and received chemotherapy. Tumor size has stabilized as demonstrated by semi-annual MRI scans.

Case 2.—An adopted boy, 17 months, had 5 café-au-lait spots and facial asymmetry, significant myopic anisometropia, and Lisch nodules in both eyes. He was given a diagnosis of NF1. Two months later, a plexiform neurofibroma was evident on CT. It was confirmed by biopsy and debulked surgically. Sixteen months later the neurofibrom[illegible] [illegible]ed. A right optic glioma was found on MRI. Vision was corrected, and further treatment was deferred by the family. Magnetic resonance imaging scans every 3 months show no change in glioma size.

Discussion.—Optic gliomas represent 66% of optic nerve tumors, 1.5% to 3% of all orbital tumors, and 0.6% to 1.5% of intracranial tumors. Most occur in children aged 10 years and younger. Although optic gliomas tend to occur more often in females, chiasmal tumors are present equally in males and females. In 10% to 70% of patients with gliomas, NF1 is also present. Although about 15% of patients with NF1 are reported to have optic gliomas, only 8% were given diagnoses of optic gliomas in this study. Most patients with optic gliomas are asymptomatic.

Conclusion.—A negative neuroimaging study does not rule out future development of optic gliomas in patients with NF1.

▶ Optic pathway gliomas are pilocytic astrocytomas that have an association with NF1. Many times patients with NF1 have screening for these lesions. Some investigators believe that these lesions are congenital hamartomas; thus, a negative CT or MRI scan might indicate freedom from subsequently having these gliomas.

The authors nicely demonstrate that this may not be the case. In addition, the report cites other cases that also note the development of optic nerve gliomas in patients with previously imaged optic pathways that were normal.

The manuscript provides interesting statistics that I will recapitulate. Optic pathway gliomas represent 66% of intrinsic optic nerve tumors, 1.5% to 3% of all orbital tumors, and 0.6% to 1.5% of all intracranial tumors. Optic nerve gliomas often occur in the first decade of life, although they have been reported in patients as old as 79 years of age. The literature is controversial with respect to what these lesions actually represent; the spectrum ranges from congenital, hamartomatous lesions to true neoplasms that invade brain tissue. Mortality is up to 50% when the lesion invades the adjacent hypothalamus; 10% to 70% of patients with optic gliomas have been reported to have NF1, whereas 15% of patients with NF1 have optic nerve gliomas. In this series, only 8% of patients with NF1 had gliomas. It is interesting that most patients with optic nerve gliomas remain asymptomatic, and only 20% have visual impairment.

These lesions can clearly grow from what appear to be normal intracranial optic nerves or chiasms. On the basis of what is reported, I believe that there is a continued risk for patients with NF1 whose initial images are normal.

R.I. Grossman, M.D.

► Once again, clinical history, findings, and judgment are "trump" over technology. Although we practice medicine in the most technologically advanced age to date, the next millennium will still be dependent on listening to patients' histories and cost-effectively using our technological firepower.

This article emphasizes the necessity to follow clinical signs and symptoms in patients' neurofibromatosis and findings of the afferent visual system. The take-home message is that if clinical symptoms indicate optic nerve or chiasmatic dysfunction, repeat MRI scanning is indicated.

R.C. Sergott, M.D.

The Role of Magnetic Resonance Imaging in Children With Intraocular Tumors and Simulating Lesions

Potter P, Shields CL, Shields JA, et al (Wills Eye Hosp, Philadelphia; Thomas Jefferson Univ, Philadelphia)

Ophthalmology 103:1774–1783, 1996 9–9

Background.—Intraocular lesions are usually diagnosed by indirect ophthalmoscopy. The role of pre- and postcontrast MRI in the assessment of children with intraocular tumors and simulating lesions was investigated.

Methods.—Forty children younger than 12 years of age with a clinical diagnosis of an intraocular lesion were studied. Lesion thickness was no greater than 2 mm. Pre- and postcontrast MR images were obtained with surface coil, with postcontrast-enhanced images obtained using fat suppression techniques.

Findings.—Twenty-two lesions were retinoblastoma; 5, Coats' disease; 2, ciliary body medulloepithelioma; 2, primary hyperplastic persistent vitreous; 3, retinal capillary hemangioma; 2, massive retinal gliosis; 1, uveal melanoma; 1, ciliary body leiomyoma; 1, retinopathy of prematurity with total retinal detachment; and 1, posttraumatic retinal gliosis. Solid intraocular lesions larger than 2 mm thick, such as retinoblastoma, ciliary body medulloepithelioma, leiomyoma, choroidal melanoma, and retinal capillary hemangioma, were hyperintense on T1-weighted images and hypointense on T2-weighted images. Regardless of the underlying causes, secondary serous or exudative retinal detachments were hyperintense in the subretinal space on T1- and T2-weighted images. Retinal gliosis was hypointense on T1- and T2-weighted images. Enhancement was minimal to marked in retinoblastoma, medulloepithelioma, retinal capillary hemangioma, leiomyoma, and choroidal melanoma on contrast-enhanced T1-weighted images with fat suppression methods. The subretinal space of Coats' disease, primary hyperplastic persistent vitreous, retinopathy of prematurity, and retinal gliosis did not enhance. Magnetic resonance sequences showed calcification in 54% of retinoblastoma tumors. On T1- and T2-weighted images, calcification showed low signal intensity, with a lack of enhancement on contrast-enhanced sequences, which differentiated it from surrounding tumor or tissue necrosis. The associated serous or exudative subretinal fluid from intraocular tumors or simulating lesions did not enhance after contrast was administered, enabling differentiation from the causative lesion.

Conclusions.—Precontrast and postcontrast MRI differentiates solid intraocular tumors from intraocular lesions with primary retinal detachment. Heterogeneity observed in retinoblastoma may indicate foci of tumor necrosis and/or calcification. The various solid tumors could not be differentiated from one another reliably based on MRI features.

▶ The authors have taken a cohort of 40 children all less than 12 years of age, the majority (n = 22) with retinoblastoma, and attempted to draw conclusions regarding the role of MRI. The purported hypothesis was to evaluate the role of pre- and postcontrast MRI studies in children with intraocular tumors and simulating lesions. Unfortunately, the authors never bothered to perform MRI evaluation in a meaningful manner. There are no blinded readings, no intra- or interobserver variability, and no control images. The authors have excluded in the Methods section all children with a clinical diagnosis of solitary intraocular tumor with "a thickness less than 2 mm due to the lack of detection of tumors with a thickness less than 2 mm." The investigators quote themselves as a reference on this issue. However, the resolving power of an MRI system is complex, depending on many factors including inherent contrast differences resulting from the tissue type and slice thickness, etc. Thus, I would take issue with the claim that MRI cannot detect tumors less than 2 mm without optimization of MRI parameters.

The particular MRI parameters used in this study varied considerably with TRS on T1-weighted images ranging between 600 and 800 msec and T2-weighted images having TRs of 1,800–2,500 msec. Such variation, of course, would have significant impact on the intensity of all tissue types. The authors never stated what effect these variations had on intensity characteristics. Fat suppression techniques also modify imaging parameters. Although the investigators state that all pre- and postcontrast-enhanced images were filmed at the same window and level, if the same pulse sequences were not applied, it would be difficult to compare intensity patterns. The authors produce a scale regarding contrast enhancement but provide no examples. The same is true for signal intensity. There are no gold standards here nor are there any variability measurements of the MR features of the lesions. Thus, it is difficult to appreciate how easy or difficult it is for one observer or multiple observers to replicate any of the purported findings.

There appears to be a conflict amongst the data that I could not understand. In the methods section, it is stated that children with the clinical diagnosis of solitary solid intraocular lesion with a thickness of less than 2 mm were not selected to undergo an MRI study. However, it appears that 10 cases with a thickness of less than or equal to 2 mm did undergo MRI. It is also interesting that calcification was identified by either US or CT or both in only 46 of the 56 tumors. I would have liked to have seen the detection of calcium broken down between US and CT.

The examples of viable retinoblastoma being hyperintense on the T1-weighted image provided in the original article are rather unconvincing. Additionally, I see no large hypointense region, rather it is isotense to vitreous. Furthermore, if CT is needed to demonstrate the calcific portion of the tumor, such need clearly detracts from the utility of MRI in detecting the hypointensity.

Another issue is the separation of T1–high intensity from regions that contrast enhanced. Without the noncontrast axial image in the same plane, it is impossible to state what enhances from what is intrinsically high signal intensity.

On Figure 7, the investigators assume that a hypointense lesion corresponds to retinal gliosis in a posttraumatic globe. The hypointensity could, of course, be calcification. Another issue is that phthisis bulbi would really not be in the differential diagnosis of retinoblastoma.

On page 1782, the observation of the lack of linear enhancement at the level of choroid in 1 patient suggested replacement of the normally markedly enhancing choroid by mass or retinoblastoma, which was confirmed histopathologically. The question to ask is, why isn't the choroid thickened and enhancing if it is retinoblastoma? Second, this appears to represent a retrospective observation after histopathologic examination and does not demonstrate the utility of MRI.

It is surprising that calcification was detected only in 82% of retinoblastoma tumors in this series. The investigators never indicate that the detection of calcification is clearly dependent on the MR pulse sequence used. Additionally, calcification may be high signal on T1. This is not discussed either. Areas of calcification can also enhance. This is not reviewed in the paper. Retinoblastoma may hemorrhage. This, too, is not elaborated in the paper.

A very significant problem with this manuscript is the references. The authors fail to reference the appropriate peer-reviewed literature in many important cases. Indeed, approximately 10 of the 24 references are from the authors' own work, many of which are chapters from books. These include the MRI features of melanoma, the appearance of hemorrhage, etc. Finally, because of a flawed methodology, the conclusion that solid neoplastic can be differentiated from nonsolid retinal detachment hemorrhage on postcontrast T1-weighted image is not sustained.

Scientific studies must have appropriate methodology if there is going to be any power attached to the conclusions. This is an essential aspect of radiologic investigation. Observations are critical and variability of the interpretation based on particular criteria provides the utility of a particular finding. This study displayed none of these characteristics, nor the methodology to answer the proposed question.

R.I. Grossman, M.D.

Magnetic Resonance Imaging in Posttraumatic Strabismus
Ward TP, Thach AB, Madigan WP Jr, et al (Walter Reed Army Med Ctr, Washington, DC; Florida Eye Inst, Vero Beach)
J Pediatr Ophthalmol Strabismus 34:131–134, 1997 9–10

Background.—MRI can provide high-resolution imaging of strabismus due to trauma. These authors report 2 cases in which MRI correctly identified posttraumatic strabismus.

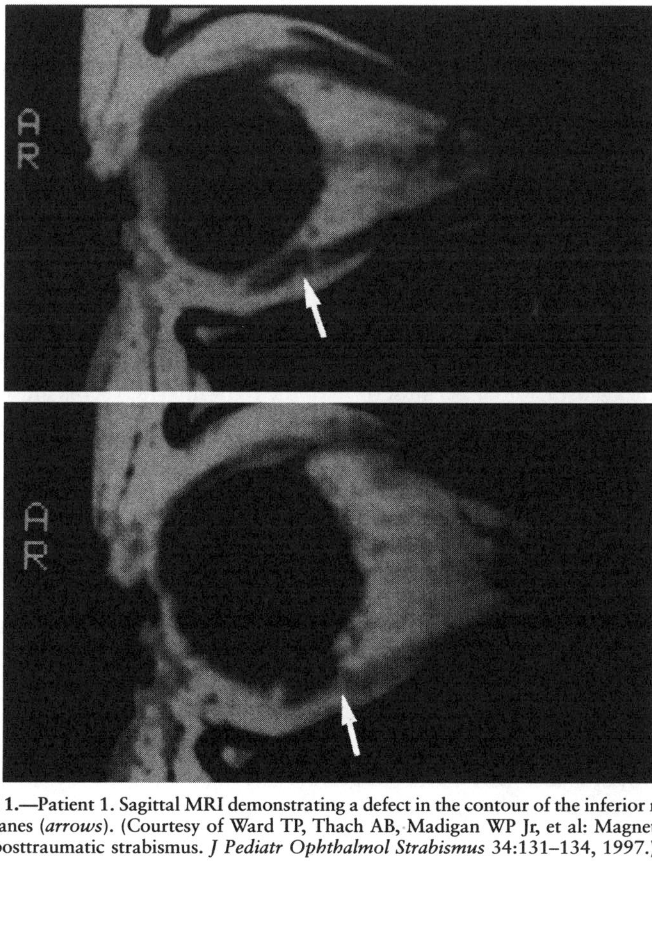

FIGURE 1.—Patient 1. Sagittal MRI demonstrating a defect in the contour of the inferior rectus muscle in several planes (*arrows*). (Courtesy of Ward TP, Thach AB, Madigan WP Jr, et al: Magnetic resonance imaging in posttraumatic strabismus. *J Pediatr Ophthalmol Strabismus* 34:131–134, 1997.)

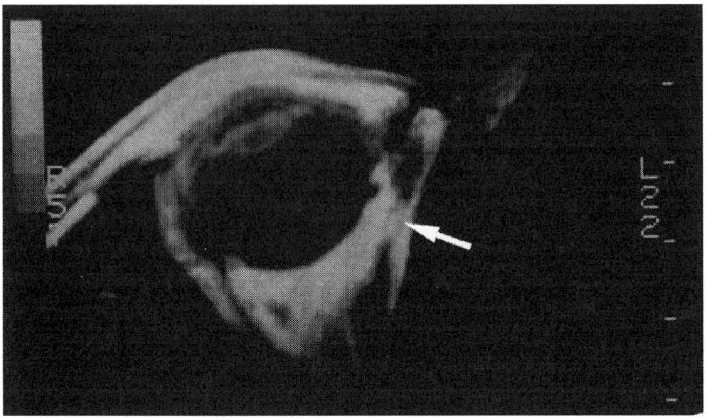

FIGURE 2.—Patient 2. Axial MRI demonstrating marked loss of muscle tissue within the belly of the right medial rectus (*arrow*). (Courtesy of Ward TP, Thach AB, Madigan WP Jr, et al: Magnetic resonance imaging in posttraumatic strabismus. *J Pediatr Ophthalmol Strabismus* 34:131–134, 1997.)

Case Reports.—Patient 1 was a 31-year-old man who 6 weeks earlier had fallen onto a standpipe and damaged his right lower eyelid. At that time, he had substantial subconjunctival bleeding over the insertion of the inferior rectus muscle, but *radiographic* imaging and CT scan did not show any fractures or foreign bodies. The patient could infraduct the right eye to about half of normal. When the authors evaluated the patient 6 weeks after the injury, the patient still had infraduction of the right eye to about half of normal. Furthermore, right hypertropia was present in the primary position and less resistance to elevation was evident in the right eye. A CT scan of the orbit was normal. However, MRI confirmed the clinical suspicion of a disinsertion of the right inferior rectus muscle (Fig 1).

Patient 2 was a 37-year-old man who had been stabbed in the right medial orbit. The medial canthus was lacerated and the optic nerve was transected, but the globe was without injury. Four months after this injury, the patient had right hypertropia in the primary position, with little adduction and no intortion in the right eye. A CT scan of the orbit was normal. However, MRI confirmed the clinical suspicion of a laceration of the right medial rectus muscle (Fig 2).

Conclusions.—The inferior and medial rectus muscles are most prone to injury after orbital trauma, probably because their insertions are so close to the limbus. Most often the diagnosis is based on history and motility examinations, and in some cases surgical exploration is necessary. MRI provides an alternative to surgical exploration that is less invasive and able to identify soft-tissue damage. Thus, in addition to its other uses in evaluating Duane's syndrome, Brown's syndrome, cranial nerve palsies, congenitally anomalous rectus muscle insertions, and trochlear trauma, MRI can be a useful tool in evaluating suspected strabismus after trauma.

Kinetic Magnetic Resonance Imaging of Orbital Blow-out Fracture With Restricted Ocular Movement

Totsuka N, Koide R (Showa Univ, Tokyo)

Orbit 16:75–83, 1997 9–11

Background.—Why eye movement is restricted in blow-out orbital fractures is not known. These authors used MRI to identify the factors involved in this dyskinesia.

Methods.—MRI was performed on patients from 1 day to 15 months after injury. (Table 1 of the original article shows the age, sex, and type of orbital fractures in the patients.) Each patient was imaged 7 times (0, 10, 20, and 30 degrees supraduction and 10, 20, and 30 degrees infraduction), and the images were reconstructed in the MRI ciné mode into an animated film.

Findings.—In normal subjects, MRI shows the shaded connective fiber septa and the adipose tissue that constitute the intermuscular membrane. In these 19 subjects, however, the adipose tissue was prolapsed, and a shadow of the connective tissue septa was near or in the prolapsed intermuscular membrane (i.e., incarcerated septa). These incarcerated septa were associated with eye movement restriction in 11 of 19 subjects. Eye movement restriction was also associated with different positions of the inferior and medial rectus muscles (i.e., deviated muscle) and with deformed or swollen muscles (i.e., deformed muscles). In particular, incarcerated septa were significantly associated with deviated muscles, which suggests that these incarcerations were at least partly responsible for the limited eye movement. Table 1 details which type of movement restriction was present in each patient. Four patients also had a deviated or deformed optic nerve, and stretched septa were evident in all 4.

Conclusions.—MRI indicates that incarcerated septa at the fracture site interfere with normal movement of the external ocular muscles. This interference results in the dyskinesia associated with blow-out fractures. Furthermore, the finding of incarcerated septa with optic nerve damage indicates another pathologic mechanism of action for these incarcerated septa.

► The bottom line of these 2 reports (Abstracts 9–10 and 9–11) is that MR is useful for localizing the results of trauma in patients with restrictive ocular movement or posttraumatic strabismus. One report uses static MR images, whereas the other use ciné MRI to analyze restricted eye movement in blow-out fractures. MRI has been advocated in the study of various ocular motility disorders including Duane's syndrome, Brown's syndrome, cranial nerve palsies, congenitally anomalous rectus muscle insertions, and trochlear trauma. In one report, imaging demonstrated defects within particular muscle bellies or insertions; the other report confirmed that incarcerated muscular septa, at the site of a fracture, interfered with contraction or relaxation of the external muscle.

These are 2 fine reports. However, I do not believe that either demonstrated the potential of high-resolution echoplanar imaging in disorders of motility or trauma. Ocular motion can be assessed by very-high speed MRI techniques. In addition, high-resolution imaging of the orbit can be performed using surface coil imaging, fat saturation, and 1-mm thick images. Multiple planes are also important in assessing the extraocular muscles.

I believe that with state-of-the-art techniques, one will have increased specificity with respect not only to muscular problems following trauma but also to the whole spectrum of strabismus. Such information may be useful in surgical planning and assessing the results of treatment. However, these two reports do demonstrate the utility of MRI in assessing functional problems of the extraocular muscles.

R.I. Grossman, M.D.

Perineural Spread of Cutaneous Squamous Cell Carcinoma via the Orbit: Clinical Features and Outcome in 21 Cases

McNab AA, Francis IC, Benger R, et al (Royal Victorian Eye and Ear Hosp, Melbourne, Australia; Prince of Wales Hosp, Sydney, Australia; Sydney Eye Hosp, Australia; et al)

Ophthalmology 104:1457–1462, 1997 9–12

Background.—Although a rare occurrence, squamous cell carcinoma can spread along nerves to infiltrate the intracranial cavity. These authors share their experiences in the perineural spread of squamous cell carcinoma.

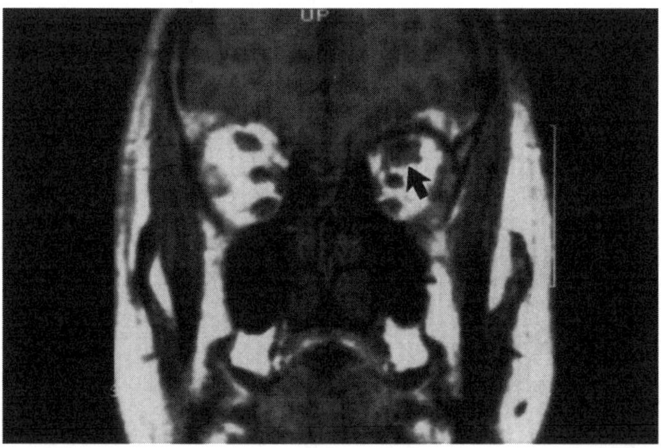

FIGURE 4.—A coronal MRI shows a moderate-sized mass in the roof of the orbit (*arrow*) in a patient with perineural spread via the supraorbital nerve of a recurrent squamous cell carcinoma in the forehead. (Published courtesy of *Ophthalmology*, from McNab AA, Francis IC, Benger R, et al: Perineural spread of cutaneous squamous cell carcinoma via the orbit: Clinical features and outcome in 21 cases. *Ophthalmology* 104:1457–1462, 1997.)

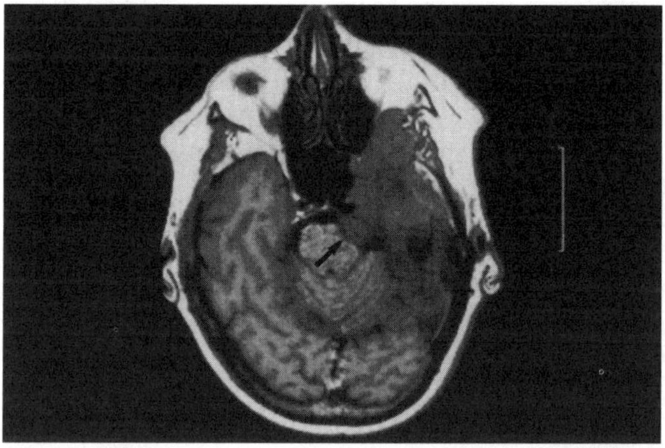

FIGURE 5.—Axial MRI shows a large tumor mass extending from the orbit into the cavernous sinus and pons (*arrow*). (Published courtesy of *Ophthalmology*, from McNab AA, Francis IC, Benger R, et al: Perineural spread of cutaneous squamous cell carcinoma via the orbit: Clinical features and outcome in 21 cases. *Ophthalmology* 104:1457–1462, 1997.)

Methods.—Record review identified 21 patients (17 men and 4 women, 38 to 82 years old) who had squamous cell carcinoma that spread perineurally via the orbit.

Findings.—The site of the primary cutaneous tumor was the forehead or brow in 11 patients, the medial canthus in 3, the cheek in 3, the temple in 2, and the upper eyelid or nasal ala in 1 patient each. In most patients, the perineural spread occurred less than 2 years after excision of the primary tumor. At presentation, all but 1 patient had dysesthesia, 14 had ophthal-

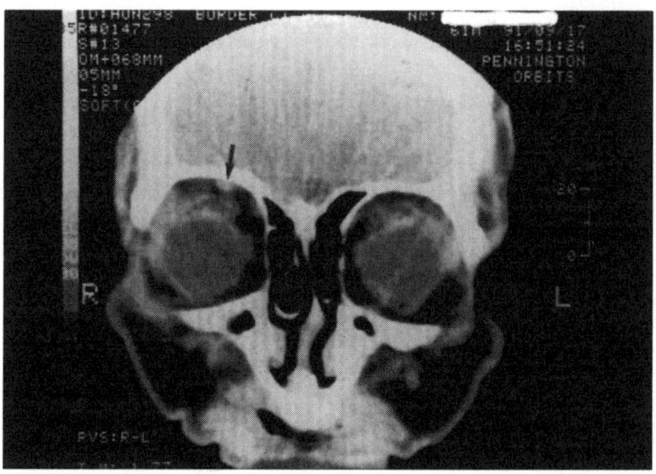

FIGURE 6.—A coronal CT scan shows subtle enlargement of the supraorbital nerve by perineural spread of cutaneous squamous cell carcinoma (*arrow*). (Published courtesy of *Ophthalmology*, from McNab AA, Francis IC, Benger R, et al: Perineural spread of cutaneous squamous cell carcinoma via the orbit: Clinical features and outcome in 21 cases. *Ophthalmology* 104:1457–1462, 1997.)

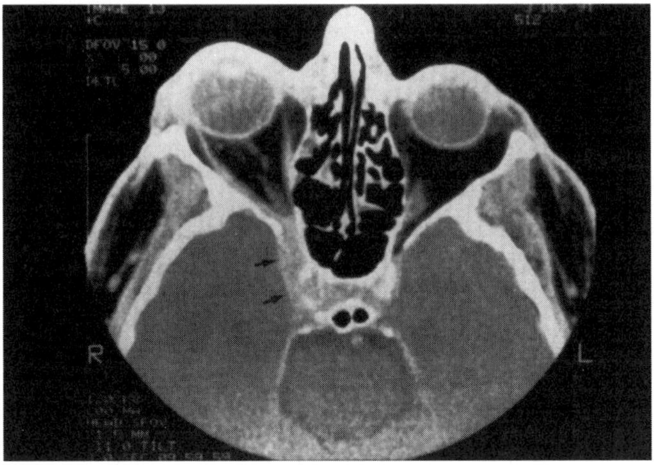

FIGURE 7.—An axial CT scan shows tumor extending through the right superior orbital fissure (note the loss of fat density compared to the other side) and into the cavernous sinus that is enlarged (*arrows*). (Published courtesy of *Ophthalmology*, from McNab AA, Francis IC, Benger R, et al: Perineural spread of cutaneous squamous cell carcinoma via the orbit: Clinical features and outcome in 21 cases. *Ophthalmology* 104:1457–1462, 1997.)

moplegia/ptosis, 14 had facial weakness, and 9 had pain. Symptoms occurred more often and with increasing intensity as follow-up progressed. Surgical resection of tumor (either radical or conservative) or radiation therapy had little effect on stopping disease progression. As of the last follow-up, 14 of 21 patients (67%) had died as a result of perineural spread of cancer, and only 4 patients were alive without evidence of disease recurrence. Most deaths (13 of 14) occurred because of local contiguous

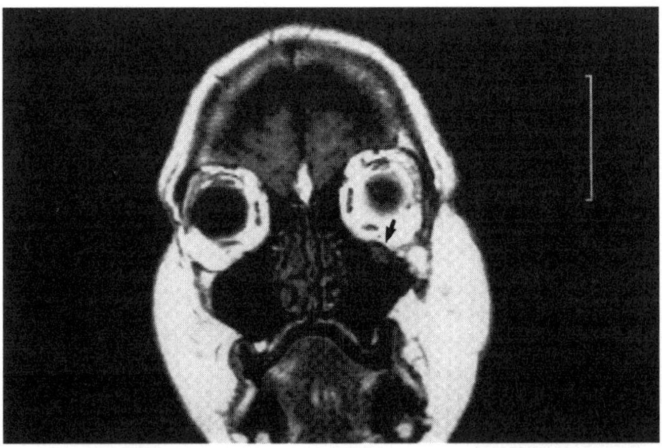

FIGURE 8.—The left infraorbital nerve is enlarged (*arrow*) by squamous cell carcinoma spreading along the nerve from a lesion on the cheek. (Published courtesy of *Ophthalmology*, from McNab AA, Francis IC, Benger R, et al: Perineural spread of cutaneous squamous cell carcinoma via the orbit: Clinical features and outcome in 21 cases. *Ophthalmology* 104:1457–1462, 1997.)

spread of the disease into the orbit, cavernous sinus, cerebrum, or brain stem. Tumor masses occurred throughout the course of the nerve (Fig 4), and even extended into the brain stem (Fig 5). Early in the course of disease, however, nerve involvement was often subtle (Fig 6). Tumor involvement often was asymmetric (Fig 7). The infraorbital nerve was enlarged within the orbit floor in patients in whom the second division of the trigeminal nerve was involved (Fig 8). As disease progressed, tumors became noticeable in the orbit, at the primary site on the face, and intracranially.

Conclusions.—Perineural spread of cutaneous squamous cell carcinoma carries a poor prognosis. Early radiation therapy can provide the best results, but once the orbit is involved, radiation therapy is probably of little use. The chance for a good outcome is improved if the clinician maintains a strong suspicion for perineural spread in evaluating patients with periorbital squamous cell carcinomas. Results of ocular motility testing and facial and trigeminal nerve function testing can be helpful in this evaluation.

Neuro-Ophthalmologic Manifestations of Adenoid Cystic Carcinoma

Lee AG, Phillips PH, Newman NJ, et al (Baylor College of Medicine, Houston; Emory Univ, Atlanta, Ga; Univ of Miami, Fla; et al)

J Neuroophthalmol 17:183–188, 1997 9–13

Background.—Intracranial adenoid cystic carcinoma is rare, and orbital involvement is typically related to spread from the lacrimal gland. These authors describe 2 patients with an unusual course of intracranial adenoid cystic carcinoma.

> *Case Report.*—Patient 1 was a 36-year-old woman 3–4 months pregnant who noted diffuse headaches, facial pain, and numbness on the right side; decreased vision in the inferior field of the right eye; and a sensation of pressure behind the right eye. During months 5–7 of her pregnancy, right visual acuity decreased and proptosis and retrobulbar pain of the right eye increased, and facial numbness continued transiently. MRI revealed a soft tissue mass in the right orbital apex that extended into the cavernous sinus. The extraocular muscles in the right orbital apex were also enlarged (Fig 1). Based on a presumptive diagnosis of orbital pseudotumor, the patient began a regimen of oral prednisone, 60 mg/day, and symptoms improved dramatically. Decreasing the prednisone dose caused symptom recurrence. During the seventh month of her pregnancy, visual field testing revealed a defect involving the inferior nerve fiber bundle in the right eye. MRI at this time showed that the soft tissue mass had grown to include the pterygopalatine fissure and skull base (Fig 2). After the patient had a vaginal delivery at 37 weeks' gestation, a right frontal craniotomy was

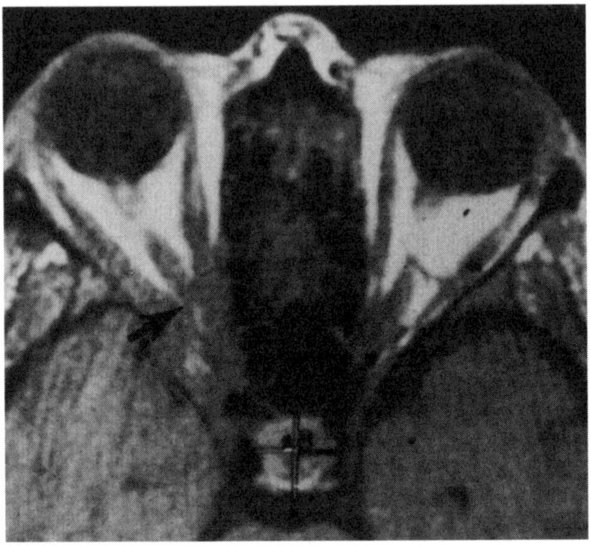

FIGURE 1.—Case 1. Axial T1-weighted MRI without contrast of the orbit reveals an isointense mass in the right orbital apex (*arrow*). (Courtesy of Lee AG, Phillips PH, Newman NJ, et al: Neuro-ophthalmologic manifestation of adenoid cystic carcinoma. *J Neuroophthalmol* 17:183–188, 1997.)

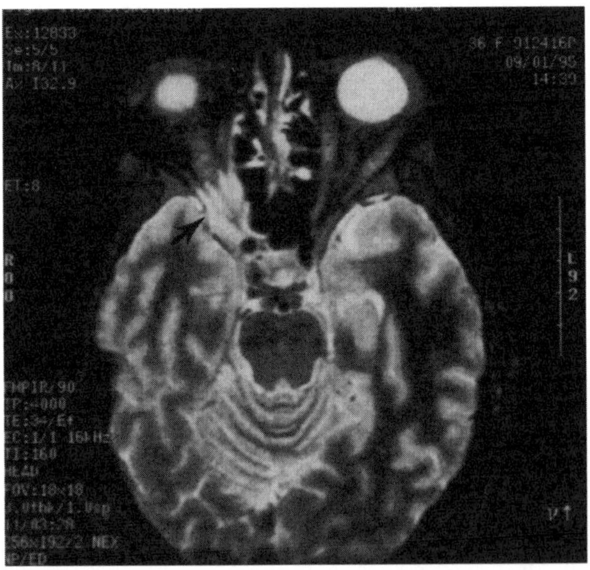

FIGURE 2.—Case 1. Axial T2-weighted MRI shows hyperintense signal intensity in the right orbital apex (*arrow*) and along the right posterior optic nerve sheath. (Courtesy of Lee AG, Phillips PH, Newman NJ, et al: Neuro-ophthalmologic manifestation of adenoid cystic carcinoma. *J Neuroophthalmol* 17:183–188, 1997.)

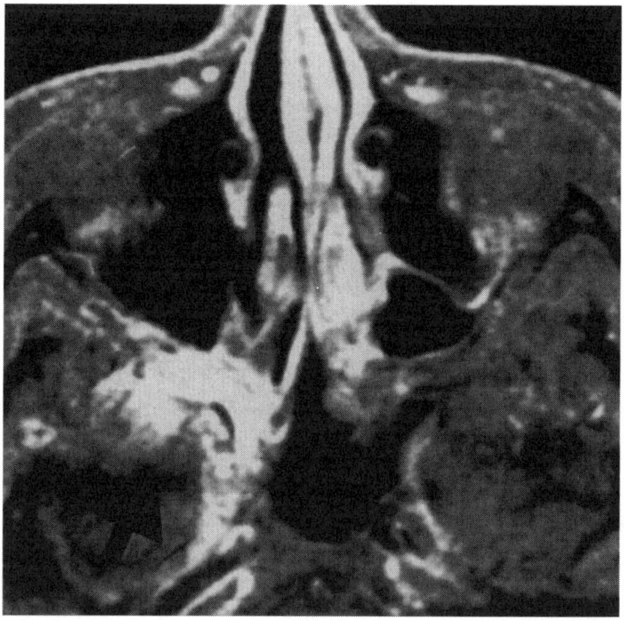

FIGURE 4.—Case 1. Axial T1-weighted MRI demonstrates contrast enhancement of lesion on the right side (*arrow*) in the area of the pterygopalatine fossa. (Courtesy of Lee AG, Phillips PH, Newman NJ, et al: Neuro-ophthalmologic manifestation of adenoid cystic carcinoma. *J Neuroophthalmol* 17:183–188, 1997.)

performed. The margin of the mass could not be grossly identified, but extended into the meninges of the cavernous sinus, the superior orbital fissure, and the greater wing of the sphenoid. Histologic diagnosis confirmed adenoid cystic carcinoma. The optic nerve appeared normal, as did the lacrimal gland tissue. The patient was administered a course of radiation therapy, and a follow-up MRI with enhancement delineated the lesion in the pterygopalatine fossa (Fig 4).

Conclusions.—Given the lack of lacrimal gland involvement, the intracranial adenoid cystic carcinoma in this patient likely developed as a result of perineural spread via involvement of the trigeminal nerve in the pterygopalatine fossa. Although steroid therapy improved visual acuity, proptosis, and the visual field defect, the numbness of the cheek remained, and this symptom prompted the biopsy. Thus, intracranial adenoid cystic carcinoma should be part of the differential diagnosis in patients with painful optic neuropathies that are responsive to steroids.

Occult Perineural Tumor Infiltration of the Trigeminal Nerve: Diagnostic Considerations

ten Hove MW, Glaser JS, Schatz NJ (Queen's Univ Kingston, Ont; Univ of Miami, Fla)

J Neuroophthalmol 17:170–177, 1997 9–14

Background.—Some patients with facial cutaneous or nasopharyngeal carcinomas experience changes in facial nerve function, even when no mass lesions are obvious. These authors report the symptoms, diagnosis, and management of 7 cases in which occult tumors invaded the trigeminal nerve.

Methods.—The 7 patients (3 men, 4 women) ranged in age from 27 to 82 years old. All but 2 had undergone previous surgery for facial or nasopharyngeal carcinomas. All patients experienced paresthesia, and many also experienced ptosis, diplopia, and pain. MRI was used to evaluate the cavernous sinus for nerve involvement.

Findings.—MRI revealed multiple cranial nerve involvement in all 7 patients, most typically cranial nerves V, III, and VI. On the basis of the nerves involved, biopsy sites were chosen to confirm the type of cavernous infiltration: 5 patients were found to have squamous cell carcinoma, 1 had basal cell carcinoma, and 1 had adenoid cystic carcinoma. T1- and T2-weighted MRI views were obtained, with and without contrast enhance-

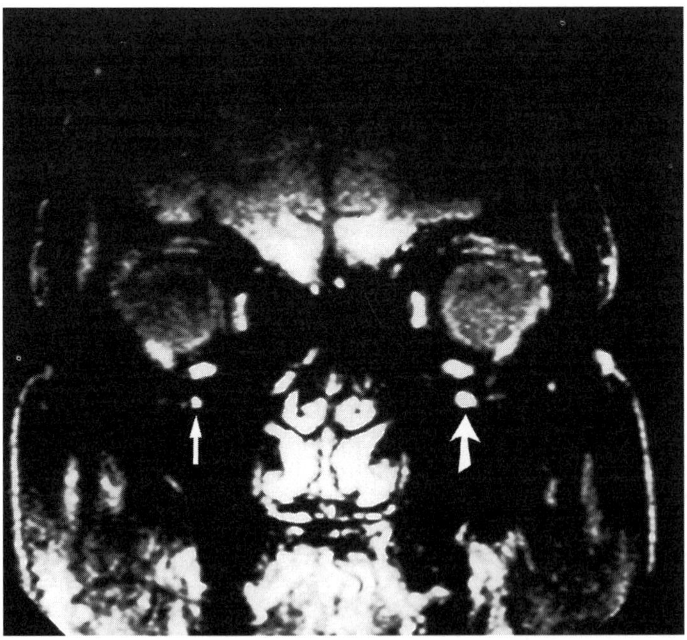

FIGURE, bottom.—T1-weighted MRI, with Gd-DPTA, coronal section. Enhancement of left infraorbital nerve is seen. (Courtesy of ten Hove MW, Glaser JS, Schatz NJ: Occult perineural tumor infiltration of the trigeminal nerve: Diagnostic considerations. *J Neuroophthalmol* 17:170–177, 1997.)

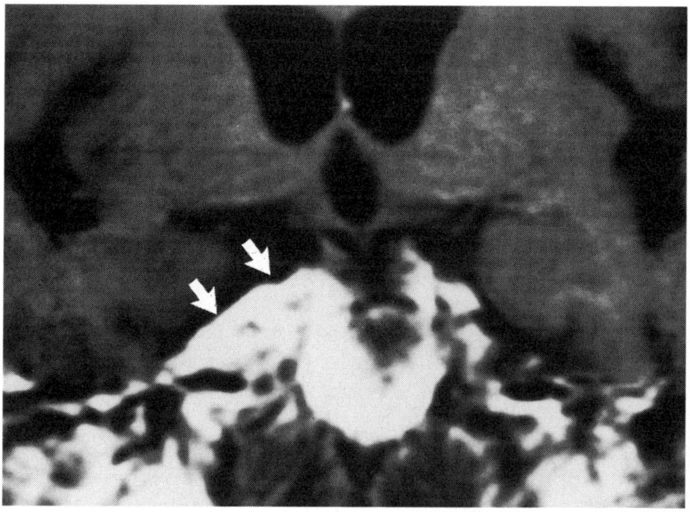

FIGURE 4.—Case 3. T1-weighted MRI, coronal section showing diffuse mass in the right cavernous sinus (*arrows*) with Gd-DPTA enhancement of the mass. (Courtesy of ten Hove MW, Glaser JS, Schatz NJ: Occult perineural tumor infiltration of the trigeminal nerve: Diagnostic considerations. *J Neuroophthalmol* 17:170–177, 1997.)

ment with gadolinium–diethylenetriamine pentaacetic acid (Gd-DPTA). In some cases, contrast enhancement helped identify nerve involvement (Fig 3), and in others it did not (Fig 4). Radiation therapy was used in all but 1 of the 7 patients, and only 1 recurrence was noted after 6 months.

Conclusions.—MRI evidence of nerve involvement and lesions indicates that the tumors in these patients spread by the means of the perineural or endoneural fascial planes. Although perineural spread of tumor is rare, it should be kept in mind when facial cutaneous or nasopharyngeal cancers are being resected. In particular, the MRI identification of the involved nerves can help choose an appropriate biopsy site, and thus lead to a quick diagnosis and the best prognosis.

► I have chosen these 3 articles (Abstracts 9–12, 9–13, and 9–14) to illustrate the diagnosis of perineural spread of tumor about the orbit. McNab et al. and Lee et al. demonstrate the manifestations of perineural spread of adenoid cystic carcinoma and squamous cell carcinoma, respectively. In the article by ten Hove et al., infiltration of the trigeminal nerve by occult tumors is described. In all examples, imaging is crucial to the diagnosis. Clinical findings are quite similar—patients in all series demonstrated symptoms including decrease or altered sensation, pain, ptosis, ophthalmoplegia, and facial weakness in a significant proportion of cases. All of the patients with squamous cell carcinoma had a sensory disturbance (numbness, altered sensation, dysesthesias).

Adenoid cystic carcinoma usually arises from the lacrimal gland; however, it can arise from the cerumen glands of the external auditory canal, ectopic lacrimal gland tissue, and other organs such as breast, bronchus pancreas, vulva, sweat glands, or genital glands. Linear meningeal thickening and enhancement similar to "a dural tail sign" has been seen with intracranial adenoid cystic carcinoma.

The first description of malignant perineural spread of tumor was described by the French pathologist, Cruveilhier in 1842.[1] One must carefully image the orbit and base of skull in two planes without and with fat saturation and contrast. Meticulous examination of all the nerves in this region, as well as the pterygopalatine fossa is essential. Asymmetry of soft tissue around skull base must arouse suspicion. Enlargement of nerves, foramen, or unusual enhancing soft tissue are suggestive of perineural spread of tumor.

The pterygopalatine fossa is a most important conduit for perineural spread. It is situated between the posterior margin of the maxillary sinus and pterygoid process, and is shaped somewhat like an ice cream cone. Superiorly, the second division of the trigeminal artery courses (a good nerve for perineural spread of tumor) to the foramen rotundum; while the vidian nerve runs through the vidian canal (in the superior aspect of the pterygoid process) to the pyterygopalatine ganglia, the greater and lesser palatine nerves also traverse (from superior to inferior) this fossa, and the distal portion of the maxillary artery. The nerves and tissue planes serve as an easy conduit for perineural spread of tumor. The propensity for tumors to progress through the perineural or endoneural fascial planes is most likely attributable to lower resistance to invasion of these potentially distensible spaces. The perineuria provide direct pathways from distal cutaneous nerve branches to the CNS. ten Hove et al. quote the series by Laine et al.[2] where trigeminal involvement manifested by (1) an enlarged foramen ovale, (2) smooth isointense enlargement of the second or third divisions of the trigeminal nerve, (3) bulging of the lateral wall of the cavernous sinus, (4) replacing of normally hypointense cistern of the Gasserian ganglion, and (5) atrophy changes in the masticatory muscles.

R.I. Grossman, M.D.

References

1. Cruveilhier J: *Maladies des Nerfs: Anatomie Pathologique du Corps Humain.* Paris, JB Bailliere, 1835–1842 (Part 2, 1935) p 3.
2. Laine FJ, Sen ME, Braun IF, et al: Perineural MR imaging. *Radiology* 174:65–71, 1990.

High Resolution Magnetic Resonance Imaging of Neurovascular Orbital Anatomy

Ettl A, Kramer J, Daxer A, et al (Gen Hosp, St Pölten, Austria; Academic Med Ctr, Amsterdam; CT and MR-Inst Schillerpark, Linz, Austria; et al)
Ophthalmology 104:869–877, 1997 9–15

Objective.—Although the resolution of CT is sufficient to visualize the ophthalmic artery and some of its branches and the frontal and oculomo-

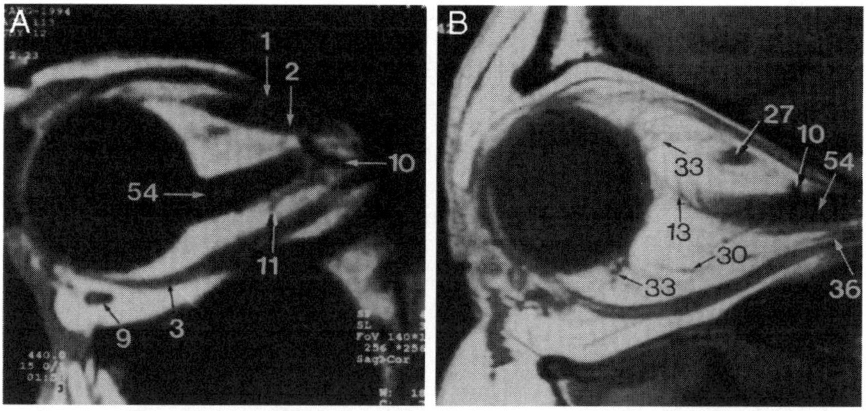

FIGURE 3.—Oblique-sagittal T1-weighted MR images of the orbit. On T1-weighted images, the orbital fat appears bright (hyperintense), whereas vitreous and cerebrospinal fluid appear dark (hypointense). Muscles, vessels, and nerves are hypointense relative to orbital fat. The numbers refer to the nomenclature of the structures (see Appendix in original article). **A,** imaging plane along the optic nerve (up-gaze, healthy research subject) showing the central retinal artery (11) originating from the knee of the ophthalmic artery (10). **B,** imaging plane along the posterior part of the optic nerve (*white arrow*) and parallel to the lateral rectus muscle. The presumed inferior division of the oculomotor nerve (36) is situated between the optic nerve and the inferior rectus muscle. The superolateral and inferolateral vorticose veins (33) are also visualized. (Patient with oculomotor nerve paralysis.) (Published courtesy of *Ophthalmology*, from Ettl A, Kramer J, Daxer A, et al: High-resolution magnetic resonance imaging of neurovascular orbital anatomy. *Ophthalmology* 104:869–877, 1997.)

tor nerves, MRI provides superior imaging of soft tissue, is capable of multiplanar imaging, and is the modality of choice for in vivo anatomical studies because it does not expose patients to ionizing radiation. The anatomy of the arteries, veins, and cranial nerves of the orbit, as demonstrated by MRI, is described.

Methods.—Magnetic resonance (1–T scanner using a surface coil) T1-weighted oblique-sagittal, coronal, and axial images of the orbit were obtained for 6 healthy volunteers, aged 29–32 years, and 1 patient, aged 54 years, with chronic oculomotor nerve paralysis on the left side. Magnetic resonance images were identified by comparing them with the collection of histologic specimens from orbits, as documented by Koornneef.

Results.—Sagittal images located the intraorbital part of the ophthalmic artery on the lateral side of the optic nerve (Fig 3). Axial images demonstrated the pathway taken by the ophthalmic artery (Fig 4). Coronal images traced the path of the supratrochlear and infratrochlear vessels (Fig 5). The superior ophthalmic vein (SOV) was visualized from its source just posterior to the superior oblique tendon and running posteriorly near the junction with the lacrimal vein to the superior orbital fissure. The estimate obtained from axial images of the diameter of the SOV in the area of the lacrimal vein ranged from 1.5 to 2.0 mm because the blood vessel margins were unclear in the images. The veine ophthalmique moyenne, identified in axial images, could not be correlated with any structure in the histologic sections. Motor nerves were difficult to distinguish from each other because of crowding, although the abducens nerve was visible between the optic nerve and the lateral rectus muscle in some axial images.

Conclusion.—Surface coil MRI, using T1-weighted images, visualizes the ophthalmic veins and their branches and orbital sensory and motor cranial nerves, enabling investigators to observe vein enlargements, arteriovenous malformations, fistulae, shunts, cavernous sinus thrombosis, and Graves' ophthalmopathy. The superior division of the oculomotor nerve and the trochlear nerve were not visualized.

► The investigators have done a very nice job correlating many of the smaller, less well-known anatomical structures of the orbit with high-resolu-

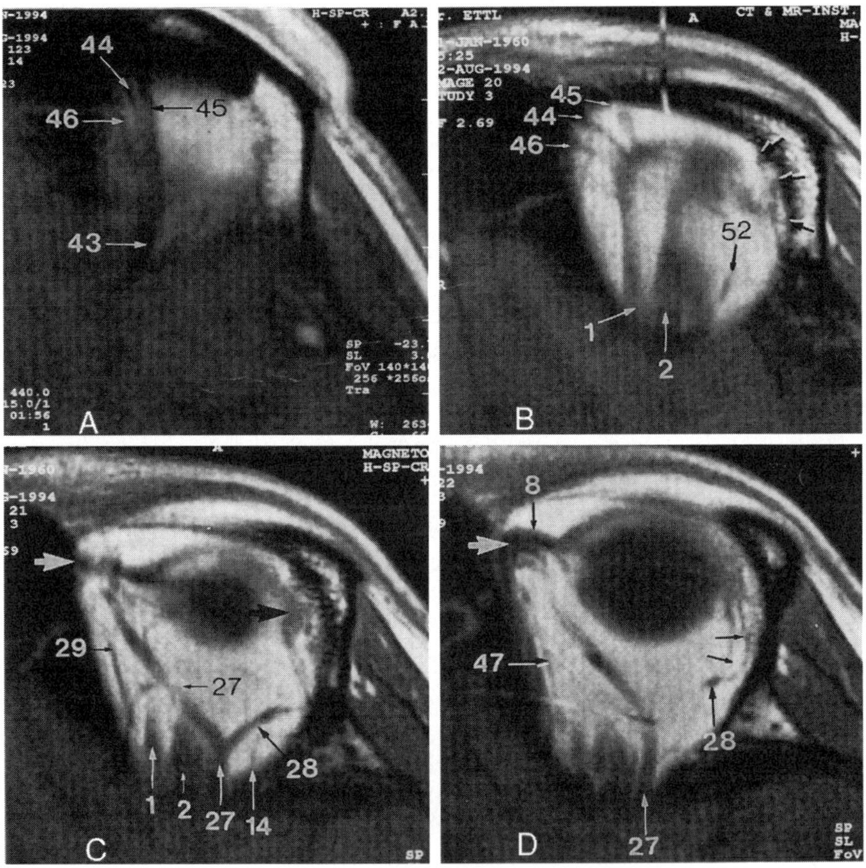

FIGURE 4.—T1-weighted axial images (left orbit, healthy research subject). The numbers refer to the nomenclature of the structures (see Appendix in original article). **A,** section inferior to the orbital roof showing the frontal nerve (43) and its branches: the supratrochlear nerve (46) and the medial (44) and lateral (45) branches of the supraorbital nerve. **B,** section just inferior to the plane of Figure 4A showing the lacrimal nerve (52) running toward the lacrimal gland (*arrows*). **C,** section 2 mm inferior to the section of Figure 4B. The superior rectus muscle (2) and the elevator muscle (1) are visible. The superior ophthalmic vein (27) traverses the orbit from the trochlea (*white arrow*) to posterolaterally inside the muscle cone. Lacrimal gland (*black arrows*). **D,** section at the level of the trochlea (*white arrow*). Lacrimal (*Continued*)

FIGURE 4 (cont.)

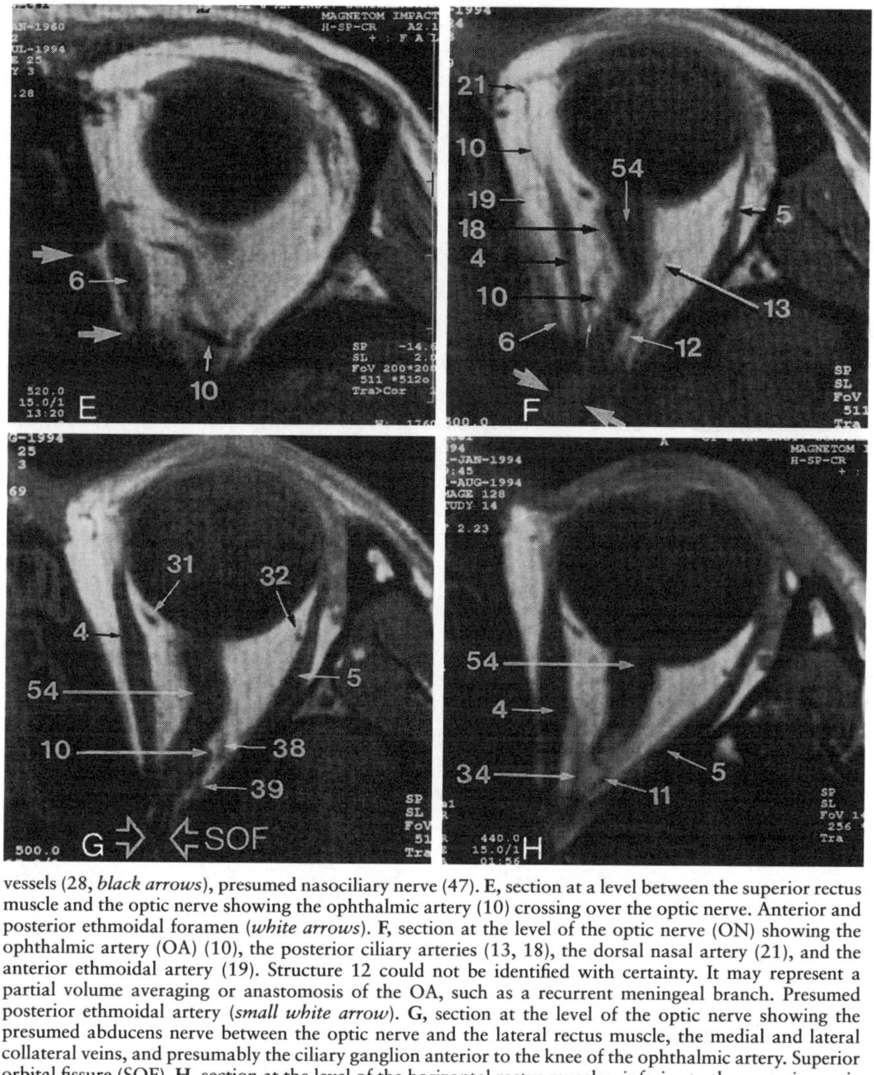

vessels (28, *black arrows*), presumed nasociliary nerve (47). **E,** section at a level between the superior rectus muscle and the optic nerve showing the ophthalmic artery (10) crossing over the optic nerve. Anterior and posterior ethmoidal foramen (*white arrows*). **F,** section at the level of the optic nerve (ON) showing the ophthalmic artery (OA) (10), the posterior ciliary arteries (13, 18), the dorsal nasal artery (21), and the anterior ethmoidal artery (19). Structure 12 could not be identified with certainty. It may represent a partial volume averaging or anastomosis of the OA, such as a recurrent meningeal branch. Presumed posterior ethmoidal artery (*small white arrow*). **G,** section at the level of the optic nerve showing the presumed abducens nerve between the optic nerve and the lateral rectus muscle, the medial and lateral collateral veins, and presumably the ciliary ganglion anterior to the knee of the ophthalmic artery. Superior orbital fissure (SOF). **H,** section at the level of the horizontal rectus muscles, inferior to the posterior optic nerve, showing the central retinal artery (11) and the presumed "veine ophthalmique moyenne" (34), a variation that originates from the medial rectus muscle to drain into the cavernous sinus. **I,** section through the posterior part of the inferior rectus muscle (3) and the inferior orbital fissure (IOF), showing the inferior ophthalmic vein (30), the medial and lateral collateral veins (31, 32), the orbital muscle of Müller (M), and the lacrimal sac (*white arrowheads*). **J,** section at the level of the IOF: the structure (36), which courses along the lateral border of the inferior rectus muscle (3), either represents the branch of the oculomotor nerve supplying the inferior oblique muscle (9) or a muscular branch of the inferior ophthalmic vein. Orbital muscle of Müller (M). (Published courtesy of *Ophthalmology*, from Ettl A, Kramer J, Daxer A, et al: High-resolution magnetic resonance imaging of neurovascular orbital anatomy. *Ophthalmology* 104:869–877, 1997.)

(*Continued*)

FIGURE 4 (cont.)

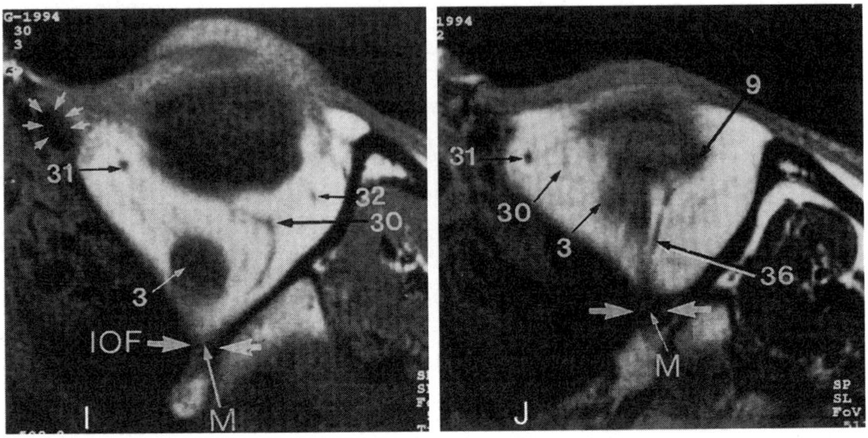

tion surface coil images of the orbit. The images presented in this study are T1-weighted, producing contrast by fat tissue interface. The anatomical detail presented in this study is excellent and, more importantly, obtainable in most centers with a standard 1.5-T magnet and surface coil technology. One interesting bit of information in this paper is the concept of vascular structures in the orbit. The authors suggest that arteries radiate in a divergent fashion from the orbital apex and traverse the adipose compartments and perforate the orbital septa. Veins are arranged in a ring-like system that incorporates them into the fibrous septa of the orbital connective tissue. The superior ophthalmic vein traverses the orbit inside the "superior ophthalmic vein hammock," which is a connective tissue septum that is located just inferior to the superior rectus muscle. The authors hypothesize that a swollen inflamed superior rectus, such as in Graves' disease or, perhaps, in orbital myositis can induce orbital soft-tissue swelling out of proportion to enlargement of the muscles.

The paper is worth spending some time reading, particularly for those individuals interested in imaging of the orbit. I must say that it is somewhat disconcerting to be switching between the Appendix, which provides a nomenclature, and the images in the text. Nevertheless, this is a very nice, detailed anatomical lesson.

R.I. Grossman, M.D.

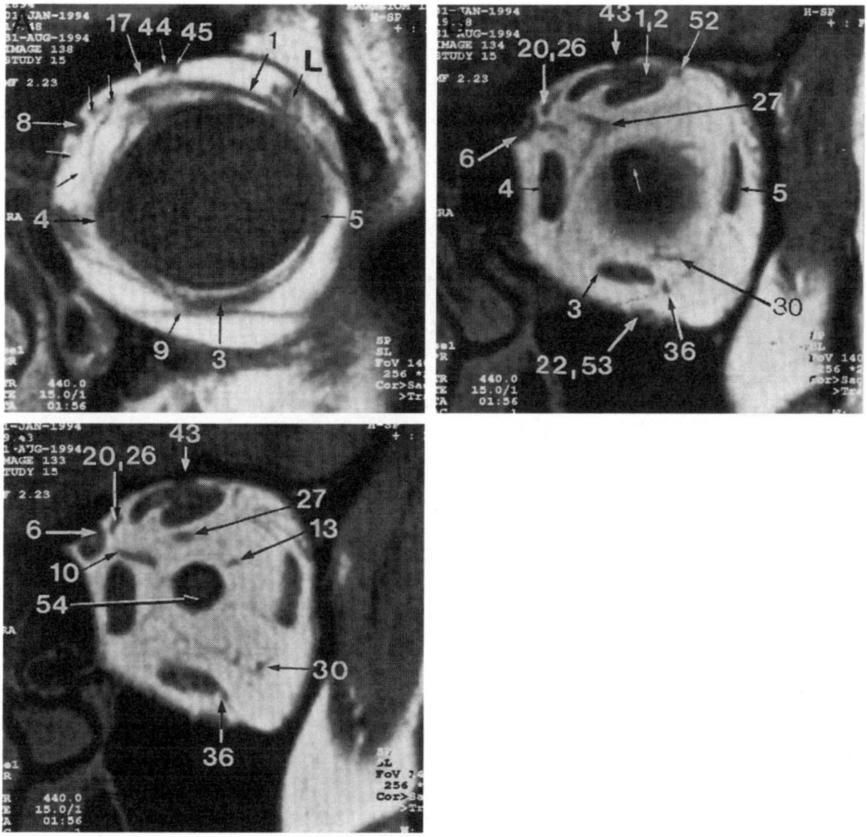

FIGURE 5.—Coronal T1-weighted MR images (right orbit, healthy research subject). The numbers refer to the nomenclature of the structures (see Appendix in original article). **A,** imaging plane at the level of the trochlea (8 indicates superior oblique tendon inside trochlea) "infracochlear" (2 *arrows inferior to trochlea*) neurovascular structures. An exact differentiation between arteries, veins, and the accompanying supratrochlear and infratrochlear nerves is not possible. Lacrimal gland (L). **B,** imaging plane through the posterior pole of the globe: the structure at the lateral border of the inferior rectus muscle most likely represents the branch of the inferior division of the oculomotor nerve (36), which supplies the inferior oblique muscle. Alternatively, it may be a muscular artery or vein. Frontal nerve (43), infraorbital neurovascular bundle (22, 53), supratrochlear vessels (20, 26), presumed lacrimal nerve (52). The hypointense signal superior to the posterior pole of the eye is caused by CSF in the subarachnoid space around the optic nerve (*arrow*). **C,** imaging plane 3 mm behind the globe showing the ophthalmic artery (10), the lateral posterior ciliary artery (13), the superior (27) and inferior (30) ophthalmic veins, the presumed inferior division of the oculomotor nerve (36), and the nasociliary nerve (47). (Published courtesy of *Ophthalmology*, from Ettl A, Kramer J, Dazer A, et al: High resolution magnetic resonance imaging of neurovascular orbital anatomy. *Ophthalmology* 104:869–877, 1997.)

Temporal Crescent Syndrome With Magnetic Resonance Correlation

Chavis PS, Al-Hazmi A, Clunie D, et al (Univ of California, San Francisco)
J Neuroophthalmol 17:151–155, 1997 9–16

Background.—Also known as half-moon syndrome, temporal crescent syndrome is characterized by a sudden loss of vision in the temporal visual field on 1 side. This case report describes the use of MRI to correlate visual field findings in a patient with temporal crescent syndrome.

> *Case Report.*—A 23-year-old woman had delivered a baby 40 days earlier. At delivery she had peripartum hypertension (blood pressure 180/10 mm Hg), severe diffuse headache, pedal edema, and a sudden loss of vision in the temporal periphery on the left. At the evaluation by these authors 40 days later, results of neurologic and laboratory testing were normal. Results of the ophthalmic examination were also normal, except for a temporal crescent peripheral field defect in the left eye. A CT scan showed a band of low focal density in the medial right occipital lobe. MRI 6 and 18 months later showed a dilated parietoccipital sulcus consistent with atrophy and gliosis in the calcarine cortex surrounding the sulcus. Disruption of the blood supply of the parietooccipital and calcarine arteries was also evident.

Conclusions.—The cresent-shaped peripheral defect affected less than 10% of the visual cortex and involved not only the parietooccipital sulcus, but also the calcarine cortex. Furthermore, parietooccipital and calcarine branches of the posterior cerebral artery, and even the temporal artery, were also affected. Thus, further cortical and arterial involvement should be sought when a patient has a visual defect mapped to the parietooccipital sulcus.

▶ The temporal crescent (half-moon) syndrome is characterized by sudden unilateral loss of vision in the temporal peripheral field. Most interesting about this syndrome is the monocular nature of this retrochiasmatic visual pathway lesion. The authors raise important points including the fact that monocular peripheral temporal visual field deficits are more often caused by retinal lesions than by cortical lesion and that a monocular retrochiasmatic field deficit in the parietal occipital sulcus can be correlated with peripheral temporal crescentic deficit. This lesion constitutes less than 10% of the striate cortex area supplied by the parietal occipital artery.

R.I. Grossman, M.D.

10 Ocular Oncology

Does Fine-needle Aspiration Biopsy Have a Role in the Diagnostic Evaluation of Small Melanocytic Choroidal Lesions?

by James J. Augsburger, M.D.

In spite of refinements in instrumentation for visualizing and imaging fundus lesions during the past 25 years, differentiating between large benign choroidal nevi and small malignant choroidal melanomas remains difficult. Various clinical features of such lesions (including larger lesion size, presence of prominent clumps of orange pigment on the surface of the lesion, absence of drusen and prominent retinal pigment epithelial alterations on the surface of the lesion, and presence of subretinal fluid overlying and around the lesion) have been identified as prognostic factors for tumor enlargement if the lesion is observed over time without treatment. The greater the number of unfavorable features exhibited by a small melanocytic choroidal lesion, the higher the probability that the lesion will enlarge if left untreated, and the greater its likelihood of being a melanoma rather than a benign nevus.

Of course, all small melanomas do not enlarge rapidly if observed, and many small nevi enlarge to a limited extent over long intervals of follow-up. Because of this, it should be obvious that the presence of unfavorable prognostic features for lesion enlargement and even documented lesion growth are not entirely satisfactory surrogate indicators of the clinical malignancy of a melanocytic choroidal lesion.

Fine-needle aspiration biopsy (FNAB) is an invasive diagnostic technique in which a surgeon attempts to obtain a small specimen of a solid lesion for cytopathologic assessment and possibly other studies. Although FNAB is used extensively in clinical oncology, it is employed rather infrequently in the evaluation of intraocular mass lesions. The major reasons for limited use of FNAB for the evaluation of presumed intraocular cancers include the following: (1) high diagnostic accuracy rate if experienced examiners evaluate a lesion and obtain and review appropriate noninvasive or minimally invasive diagnostic tests; (2) unfamiliarity or lack of experience with the techniques of intraocular FNAB; (3) lack of cytopathologists experienced in the diagnosis of intraocular neoplasms and simulating lesions; (4) concern that FNAB may liberate tumor cells into the venous blood or seed tumor cells along the needle tract and thereby promote metastasis or reimplantation growth of a primary intraocular malignant neoplasm; and (5) concern that FNAB will cause uncorrectable visual loss in the affected eye. Studies reported to date provide rather compelling evidence that the concerns mentioned above are not justified on the basis of clinical experience.

In spite of these reasons, FNAB appears to be an attractive option for evaluating selected intraocular tumors in ocular oncology referral centers in which experienced clinicians perform the biopsies and experienced cytopathologists interpret them. FNAB has proven useful for confirming metastatic carcinoma in patients with a presumed choroidal metastasis but no evidence of a primary tumor or other metastatic lesions on comprehensive systemic evaluation, for confirming the pathologic nature of atypical fundus lesions in patients with known systemic cancer, and for confirming the diagnosis of choroidal melanoma prior to enucleation in patients who refuse recommended treatment in the absence of pathologic confirmation of the diagnosis.[1–3] But FNAB for the evaluation of small but worrisome melanocytic choroidal lesions (i.e., ones that could be either large benign nevi or small malignant melanomas) is controversial. There are several reasons why this is so. First, FNAB is rather frequently associated with a "QNS" (quantity not sufficient) sample result. Second, there is no published evidence indicating how well a cytologic diagnosis of nevus vs. melanoma correlates with the histopathologic diagnosis of such lesions. There is clearly considerable difficulty in distinguishing atypical nevus cells from low-grade melanoma cells. Third, there is an indeterminate risk of sampling error. Unless the cytopathologic diagnostic accuracy rate can be shown to be high, we may well be deluding ourselves if we believe the cytopathologic report without reservation and act upon that cytopathologic diagnosis.

We are currently reviewing our experience with FNAB of small melanocytic choroidal tumors in an attempt to assess the validity of some of these criticisms. As a result of our analyses, we hope to be able to provide better insight into the role of FNAB in such lesions in the near future.

References

1. Augsburger JJ, Shields JA: Fine needle aspiration biopsy of solid intraocular tumors: Indications, instrumentation and techniques. *Ophthalmic Surg Lasers* 15:34–40, 1984.
2. Augsburger JJ, Shields JA, Folberg R, et al: Fine needle aspiration biopsy in the diagnosis of intraocular cancer: Cytologic-histologic correlations. *Ophthalmology* 92:39–49, 1985.
3. Augsburger JJ: Fine needle aspiration biopsy of suspected metastatic carcinomas to the posterior uvea. *Trans Am Ophthalmol Soc* 86:499–560, 1988.

Orbital Metastases: Diagnosis and Course
Char DH, Miller T, Kroll S (Univ of California, San Francisco)
Br J Ophthalmol 81:386–390, 1997 10–1

Background.—Orbital metastases are an uncommon cause of proptosis in adults. Metastatic orbital tumors are significantly less common than uveal metastases. Several studies have reported a relative incidence of 1:8. The authors sought to answer 3 questions about orbital metastases based on their experience with 31 patients. These questions involved the accuracy of current diagnostic techniques, survival rates associated with orbital metastases, and the correlation of clinical factors and prognosis.

Methods.—In a retrospective study, 31 outpatients with orbital metastases treated during a 20-year period (1976–1995) in the authors' center were analyzed. All patients had CT, MR, or both types of imaging. The patient group consisted of 15 men and 16 women, and the median patient age was 57 years.

Results.—Of the 31 patients, 11 had no known primary tumor at the time of diagnosis. The predominant orbital symptoms were diplopia in 48% of patients, proptosis in 26%, and decreased vision in 16%. All 31 lesions were detected by CT, MRI, or both. Interestingly, the authors did not find a single case in which MR was superior to CT for establishing a diagnosis of metastasis. Several imaging patterns were believed to be typical of orbital metastases, including intramuscular focal masses, bone

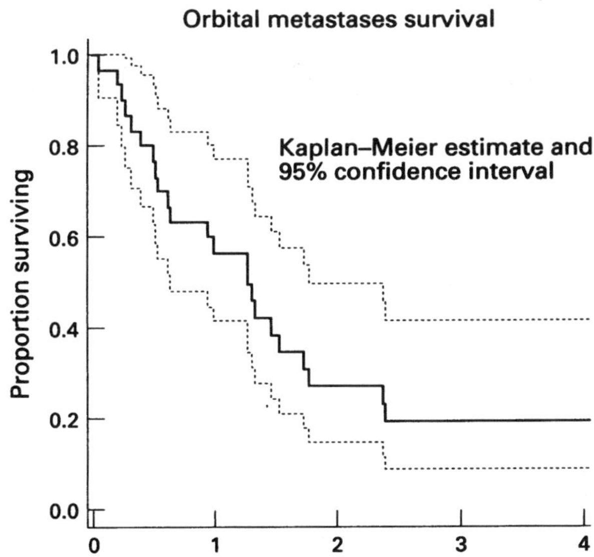

FIGURE 5.—Kaplan-Meier survival curve of patients with orbital metastases. The mean survival time for patients with orbital metastases was 1.3 years. The 2-year survival rate was 27% (31 patients). (Reprinted with permission of the BMJ Publishing Group, from Char DH, Miller T, Kroll S: Orbital metastases: Diagnosis and course. *Br J Ophthalmol* 81:386–390, 1997.)

destruction plus contiguous mass, and diffuse intraconal lesions. Fine-needle aspiration biopsy established the diagnosis in 15 patients. Treatment options were tumor debulking, photon or heavy charged particle irradiation (for metastatic cutaneous melanoma), and chemotherapy (for patients with widespread systemic disease). Median survival was 1.3 years. Survival at 2 years was 27% (Fig 5).

Discussion.—Orbital metastases can be difficult to diagnose, even with current diagnostic methods. The management of these patients was based on the location and extent of orbital and systemic disease and vision. Orbital symptoms were palliated in most patients, but survival was low. There was no correlation between any clinical factor and outcome.

► This article provides a nice overview of the current status of diagnosis and treatment of patients with metastatic carcinoma to the orbit from various primary cancers. The diagnostic approach described by the authors includes comprehensive clinical examination; detailed review and consideration of the patient's prior medical–surgical history; imaging of the orbit by CT, MRI, or both; and biopsy of the orbital mass by fine-needle aspiration or incisional techniques for patients in whom the diagnosis remains uncertain. Treatment of orbital metastases consists of debulking large lesions, radiation therapy, chemotherapy, or a combination of these techniques. Although this treatment approach is usually effective in controlling local disease, the survival prognosis of patients with orbital metastasis is generally quite poor, as indicated in Fig 5.

J.J. Augsburger, M.D.

Mortality in Patients With Small Choroidal Melanoma: COMS Report No. 4

Melia BM, and The Collaborative Ocular Melanoma Study Group (Kellogg Eye Ctr, Ann Arbor, Mich)

Arch Ophthalmol 115:886–893, 1997 10–2

Background.—The Collaborative Ocular Melanoma Study consists of 2 randomized clinical trials, 1 for large tumors and another for medium size tumors, and a nonrandomized longitudinal study of small tumors. The purpose of this work was to describe the baseline clinical characteristics and survival experience of the patients in the small tumors group.

Methods.—There were 204 patients enrolled in this study, in which small choroidal melanomas were defined as 1.0–3.0 mm in apical height and at least 5.0 mm in basal diameter. Patients were followed up annually, for at least 3 years and then 2 additional assessments of treatment status and mortality were performed 4 and 5 years later. Ninety-two months was the median length of follow-up. At the time of study enrollment, 8% of patients were treated; during follow-up, an additional 33% were treated.

Results.—Death occurred in 27 patients, six of these deaths were caused by metastatic melanoma. Four of the 6 deaths occurred more than 5 years after enrollment. Patients with tumors that had been diagnosed within 180 days before enrollment, were observed initially, and were subsequently treated during followup, comprised the pool from which all 6 deaths from metastatic melanoma occurred. The 5-year all-cause mortality rate was 6%, and the 8-year all-cause mortality rate was 14.9%. An increased risk of death was seen among older patients, patients with a history of diabetes, and patients with more anteriorly located tumors and more recently diagnosed tumors.

Conclusions.—There is a low risk of dying within 5 years among otherwise healthy patients with an average age of 60 years, without a previous diagnosis of malignant disease who have small choroidal lesions. A small choroidal melanoma treatment trial should be conducted with a follow-up of at least 10 years and a large sample size.

▶ Although the information presented in this report is interesting, I find the principal conclusion reached by the authors (that "a small choroidal melanoma treatment trial is feasible") frankly astonishing. The authors acknowledge that the 5-year melanoma-specific mortality rate is low, that a randomized clinical trial of alternative treatment options for such small choroidal melanomas would require a very large sample size, and that all enrolled patients would need to be followed for at least 10 years just to see whether a significant difference in mortality rates occurred with the different treatments. The authors do not specify the magnitude of a difference in 10-year melanoma-specific mortality distributions they would consider significant or provide values of alpha and beta they believe to be appropriate for a study of this type. Without this information, readers can only guess at what the authors mean when they mention that a "large sample size" will be required. Furthermore, the authors do not indicate the methods of treatment they think would be appropriate to compare in such a trial or comment on the expected cost of such a study. As many readers probably know, I have frequently criticized the COMS randomized clinical trials for medium-size and large choroidal melanomas because of sample size issues. I think that the likelihood of a successful randomized treatment trial for small choroidal melanomas is between slim and none.

J.J. Augsburger, M.D.

Surgical Management of Conjunctival Tumors

Shields JA, Shields CL, De Potter P (Wills Eye Hosp, Philadelphia)
Arch Ophthalmol 115:808–815, 1997 10–3

Background.—There are no clear guidelines for the management of conjunctival neoplasms. Nor are there any specific, step-by-step instructions for surgical resection of these tumors, whether premalignant or malignant. The authors detailed their surgical approach to conjunctival neoplasms.

Conjunctival Tumors Arising at the Limbus.—For patients with conjunctival tumors arising at the limbus, the conjunctiva, cornea, and scleral tissues affected should be excised completely. The tumor is removed completely in a single procedure. Incisional biopsy is rarely needed to establish the diagnosis of carcinoma or melanoma, except when orbital exenteration of an extensive tumor is planned. Frozen sections are not needed for localized conjunctival malignancies, as the excisional borders will be adequate and the tumor margins are frozen after excision. If tumor extension to the resection margin is a possibility, a biopsy specimen of the margin can be obtained before cryotherapy is applied.

> *Technique.*—Surgical removal of tumors arising from the limbus begins with localized alcohol corneal epitheliectomy, with absolute alcohol applied using a cotton swab. The alcohol is applied to the corneal epithelium and to the tumor adjacent to the limbus. The next step is wide resection of the tumor using a no-touch technique. The surgeon uses the blade to scroll the epithelium, attempting to remove it intact. Next, the conjunctival part of the tumor is removed by partial lamellar scleroconjunctivectomy. The incision should include at least 4–5 mm of normal conjunctiva. A thin base of sclera is removed from beneath the tumor. The base is grasped with fine-toothed forceps. The tumor can then be removed, along with the scleral base. After the specimen is treated and bleeding is controlled, cryotherapy is applied to the margins of the exposed bulbar conjunctiva. Finally, the wound is closed using running or interrupted 6-0 or 7-0 absorbable suture.

Tumors Arising from the Extralimbal Bulbar and Forniceal Conjunctiva.—Some malignancies arise from extralacrimal locations in the bulbar, forniceal, or palpebral conjunctiva. They carry an increased danger of orbital invasion or regional lymph node metastasis, especially if the tumor is a melanoma. Patients with suspected orbital involvement should undergo MRI. If orbital involvement is absent, alcohol is applied around the tumor and a circular conjunctival incision with a margin of at least 5 mm is made. The incision continues down into bare sclera, and the tumor is removed along with a thick pseudocapsule of Tenon fascia. Cryotherapy and closure are carried out as for limbal tumors. For larger defects, flaps or grafts may be needed for closure. Care must be taken to avoid seeding tumor cells to the fellow eye or the buccal mucosa.

Discussion.—Based on long experience, the authors present the first detailed approach to surgical management of conjunctival tumors. They emphasize the importance of minimal manipulation, or a "no-touch" technique. Especially for tumors near the limbus and adherent to underlying structures, scleral dissection is an important part of the resection. Cryotherapy helps avoid tumor recurrence. The techniques described appear to offer good results in the management of conjunctival malignancies, especially squamous cell tumors, melanomas, and primary acquired melanosis.

► The approach to excision of solid epithelial neoplasms of the limbal conjunctiva described by the authors is generally quite good. However, I disagree with them regarding their almost routine use of lamellar sclerokeratectomy as an adjunct to excision of limbal lesions at the limbus. Part of my disagreement stems from the fact that even normal conjunctiva is usually quite strongly adherent to the sclera at the limbus. Consequently, using apparent adherence of the lesion at the limbus as a determining factor in favor of lamellar sclerokeratectomy means that virtually all cases will require this step.

Another part of my disagreement on this point stems from the fact that lamellar sclerokeratectomy thins the sclera in cases with deep scleral invasion but does not remove all of the tumor. If histopathologic study of the excised superficial layers of limbal cornea and sclera reveals tumor cells extending to the innermost surface, some form of supplemental treatment will be required. The thin sclera will make subsequent treatments such as ^{90}Sr applicator radiotherapy or epibulbar ^{125}I or ^{106}Ru plaque radiotherapy potentially much more dangerous because it increases the risk of eye wall necrosis at the site of thinning.

I also disagree with the authors regarding the value of routine conjunctival cryotherapy around the margins of the excised site. To my knowledge, the most important predictor of satisfactory local tumor control after excision of a limbal lesion is adequate surgical margins confirmed by histopathologic study. In a center that specializes in treatment of ocular tumors, it is hoped that the surgeons will take great care to map out the extent of the lesion clinically before surgery and to then use that information to ensure adequate margins around the lesion. In my opinion, most eyes managed in this way will not benefit from supplemental cryotherapy, and this added step will increase conjunctival swelling and, thereby, prolong healing in most of them.

Another criticism of the techniques described by the authors concerns the limited attention they devote to conjunctival closure after resection. The authors indicate that primary conjunctival closure is simply a matter of extending the conjunctival incision around the limbus, undermining the conjunctiva and separating Tenon's fascia and deep substantial propria from the epithelium and superficial substantia propria, mobilizing the thin superficial conjunctiva toward the surgical defect, and placing and tying several interrupted or running absorbable sutures.

Anyone who has excised numerous conjunctival tumors knows that nice conjunctival closure (shown in the illustrations in the original article) simply does not happen. Primary closure, as described, would cause substantial overriding of the limbus by a ridge of conjunctiva at both margins of the defect, as well as a bulky fold of conjunctiva at the forniceal margin of the closed defect. In my surgery, I stress cosmetic methods of conjunctival closure to the residents and fellows and emphasize techniques including relaxing excision, excision of Burrow's-type triangles to prevent ridges and folds, and even the use of pedicle flaps and bridge transposition flaps.

J.J. Augsburger, M.D.

Ocular Non-Hodgkin's Lymphoma: A Clinical Study of Nine Cases

Verbraeken HE, Hanssens M, Priem H, et al (Univ Hosp of Ghent, Belgium)
Br J Ophthalmol 81:31–36, 1997 10–4

Background.—The number of reported cases of ocular non-Hodgkin's lymphoma is increasing. Ocular involvement is rare in Hodgkin's lymphoma but common in non-Hodgkin's lymphomas. There are 2 recognized forms of disease: primary oculo-central nervous system non-Hodgkin's lymphoma and systemic non-Hodgkin's lymphoma with secondary metastatic ocular involvement. Primary ocular non-Hodgkin's lymphoma used to be called ocular reticulum cell sarcoma, but it is now considered a large-cell non-Hodgkin's lymphoma. Primary ocular non-Hodgkin's lymphoma is often followed by CNS non-Hodgkin's lymphoma, although primary CNS lymphoma is only associated in 12% to 15% of cases with ocular involvement. Patients with primary oculo-central nervous system large-cell non-Hodgkin's lymphoma have limited life expectancy. Treatment can improve the quality of life.

Methods.—The medical records of all patients with non-Hodgkin's lymphoma with ocular involvement between 1984 and 1993 were reviewed. Complete hematologic staging was done in all patients with suspected non-Hodgkin's lymphoma.

Results.—The medical records of 9 patients were examined. There were 6 men and 3 women, and the age range was 36 to 75 years. Eight patients had oculo-cerebral large-cell non-Hodgkin's lymphoma, and 1 patient had small-cell non-Hodgkin's lymphoma. The first symptoms of disease were ocular manifestations in 4 patients. In 1 patient, ocular and CNS localizations were diagnosed simultaneously. Central nervous system involvement was present when ocular symptoms occurred in 2 patients. In 5 patients with pure ocular localization, steroid treatment for intermediate uveitis had been administered. The diagnosis was made by CNS biopsy in 3 patients, anterior chamber tap in 1, vitreous aspirate in 3, hematology in 1, and necropsy in 1.

Discussion.—Primary ocular non-Hodgkin's lymphoma is difficult to diagnose and is often misdiagnosed as uveitis; a high degree of suspicion is essential. In most cases, vitrectomy permits a cytologic diagnosis. Remission can often be achieved with radiotherapy, steroids, and chemotherapy, alone or in combination. Recurrences are common and patients die of their lymphoma within a few years of diagnosis. Treatment can improve the patient's quality of life between recurrences. Steroid treatment, vitrectomy, radiotherapy, chemotherapy or a combination of those modalities can save the vision of most patients.

▶ This timely article serves as a reminder regarding the poor survival prognosis in patients with primary non-Hodgkin's lymphoma of the retina and CNS. The median survival after initial ocular manifestations in this group of patients was between 2 and 3 years. Hopefully, new forms of combination chemotherapy or other methods of treatment that improve this prognosis will become available in the not-too-distant future.

J.J. Augsburger, M.D.

Long-term Results After Low Dose Ocular Irradiation for Choroidal Haemangiomas

Schilling H, Sauerwein W, Lommatzsch A, et al (Univ Eye Hosp, Essen, Germany; Univ Essen, Germany)

Br J Ophthalmol 81:267–273, 1997 10–5

Introduction.—Choroidal hemangiomas (CH) have generally been treated by surface photocoagulation. However, in eyes with an extensive exudative retinal detachment, this approach frequently requires repeated treatments or additional invasive interventions. A possible alternative approach is low-dose external beam irradiation. This low-dose irradiation approach to the treatment of CH was studied.

Methods.—The study group consisted of 48 patients (51 eyes) with symptomatic CH. Thirty-six eyes had a circumscribed CH of the posterior pole, and 15 had a diffuse CH as part of the Sturge-Weber syndrome. All patients were treated because of exudative retinal detachment that included or was threatening the fovea. Treatment consisted of external irradiation with high-energy photons via a lateral field. The standard total absorbed dose was 20 Gy given in 10 fractions of 2 Gy each. Mean follow-up was 4.5 years in the patients with circumscribed CH and 5.3 years in those with diffuse CH. Reliable information on symptom onset was available for 33 patients, 17 of whom had symptoms longer than 6 months.

Results.—Treatment resulted in complete resolution of subretinal fluid in 64% of eyes with a circumscribed CH. The other 36% of eyes were left with some serous detachment located away from the fovea. Thirty-nine percent of patients in this group had their visual acuity improve by 2 lines or more, 39% had stable acuity, and 22% had reduced acuity. The functional results depended largely on the duration between the patient's first symptoms and treatment.

The eyes with diffuse CH showed similar morphological results. Visual acuity improved in 47% of eyes and was unchanged or worsened in the rest. The poor functional outcomes in this group were largely related to secondary glaucoma.

Conclusions.—Low-dose external beam irradiation appears to be an effective, noninvasive treatment alternative for patients with CH. The visual results depend on how soon after initial symptoms the treatment begins. For patients with CH associated with Sturge-Weber syndrome, the occurrence of subretinal fibrosis is also associated with poor visual results.

► Treatment of CH by low-dose fractionated external beam radiation therapy is not new. However, it has taken most of the last 20 years for ophthalmologists to become aware that such treatment is effective against these benign choroidal vascular tumors and the serous retinal detachments they produce. In retrospect, it appears that most of us have been so worried about the potential long-term adverse consequences of ocular radiation therapy that we have withheld this treatment until too late. Consequently, many eyes in the current series and in my own experience have not regained any vision even though the hemangioma regressed and the associated retinal detachment diminshed or resolved. In a concurrent editorial by Plowman and Hungerford[1] from London, England, radioactive plaque brachytherapy is emphasized as an alternative to low-dose fractionated external beam radiotherapy for eyes with diffuse or circumscribed CH. The precise relative benefits vs. risks of these 2 radiotherapy approaches are uncertain but appear to warrant further study.

J.J. Augsburger, M.D.

Reference

1. Plowman PN, Hungerford JL: Radiotherapy for ocular angiomas (editorial). *Br J Ophthalmol* 81:258–259, 1997.

Cost Comparison of Molecular Versus Conventional Screening of Relatives at Risk for Retinoblastoma

Norrani HZ, Khan HN, Gallie BL, et al (Univ of Toronto; Hosp for Sick Children, Toronto; Eye Research Inst of Canada, Toronto; et al)

Am J Hum Genet 59:301–307, 1996 10–6

Purpose.—Retinoblastoma (RB) is a frequent childhood cancer that has hereditary and nonhereditary forms. Because parents and grandparents can be unaffected carriers of RB1 gene mutations, children who are relatives of affected patients are routinely screened for RB. This is generally done by repeated ophthalmologic examination under general anesthesia. It is now possible to detect the RB1 mutation by molecular analysis. The costs of genetic and conventional screening for relatives at risk of RB were compared.

Methods.—The study used a decision-analysis model to compare the 2 strategies. The direct health care costs associated with each approach were ascertained. Sensitivity analysis was performed to test the assumptions made in the analytical model.

Results.—The expected costs of conventional RB screening for a prototypical family with 7 relatives at risk were $31,430, in 1994 Canadian dollars. This included 3 clinical examinations and 8 examinations under general anesthesia over the first 3 years of life for each relative at risk. For the genetic approach, the expected cost was only $8,674. This approach included identification of the RB1 gene mutation in the proband, testing relatives at risk for the mutation, and performing clinical follow-up in relatives with the mutation. Molecular screening was more economical across the range of assumptions in the study model.

Conclusions.—Molecular screening appears to be less expensive than conventional screening for at-risk relatives of patients with RB. The results of this decision-analysis study suggest that resources are better directed toward the molecular strategy for identification of mutations in the RB1 gene. The clinical outcomes of the two approaches were not analyzed.

► In this article, the authors use multiple assumptions to derive comparative estimated costs of "molecular" vs. "conventional" screening of relatives at risk for RB. Several of their assumptions are not necessarily correct. For example, the authors indicate that 'at risk infant relatives' of children with RB *must* undergo ophthalmic examinations under anesthesia at 5, 7, 9, 12, and 16 months of age and every 6 months thereafter up to age 3 years. To my knowledge, there has never been a comparative clinical study evaluating the relative effectiveness of unanesthetized ophthalmic examinations in the office (with sedation and restraint of the child, as needed) vs. ophthalmic examinations under anesthesia in young at risk relatives performed by the same qualified examiners for detecting new RB lesions of a locally controllable size and extent.

Unlike the authors, I perform almost all examinations on young at risk relatives in the office. I use topical anesthesia and a lid speculum and perform scleral depression to see the ora serrata if that anatomical site cannot be visualized without this manuever. Only if I am unable to obtain a satisfactory view or detect a potentially treatable lesion do I proceed to examination under anesthesia EUA. There is no question that outpatient examinations of such children in the office are much less expensive than EUAs. The question then appears to be whether the substantially more costly EUAs provide meaningfully higher rates of local tumor control, visual preservation, and ocular preservation than do outpatient ophthalmic examinations in the office.

Another bothersome assumption of this analysis is that young relatives of children with RB who are evaluated by molecular methods and determined to be at no apparent increased risk of RB relative to background need not be monitored ophthalmically. If prediction of risk of RB on the basis of molecular studies were a completely reliable technique, then this might be true. However, there are enough cases of RB that were not predicted by genetic analysis to warrant continued outpatient examination of such children. The costs of such evaluations must be added to the equation.

Other factors not addressed in this article but of great importance clinically include the length of time required to complete the family genetic analysis and the medicolegal implications of risk predictions based on genetic testing. With regard to the former point, complete genetic analysis of a prototype RB family (as defined by the authors) usually requires about 6–12 months at present. Because of the length of this testing interval, the authors would need to perform several examinations using anesthesia (according to their schedule) on some children who do not prove to be genetically at risk of developing RB before to completion of testing. The costs of these examinations must be added to their molecular screening estimate. With regard to the second point, if a laboratory predicts that an infant or young child is not at risk but, in spite of the prediction, that child develops RB, then the laboratory and individuals in that laboratory are subject to suit for erroneous prediction and possible resultant delay in diagnosis. Most laboratories involved in genetic testing get around this point by insisting that their predictions are for research purposes only and should not be used in clinical decision making. Of course, use of risk predictions based on genetic testing for clinical decision making is exactly what the authors of this paper suggest should be done. Several laboratories in the United States no longer provide risk predictions to families because of such medicolegal considerations.

J.J. Augsburger, M.D.

Transvitreal Retino-choroidal Biopsy of Suspected Malignant Lesions of the Choroid: Follow-up of Cases Over 7 Years

Jensen OA, Prause JU, Scherfig E (Univ of Copenhagen; Rigshospitalet, Copenhagen)

Acta Ophthalmol Scand 75:409–411, 1997 10–7

Objective.—The authors perform transvitreal retino-choroidal (TVRC) biopsy in malignant melanomas of the choroid and other suspected neoplastic lesions. The efficiency, side effects, and outcomes of this technique were studied.

Patients and Findings.—The 7-year experience included 92 patients undergoing TVRC biopsy: 51 men and 41 women, aged 16–88 years. Ninety-one biopsies produced sufficient material for diagnosis. A malignant neoplasm was detected in 87% of biopsies, almost always malignant melanoma of the choroid. The biopsy was negative in 10 cases and unsuccessful in 2. Brachytherapy was used for tumors of suitable size. In 23 cases, the tumor was so large as to require primary enucleation. Another 8 eyes had to be removed after radiation therapy. These 31 eyes were analyzed for changes caused by the biopsy, and to assess the results of biopsy typing with those of whole-tumor typing. In eyes examined after radiation therapy, viable tumor cells were found mainly in the inner part of the tumor. There was no evidence of scleral necrosis.

Conclusions.—Transvitreal retino-choroidal biopsy appears to be a safe and efficient procedure. It effectively ensures that the irradiated lesion is malignant; such verification is needed before any conservative therapy is given. The biopsy procedure appears to have no effect on prognosis. The authors apply argon endolaser around the puncture through the retina to ensure that the biopsy procedure does not cause retinal detachment.

► The results of this study confirm the previously reported clinical value of fine-needle aspiration biopsy in selected patients with a presumably malignant choroidal neoplasm. They also confirm the apparent long-term clinical safety of the technique. However, this work does not provide any useful information about which lesions *should* have a biopsy performed on them. According to the authors, they performed fine-needle aspiration biopsy on all presumed choroidal melanomas and other possibly malignant intraocular lesions referred to their center during the reported study interval. Given the high accuracy rate of intraocular tumor diagnosis (except for small melanocytic choroidal tumors) in major ocular oncology centers around the world, it is unclear why the authors felt the need to biopsy each and every lesion. The authors' decision to biopsy all *possibly* malignant intraocular lesions probably also explains how they could have performed a biopsy on a choroidal osteoma, 2 circumscribed choroidal hemangiomas, and a disciform macular lesion: the correct clinical diagnosis is usually not difficult in lesions of these types. It is also unfortunate that the authors did not provide more detailed descriptive statistics on the lesions in which they performed a biopsy. The available information does not, for example, allow readers to know how many biopsies of small tumors (i.e., less than 3 mm thick) were performed.

J.J. Augsburger, M.D.

Choroidal Hemangiomas: Visual and Anatomic Results of Treatment by Photocoagulation or Radiation Therapy

Madreperla SA, Hungerford JL, Plowman PN, et al (St Bartholomew's Hosp, London; Moorfields Eye Hosp, London)

Ophthalmology 104:1773–1779, 1997 10–8

Background.—In patients with choroidal hemangioma, subretinal fluid can accumulate, causing visual loss. The subretinal fluid collection can be treated with photocoagulation; however, fluid may recur and patients may be left with poor visual acuity. The results of radiation therapy vs. photocoagulation were retrospectively compared in patients with choroidal hemangiomas causing visual loss.

Methods.—Participants included 28 patients with choroidal hemangiomas with subretinal fluid accumulation causing visual loss. Twenty-three patients had circumscribed choroidal hemangiomas (CCH), and 5 had diffuse choroidal hemangiomas (DCH). In the CCD group, treatment consisted of photocoagulation for 13 patients, plaque brachytherapy for 8, and lens-sparing external beam radiotherapy (LSRT) for 2. All DCH patients were treated with LSRT. The visual and anatomical results of radiation therapy and photocoagulation were compared.

Findings.—One year after treatment, 75% of CCH patients treated with brachytherapy had visual acuity of 6/12 or better, and all were free of subretinal fluid. Of CCH patients treated with photocoagulation, 38% had visual acuity of 6/12 or better and 46% were free of subretinal fluid. Neither CCH patient treated with LSRT achieved visual acuity of 6/12 or better, although 1 was free of subretinal fluid. In the DCH group, LSRT eliminated subretinal fluid in all patients, improved vision in 2, and stabilized vision in 3.

Conclusions.—For patients with visual loss caused by subretinal fluid related to CCH, plaque brachytherapy is a useful treatment alternative. It provides good visual and anatomical results, compared with photocoagulation. For patients with DCH, good results are achieved with LSRT.

▶ These authors found that plaque radiotherapy provided substantially better visual outcomes than did laser therapy in eyes with CCH, provided that the irradiation was not delayed until irreversible retinal degeneration had occurred. This information is important because laser therapy is generally regarded as the standard treatment for eyes with CCH. The authors also confirmed the previously reported utility of relatively low-dose external beam radiation therapy in eyes with visual impairment caused by DCH. These results suggest that plaque and external beam radiotherapy should at least be considered as primary treatment for patients with symptomatic visual loss caused by a choroidal hemangioma.

J.J. Augsburger, M.D.

Cancer Incidence After Retinoblastoma: Radiation Dose and Sarcoma Risk

Wong FL, Boice JD Jr, Abramson DH, et al (NIH, Bethesda, Md; Univ of Texas, Houston; New York Hosp; et al)

JAMA 278:1262–1267, 1997 10–9

Introduction.—Although children with nonhereditary retinoblastomas do not appear to be at increased risk for second cancers, the risk for subsequent primary tumors is quite high among those with hereditary retinoblastoma. Children in the latter group have germline mutations in the retinoblastoma tumor suppressor gene, and their risk of a second cancer is further increased by radiotherapy. A study of survivors of childhood retinoblastoma examined their long-term risk of new primary cancers.

Methods.—A review of medical records of hospitals in Boston and New York identified a cohort of 1,729 retinoblastoma patients treated between 1914 and 1984. The study group consisted of 1,604 patients who survived at least 1 year after diagnosis. Patients whose retinoblastoma was classified as hereditary had bilateral tumors or unilateral tumor with a family history of retinoblastoma. To collect information on new cancers and family history, telephone interviews were conducted during 1987 to 1988 and in 1993. A nested case-control study investigated the radiation dose-response relationship for bone and soft tissue sarcomas.

Results.—The study cohort included 1,150 members diagnosed before the age of 2 years and 961 (60%) with hereditary retinoblastoma. Median follow-up duration was 22 years. Radiotherapy had been administered to

88% of hereditary patients and 18% of nonhereditary patients. A total of 199 additional cancers developed in 188 survivors at a median of 15.0 years after diagnosis of retinoblastoma. All but 9 of these cancers occurred in the hereditary group, and the incidence of subsequent cancers was statistically significantly elevated in this group (relative risk = 30). Fifty years after retinoblastoma was diagnosed, the cumulative incidence of second primary cancer was 51.0% in hereditary cases versus 5.0% in nonhereditary cases. Radiotherapy in hereditary patients increased risk of second cancer by 58.3% at 50 years of follow-up; the corresponding risk for nonirradiated hereditary patients was 26.5%. All 114 sarcomas occurred in the hereditary group, and a radiation risk for all sarcomas appeared at doses greater than 5 Gy.

Conclusion.—By age 40, survivors of childhood retinoblastoma were at exceptionally high risk for sarcoma, brain tumor, cutaneous melanoma, and pineoblastoma, confirming that germline mutations in the retinoblastoma gene exert a powerful carcinogenic effect on other tissues. The risk of second cancer is further increased by radiotherapy.

▶ Although several articles dealing with the increased incidence of second malignancies in survivors of hereditary retinoblastoma have been published, this is the first article to address specifically the relationship between radiation dose and subsequent development of soft tissue and bony sarcomas in this patient group. The authors found not only that the incidence of soft tissue and body sarcomas was increased substantially in these patients but also that the incidence of such tumors in the field of radiation was positively influenced by increasing radiation dose. One surprise in this data set was the finding that younger age of the affected patient at the time of treatment (younger than vs. older than 1-year-old) did not simultaneously influence the incidence of such tumors. The good news in this report is that most of the radiation-induced sarcomas appeared in patients who had undergone ocular-orbital radiotherapy by means of techniques employed a generation ago: these techniques included use of low-energy photon beams or electron beams and delivery of a relatively high dose of radiation. We hope long-term studies of retinoblastoma survivors treated by higher-energy photon beams and receiving a total dose less than 50 Gy will reveal substantially reduced frequencies of radiation-induced bony and soft tissue sarcomas.

J.J. Augsburger, M.D.

Metastatic Risk for Distinct Patterns of Postirradiation Local Recurrence of Posterior Uveal Melanoma

Harbour JW, Char DH, Kroll S, et al (Univ of California, San Francisco; Washington Univ, St Louis)

Ophthalmology 104:1785–1793, 1997 10–10

Introduction.—Local recurrence of posterior uveal melanoma is a potential complication after radiation therapy. These recurrences may occur

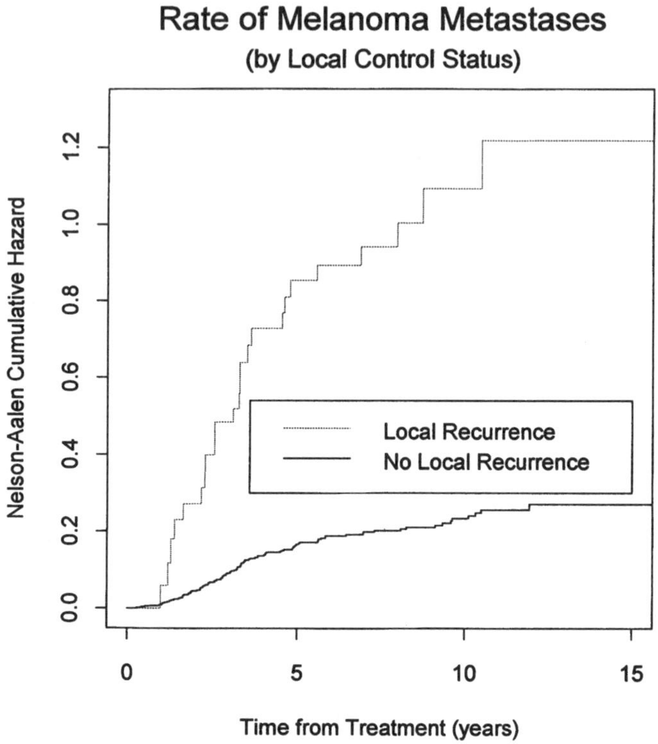

FIGURE 3.—Nelson-Aalen Cumulative Hazard plot of rate of systemic metastasis in patients with and without local recurrence. (Published courtesy of *Ophthalmology*, from Harbour JW, Char DH, Kroll S, et al: Metastatic risk for distinct patterns of postirradiation local recurrence of posterior uveal melanoma. *Ophthalmology* 104:1785–1793, 1997.)

in a horizontal/marginal or vertical/diffuse pattern. There have been no thorough analyses of the risk factors, treatment, or prognostic significance of these recurrence patterns. The prognostic implications of a horizontal/marginal or vertical/diffuse pattern of local recurrence of posterior uveal melanoma were examined.

Patients and Findings.—Participants included 766 patients treated with iodine-125 plaque or helium ion plaque radiation therapy for posterior uveal melanoma. At a median follow-up of 52 months, 66 patients had local recurrences. The recurrence was classified as horizontal/marginal in 27 patients and vertical/diffuse in 39. Corresponding 5-year actuarial recurrence rates were 4.6% and 5.6%, respectively. Nineteen percent of patients with horizontal/marginal recurrence had systemic metastases, compared with 49% of those with vertical/diffuse recurrence. The risk of metastases was elevated twofold for patients with horizontal/marginal recurrence and fivefold for those with vertical/diffuse recurrence. The actuarial rate of systemic metastases was 2.9% per year overall, 6.3% per year for patients with horizontal/marginal recurrence, and 15.5% per year for those with vertical/diffuse recurrence (Fig 3).

Conclusions.—Patients with local recurrence of posterior uveal melanoma after radiation therapy are at increased risk of systemic metastases. More aggressive melanomas may be more likely to recur, or inadequate treatment may increase the risk of metastasis as well as recurrence. The risk of metastases appears to be higher for patients with vertical/diffuse recurrences than with horizontal/marginal recurrences.

► This is an interesting paper, but the significance of the results is not obvious. The authors ostensibly evaluated the relationship between "pattern of postirradiation local recurrence of posterior uveal melanomas" and actuarial probability of postirradiation metastatic melanoma in a group of 766 patients. They showed, as others have shown previously, that the rate of melanoma metastasis was substantially higher among patients who experienced local tumor relapse. They did not show whether this relationship was attributable to an intrinsically greater potential of certain choroidal melanomas to recur locally and also metastasize, or whether local persistence of tumor gave rise to the subsequent metastasis in a substantial proportion of these patients who had metastasis. Given the limited number of cases with each type of local recurrence, the low postirradiation rates of metastatic disease in each recurrence pattern group, and the exploratory nature of this study, these findings must be regarded as preliminary and in need of confirmation on other groups of patients and by other investigators.

J.J. Augsburger, M.D.

Diagnosis of Intraocular Lymphoma by Flow Cytometry

Davis JL, Viciana AL, Ruiz P (Bascom Palmer Eye Inst, Miami, Fla; Univ of Miami, Fla)

Am J Ophthalmol 124:362–372, 1997 10–11

Introduction.—Diagnosis of intraocular lymphoma by cytopathologic examination of vitreous cells is frequently difficult. The skill of the observer and adequate preservation of numerous cells are necessary for success, along with repeated biopsies. A possible alternative to immunocytochemical techniques for immunophenotyping vitreous cells is cytofluorographic analysis, or flow cytometry. Several advantages are provided with flow cytometry such as minimizing the impact of morphologic preservation. For clinicians who have no access to immunocytochemical laboratories with experience processing vitreous specimens, diagnosis may be facilitated with flow cytometry.

Methods.—Twenty-one patients who had diagnostic vitrectomy and flow cytometry for suspected intraocular lymphoma during a 4-year period were retrospectively studied. Vitrectomy was performed with the vitreous specimens being delivered to pathology and the cytofluorographic laboratory at room temperature as rapidly as possible, usually within 20 minutes of collection. For the flow cytometry procedure, cells were counted and stained with antibodies selected from a leukemia and lymphoma panel generally used for white blood cells from peripheral blood or bone marrow and for cell suspensions of solid tissue. A single slide of cells prepared from the cell pellet and stained with Wright-Giemsa stain was used for cytopathology characteristics to be examined.

Results.—Ten of the 20 patients evaluated had a final diagnosis of intraocular lymphoma. Four of the 10 patients had a prior diagnosis of extraophthalmic lymphoma. In 2 confirmed patients, flow cytometry was diagnostic and in 2 other confirmed patients, it was not diagnostic. No prior lymphoma diagnoses were given for 6 patients with lymphoma. In 5 of the 6 patients, flow cytometry indicated intraocular lymphoma. The flow cytometry results of 10 patients with uveitis or intraocular inflammation indicated a heterogenous inflammatory infiltrate in all of them.

Conclusions.—In 7 of 10 patients who had final diagnoses of lymphoma, cytofluorography was considered diagnostic of a B-lymphocyte or T-lymphocyte lymphoproliferative process. Abnormal morphologic characteristics would have permitted the diagnosis of lymphoma in only 3 of 10 patients, despite the fact that a smear of each specimen was examined by a pathologist. In only 30% of the patients, a diagnosis of lymphoma would have been made by cytopathologic features. For defining the character of vitreous cells, flow cytometry is an excellent technique. Clinicians may wish to consider this technique as an alternative or adjunctive technique to cytology alone.

► The concept described by these authors is certainly worthy of consideration. The authors are correct in their assertion that cytopathologic diagnosis of lymphoma vs. inflammatory process based on microscopic analysis of vitreous specimens is difficult. While cytopathologic diagnosis is based on subjective appreciation of nuclear and cytoplasmic characteristics of cells contained in a fluid specimen, flow cytometric diagnosis is based on a quantitative analysis of the various cell types in the specimen that are labeled by different immunocytochemical stains. As shown in this series of patients, neither method of diagnosis is completely reliable. Because flow cytometry requires rather expensive equipment that is well calibrated and regularly serviced, the availability of several different immunocytochemical stains, experienced technicians to process the specimens and operate the instrument, and a pathologist experienced in the use of flow cytometry for the diagnosis of hematologic malignancies, it is an expensive technology that is not used widely at present for the analysis of ocular fluid specimens in most centers. In fact, Wills Eye Hospital gave up its flow cytometer a number of years ago because the cost of maintaining and operating the instrument was prohibitive. In view of this, it seems likely that cytopathologic techniques will remain the standard method of diagnosis of intraocular lymphoma from vitreous specimens in most centers, and that flow cytometry will remain an informative adjunct in a few research centers.

J.J. Augsburger, M.D.

The Polymerase Chain Reaction (PCR) in the Routine Genetic Characterization of Retinoblastoma: A Tool for the Clinical Laboratory

Mastrangelo D, Squitieri N, Bruni S, et al (Univ of Siena, Italy)

Surv Ophthalmol 41:331–340, 1997 10–12

Objective.—Retinoblastoma (RB), the most frequent primary malignant intraocular neoplasm of children, is an important tumor to diagnose and treat. The causative gene, the RB1 gene, has been identified and characterized. The polymerase chain reaction (PCR), an innovative technique that can produce large amounts of specific DNA fragments from a very small amount of DNA, has proved very useful in studying the molecular genetics of many different ocular disorders. The use of the PCR to perform genetic analyses of patients with RB was reviewed.

Polymerase Chain Reaction Analysis of the RB1 Gene.—The routine use of PCR for genetic characterization of the RB1 gene in the clinical laboratory is advocated. Polymerase chain reaction can perform RB1 gene sequence polymorphism analysis to determine the genetic "fingerprint" of the gene. In addition, PCR permits analysis of the variable number of tandem repeats and short tandem repeats, as well as multiplex analysis. It also can detect loss of heterozygosity in RB and single-strand conformation analysis of the RB1 gene. With new equipment, the average PCR amplification time has been reduced to 15–20 minutes. New technologies permit increased efficiency and automation. These and future advances will make genetic testing of RB1 and other complex genes clinically practical.

Discussion.—Recent advances in PCR technique provide a greatly simplified approach to genetic characterization of patients with RB and their families. The genetic testing techniques described by the authors can provide the clinician with an accurate genetic map of each patient with RB.

► The authors of this review article suggest that PCR can and should be used in most ophthalmic laboratories to determine the precise nature of the genetic defect in RB and other ophthalmic disorders. I suspect that they are being more than a little overoptimistic about the potential for such investigation. In spite of the use of PCR, genetic testing for RB remains labor-intensive and complex. It is also very expensive. In my opinion, it would make much more sense to have a few laboratories doing such analyses routinely than to have multiple small laboratories trying to duplicate each other's work.

J.J. Augsburger, M.D.

11 Pathology

Ectopia Lentis in Heritable Disorders of Connective Tissue

by Ralph C. Eagle, Jr., M.D.

Ectopia lentis, or spontaneous dislocation of the lens, occurs in a variety of heritable diseases of connective tissue. The ophthalmologist must be familiar with these disorders because patients may exhibit ocular complications, or the ophthalmologist may be asked to evaluate the ocular status of affected patients. Most patients who have heritable ectopia lentis have homocystinuria, Marfan's syndrome, or Weill-Marchesani syndrome.

In the first edition of his textbook *Heritable Disorders of Connective Tissue,* published in 1956, Dr. Victor McCusick stated, "What the suspensory ligament of the lens has in common with the tunica media of the aorta is obscure. If this common factor were known the basic defect of Marfan Syndrome might be understood."[1] Forty years after McCusick's prophetic comment, it has been determined that the common factor shared by the zonule and the elastic tissue of the aorta is an extracellular matrix glycoprotein called fibrillin-1.[2–4] Furthermore, more than 50 mutations in the gene for fibrillin-1 have been identified in patients with Marfan's syndrome, and there is strong evidence that the syndrome's many manifestations are caused by fibrillin abnormalities.[4]

Fibrillin-1 is a major constituent of the zonular fibers. This 350 kd glycoprotein also constitutes the microfibrillar framework involved in the formation of elastic tissue throughout the body. The gene for fibrillin-1 is located on the long arm of chromosome 15. Like many extracellular matrix proteins, fibrillin 1 is composed of numerous small protein subunits called domains. Fibrillin-1 is especially rich in domains that resemble epidermal growth factor (EGF).[5] These EGF-like domains bind calcium. Calcium binding by the EGF-like domains plays an important role in determining the size and conformation of fibrillin molecules and their aggregation into larger fibrils.[6] Most of the fibrillin mutations that have been identified in kindreds with Marfan's syndrome involve calcium binding EGF-like domains.[4] The structure of these domains includes important disulfide bonds.

Fibrillin-1 is the key molecule in heritable ectopia lentis. Recently, it has become evident that other heritable disorders of connective tissue that are complicated by lens dislocation are either caused by mutations in the fibrillin-1gene or by metabolic defects that affect the structure of fibrillin secondarily, generally by interfering with the formation of disulfide bonds. Homocystinuria is the most important disorder in the latter category.

About 70% of patients with heritable ectopia lentis have Marfan's syndrome.[7] The major manifestations of Marfan's syndrome are ocular, skeletal, and cardiovascular. Patients with this syndrome are usually tall and have arachnodactyly and other skeletal abnormalities such as scoliosis and pectus excavatus or carinatum. Aortic dilatation and fatal dissecting aortic aneurysms are caused by an abnormal elastic layer in the aorta.

Ocular manifestations that occur with varying frequency in patients with Marfan's syndrome include ectopia lentis, high myopia, a propensity to develop retinal detachment, large flat corneas, peripheral iris transillumination, and glaucoma caused by incomplete angle development.[7] Ectopia lentis usually is bilateral and occurs in about 50% to 80% of cases. The lens typically dislocates superiorly or superotemporally in patients with Marfan's syndrome. Biomicroscopy discloses segmental defects in the inferior part of the zonule. The zonular fibers may appear stretched or broken, and the zonular bundles thin and scanty. Superior dislocation of the lens never occurs in patients with homocystinuria. This is an extremely important differential point because patients with homocystinuria may have a marfanoid habitus.

Fibrillin-1 mutations have been identified in some families who inherit simple or isolated ectopia lentis as an autosomal dominantly inherited trait.[8] These fibrillin-1 mutations are relatively innocuous and do not affect the cardiovascular system.

The autosomal dominant type of Weill-Marchesani syndrome recently was linked to the fibrillin-1 gene on chromosome 15.[9] Weill-Marchesani syndrome is the antithesis of Marfan's syndrome.[10] Patients with this disorder are short and muscular and have short fingers, broad hands, hearing defects, and limited joint mobility. The syndrome's classic manifestations are microspherophakia and brachydactyly.

The most debilitating complications of Weill-Marchesani syndrome are ocular. Patients frequently exhibit 15 or 20 diopters of myopia, caused by the microspherophakic lens, whose volume is 20% to 40% less than normal. Lens dislocation develops in the second decade. The dislocation is often axial and may produce pupillary block glaucoma. The term *inverse juvenile glaucoma* has been applied to this type of glaucoma because pupillary mydriasis lowers the intraocular pressure.

The second major category of heritable ectopia lentis is caused by metabolic disorders that have a secondary effect on the structure of fibrillin. These include homocystinuria, sulfite oxidase deficiency, and molybdenum cofactor deficiency. All are disorders of sulfur containing amino acids.

Homocystinuria is caused most often by a deficiency in the enzyme cystathionine β synthase, which normally catalyses the condensation of homocysteine with serine to form cystathionine, an important precursor of cysteine and cystine.[11] The resultant cysteine deficiency in affected patients is thought to interfere with the formation of the disulfide bonds that are important determinants of fibrillin structure and aggregation.

Patients who have homocystinuria typically are tall and have a marfanoid habitus. Many are blonde with fair skin and a malar flush. About 50% develop progressive mental retardation. Patients with this disorder are at major risk for the development of arterial and venous thromboses, which markedly diminish their life expectancy. 75% die by 30 years of age. The thromboembolic complications of homocystinuria may be related to secondary defects in an endothelial protein thrombomodulin, which like fibrillin contains multiple EGF-like domains with disulfide bonds.[12] Ophthalmic surgeons must remember that homocystinuric patients are at greater risk for thromboembolic complications during general anesthesia.

Lens dislocation occurs in about 90% of patients with homocystinuria. The entire zonule is defective. The lens usually dislocates inferiorly, or into the anterior chamber. Patients may have acute pupillary block glaucoma. Other ocular manifestations include high myopia, retinal detachment, and peripheral retinal pigment epithelium degeneration.

Sulfite oxidase deficiency is another rare cause of lens dislocation. Patients with sulfite oxidase deficiency are unable to convert sulfite to sulfate, which leads to an accumulation of sulfite.[13] Sulfite destroys structurally important sulfhydryl groups and disulfide bonds. Patients with sulfite oxidase deficiency typically have seizures in early infancy and have severe neurological abnormalities. Lens dislocation occurs in about 50%. Most patients with sulfite oxidase deficiency actually have a deficiency in a molybdenum cofactor that is shared by three enzymes: sulfite oxidase, xanthine dehydrogenase, and aldehyde oxidase.[14] The clinical manifestations of the latter two enzyme deficiencies are relatively innocuous.

Ectopia lentis does occur rarely in other systemic disorders. Hyperlysinemia and Ehlers-Danlos syndrome are often listed as causes of heritable lens dislocation, but the association of ectopia lentis with each of these disorders is extremely tenuous. Only one of seven reported cases of hyperlysinemia had ectopia lentis, and many authorities doubt the association.[15, 16] Similarly, only a single case of lens dislocation in Ehlers-Danlos syndrome has been reported.[17] The ocular manifestations of the ocular-scoliotic type of Ehlers-Danlos syndrome include retinal detachment and scleral rupture after mild trauma, not ectopia lentis. This type of Ehlers-Danlos syndrome is caused by an autosomal recessive deficiency in the enzyme lysyl hydroxylase which is involved in collagen synthesis.[18]

In conclusion, Marfan's syndrome, the most common cause of heritable lens dislocation, is caused by more than 50 mutations in the gene for fibrillin-1, a major constituent of zonule fibers. Most of the other heritable disorders associated with ectopia lentis are also caused by fibrillin mutations, or by metabolic defects that affect the structure of fibrillin secondarily by interfering with the formation of disulfide bonds.

References

1. Godfrey M: The Marfan syndrome, in Beighton P (ed): *McCusick's Heritable Disorders of Connective Tissue.* St Louis, Mosby, 1993, p 105.
2. Hollister DW, Godfrey M, Sakai LY, et al: Immunohistologic abnormalities of the microfibrillar-fiber system in the Marfan syndrome. *N Engl J Med* 323:152–159, 1990.
3. Maumenee IH: The Marfan syndrome is caused by a point mutation in the fibrillin gene. *Arch Ophthalmol* 110:472–473, 1992.
4. Hayward C, Brock DJ: Fibrillin-1 mutations in Marfan syndrome and other type-1 fibrillinopathies. *Hum Mutat* 10:415–423, 1997.
5. Downing AK, Knott V, Werner JM, et al: Solution structure of a pair of calcium-binding epidermal growth factor-like domains: Implications for the Marfan syndrome and other genetic disorders. *Cell* 85:597–605, 1996.
6. Reinhardt DP, Mechling DE, Boswell BA, et al: Calcium determines the shape of fibrillin. *J Biol Chem* 272:7368–7373, 1997.
7. Maumenee IH: The eye in the Marfan syndrome. *Trans Am Ophthalmol Soc* 79:684–733, 1981.
8. Edwards MJ, Challinor CJ, Colley PW, et al: Clinical and linkage study of a large family with simple ectopia lentis linked to FBN1. *Am J Med Genet* 53:65–71, 1994.
9. Wirtz MK, Samples JR, Kramer PL, et al: Weill-Marchesani syndrome: Possible linkage of the autosomal dominant form to 15q21.1. *Am J Med Genet* 65:68–75, 1996.
10. Maumenee IH: The Weill-Marchesani syndrome, in Beighton P (ed): *McCusick's Heritable Disorders of Connective Tissue.* St Louis, Mosby, 1993, pp 179–187.
11. Pyeritz RE: Homocystinuria, in Beighton P (ed): *McCusick's Heritable Disorders of Connective Tissue.* St Louis, Mosby, 1993, pp 137–178.
12. Schienle HW, Seitz R, Nawroth P, et al: Thrombomodulin and ristocetincofactor in homocystinuria: A study in two siblings. *Thromb Res* 77:79–86, 1995.
13. Shih VE, Abroms IF, Johnson JL, et al: Sulfite oxidase deficiency: Biochemical and clinical investigations of a hereditary metabolic disorder in sulfur metabolism. *N Engl J Med* 297:1022–1028, 1997.
14. Lueder GT, Steiner RD: Ophthalmic abnormalities in molybdenum cofactor deficiency and isolated sulfite oxidase deficiency. *J Pediatr Ophthalmol Strabismus* 32:334–337, 1995.
15. Smith TH, Holland MG, Woody NC: Ocular manifestations of familial hyperlysinemia. *Trans Am Acad Ophthalmol Otolaryngol* 75:355–360, 1971.
16. Hyperlysinemia [lysine:alpha-ketoglutarage reductase deficiency], in McCusick VA: *Mendelian Inheritance in Man: Catalogs of Autosomal Dominant, Autosomal Recessive, and X-linked Phenotypes.* Baltimore, Md, Johns Hopkins University Press, 1990, pp 1257–1258.
17. Thomas C, Cordier J, Algan B: Les altérations oculaires de la maladie d'Ehlers-Danlos. *Arch Ophtalmol* 14:691–697, 1954.
18. Beighton P: The Ehler-Danlos syndromes, in Beighton P (ed): *McCusick's Heritable Disorders of Connective Tissue.* St Louis, Mosby, 1993, pp 189–251.

Giant Cell Arteritis: New Concepts in Pathogenesis and Implications for Management

Weyand CM, Bartley GB (Mayo Clinic and Found, Rochester, Minn)
Am J Ophthalmol 123:392–395, 1997 11–1

Background.—In a recent prospective study of clinical and laboratory predictors of vasculitis in temporal artery biopsies, a positive temporal artery biopsy was associated with the presence of jaw claudication, anorexia, and neck pain in a cohort of 363 patients. Marked acute phase reactant responses appeared to be strongly predictive of patients with giant cell arteritis. New concepts in pathogenesis and implications for management of giant cell arteritis were reviewed.

Discussion.—Giant cell arteritis, an inflammatory vasculopathy preferentially targeting medium-sized and large arteries, initially manifests as constitutional symptoms, such as fever, anorexia, weight loss, night sweats, depression, fatigue, and malaise in many patients. It appears to be an autoimmune syndrome, resulting from a response directed toward antigens in the arterial wall of selected blood vessels. Tissue destruction is conceptualized as a "downstream" effect of a chronic, persistent immune process in this model. Clonal expansion occurs in T lymphocytes infiltrating the temporal artery wall. A selected group of T cells is recruited to independent sites of arteritis, where they proliferate in situ, suggesting the presence of an immunogenic antigen in the artery. Full-blown vasculitis and giant cell formation are related directly to the tissue production of interferon-gamma, a key cytokine in the disease process. Interferon-gamma–producing T cells are found in the adventitia of inflamed arteries. The immunologic injury appears to occur in the adventitial layer in patients with giant cell arteritis. Macrophages also play a key role in giant cell arteritis. Circulating macrophages secrete interleukin-6 and interleukin-1β, thereby contributing to the disease. Inflammatory infiltrates have a defined topographic distribution in the blood vessel wall. The functional commitment of tissue-infiltrating macrophages is strongly associated with their localization in the artery.

The clinical presentation of giant cell arteritis can vary. Some patients have signs of cranial ischemia manifesting as ocular involvement and jaw claudication, and some have polymyalgia rheumatica. Giant cell arteritis may also be diagnosed in patients assessed for systemic inflammatory disease manifesting as fever of unknown origin. The distinct clinical phenotypes of giant cell arteritis appear to be associated with molecular events in the vascular lesions. Ischemic complications typically occur in patients with high transcription of interferon-gamma in the tissue. Polymyalgia rheumatica is correlated with T-cell cytokine interleukin-2 dominance, and fever as an initial symptom occurs in patients with low levels of interferon-gamma transcription in temporal artery tissue extracts. High in situ production of interferon-gamma predicts the finding of giant cells in the temporal artery lesions.

► This excellent and informative editorial on the pathogenesis and immunopathology of giant cell arteritis accompanies Hayreh's report in the *American Journal of Ophthalmology*[1] on the validity and reliability of various diagnostic criteria in that disease. Giant cell arteritis should be excluded by an expedient temporal artery biopsy in all elderly patients who are seen with ischemic optic neuropathy or central retinal artery occlusion and have elevated erythrocyte sedimentation rates and C -reactive protein values. The biopsied segment of artery should be at least 2 cm long, and the pathologist should divide it into multiple transverse segments to ensure adequate sampling and lessen the possibility of missing skip lesions (which do occur). If the initial result biopsy is negative and clinical suspicion remains high, the second side should be biopsied. Nine percent of such biopsies proved positive in Hayreh's series. If giant cell arteritis is suspected clinically, high-dose corticosteroid therapy should be initiated immediately *before the biopsy* to prevent visual loss in the remaining eye. A short course of steroids will not adversely affect the histopathology.

R.C. Eagle, Jr., M.D.

Reference

1. Hayreh SS, Podhajsky PA, Raman R, et al: Giant cell arteritis: Validity and reliability of various diagnostic criteria. *Am J Ophthalmol* 123:285–296, 1997.

Pneumocystis carinii **Infection of the Conjunctiva in a Patient With Acquired Immune Deficiency Syndrome**

Ruggli GM, Weber R, Messmer EP, et al (Univ Hosp of Zürich, Switzerland; Baylor College of Medicine, Houston)
Ophthalmology 104:1853–1856, 1997 11–2

Introduction.—Pulmonary *Pneumocystis carinii* is the most frequently occurring life-threatening complication in patients with congenital or acquired AIDS. *P. carinii* is an opportunistic monocellular parasite that is exclusively present in the extracellular space. It has several morphological features of protozoa, but is considered a fungus by some investigators. The most common ophthalmic manifestations of AIDS-associated *P. carinii* include *Pneumocystis* choroidopathy, retinal manifestations, and orbital involvement. Clinical features and histologic findings of a unique *P. carinii* infection with conjunctival involvement in a homosexual man were described.

Case Report.—Man, 33, tested HIV-antibody positive in February 1990 and AIDS was diagnosed in April 1995. Aerosolized pentamidine was started prophylactically for *P. carinii* pneumonia in January 1994 and he never experienced signs or symptoms of pulmonary infection from this organism. In January 1996, he reported an irritation in his right eye. The tarsal conjunctiva of the right eye had a slightly elevated, placoid, white avascular lesion with well-defined borders. About half of the subtarsal area and the margin of the upper lid were involved. Two punch biopsy samples were obtained from the lesion of the tarsal conjunctiva using local anesthesia. Microscopic examination revealed that the tissue of the affected area was partly covered by normal conjunctival mucosa. The underlying stroma had confluent lakes of amorphous eosinophilic frothy and vacuolated material with remnants of fibrovascular tissue. The deposits were surrounded by areas of reactive fibroblastic proliferation and capillary sprouting. No inflammatory infiltrates were detected. Gomori methenamine silver stain revealed numerous round-to-oval cysts within the necrotic tissue, some which resembled ping-pong balls measuring 3–7 µm in diameter. Numerous toluidine blue-positive cysts were seen with light microscopy of a conjunctival smear specimen. Indirect immunofluoresence using monoclonal mouse anti-*P. carinii* antibodies revealed *P. carinii* cysts. The patient was given oral treatment with dapsone and trimethoprim for diagnosis of extrapulmonary *P. carinii* infection.

Conclusion.—White placoid conjunctival lesions in patients with AIDS may suggest an infection caused by *P. carinii*. Pneumocystosis in patients with immunologic disorders seems to result from activation of latent disease because there is serologic documentation of widespread (nearly 100%) acquisition of anti-*P. carinii* antibodies in early childhood.

▶ This unusual conjunctival infection by *P. carinii* occurred in a moribund AIDS patient who had been receiving extended prophylaxis for pulmonary pneumocystosis with aerosolized pentamidine. Although this therapy prevents *P. carinii* pneumonia which is the most common life-threatening infectious complication of AIDS, it has little or no effect on extrapulmonary pneumocystosis. An association between aerosolized pentamidine therapy and *Pneumocystis* choroidopathy has been noted previously.

R.C. Eagle, Jr., M.D.

Adenoid Cystic Carcinomas of the Lacrimal Gland in Childhood and Adolescence

Tellado MV, McLean IW, Specht CS, et al (Armed Forces Inst of Pathology, Washington, DC; Naval Hosp, Charleston, SC)

Ophthalmology 104:1622–1625, 1997 11–3

Introduction.—Adenoid cystic carcinoma of the lacrimal gland is rare. It is the second most commonly occurring epithelial neoplasm of the lacrimal gland after benign mixed tumor and is the most common malignant epithelial neoplasm of the lacrimal gland. This tumor may be classified into different histologic types—tubular, cribriform, sclerosing, comedocarcinoma, and basaloid—depending on the most dominant histologic pattern. The basaloid pattern may be identified by solid lobules or small nests completely filled with neoplastic cells. Basaloid pattern tumors are likely to recur and metastasize quickly. Patients usually die of disease within 3 years. The relation between histologic features and behavior of a series of adenoid cystic carcinomas of the lacrimal gland in children and adolescents was examined.

Methods.—Eleven patients 18 years of age or younger with adenoid cystic carcinoma were identified in the Registry of Ophthalmic Pathology. Of 11 surgical specimens available for review, 5 were orbital exenterations and 6 were tumor excisions. Grading for the proportion of basaloid histologic pattern was as follows: grade I, 0%; grade II, less than 25%; grade III, 25% to 50%; grade IV, greater than 50%. Surgical specimens were also examined for mitotic count, presence or absence of necrosis, hemorrhage, and invasion of surrounding tissues.

Results.—The mean age of 9 girls and 2 boys was 14 years. Mean follow-up period after treatment of 8 of 11 available patients was 10 years. Five of 8 patients (62.5%) survived. Four of 5 patients were disease-free and 1 had orbital recurrence at last follow-up. Of 5 known survivors, 4 had grade I tumors and 1 had a grade II tumor. The estimated survival rate at 15 years was 58%. Mean mitotic count of 5 tumors was 3.4 per 20 40× fields. Of patients known to die of disease, 1 had grade I tumor, 1 had grade II tumor, and 1 had grade III tumor. Mean mitotic count of 3 tumors was 8 per 20 40× fields. Other findings in these 3 tumors included necrosis in 2, intralesional hemorrhage in 3, perineural invasion in 2, and vascular invasion in 2.

Conclusion.—The presence of a basaloid pattern in adenoid cystic carcinomas is correlated with poor prognosis. Young patients tended to have low-grade tumors. When necrosis, hemorrhage, perineural invasion, and high mitotic count were observed, they were usually associated with fatal outcome. Young patients with no basaloid pattern and less aggressive histologic features may have better prognosis.

► I have seen 2 children with adenoid cystic carcinoma of the lacrimal gland during the last decade. The most recent case was unsuspected clinically because the tumor was cystoid and was misdiagnosed as a dermoid cyst in imaging studies. Similar to most of the pediatric cases reported in this series, that tumor was a relatively low-grade, totally cribriform lesion that lacked a solid basaloid pattern.

This encouraging article indicates that there may be some hope for children with this lacrimal gland malignancy. In the past, a dismal prognosis generally has been assigned to adenoid cystic carcinoma of the lacrimal gland.

R.C. Eagle, Jr., M.D.

TUNEL-Positive Ganglion Cells in Human Primary Open-angle Glaucoma

Kerrigan LA, Zack DJ, Quigley HA, et al (Johns Hopkins Univ, Baltimore, Md)
Arch Ophthalmol 115:1031–1035, 1997 11–4

Background.—The mechanisms of ganglion cell death in glaucoma are uncertain, though high intraocular pressure and differing susceptibility of ganglion cells may play a role. Apoptotic cell death may result from blockage of axoplasmic flow at the lamina cribrosa, in turn leading to blockage of neurotrophic signaling from axon terminals to cell bodies. Under this hypothesis, the process of apoptosis may be initiated by neurons that have not received the appropriate chemical signal from their target neurons. There is in vitro evidence to suggest neurotrophin withdrawal as an initiating mechanism of apoptosis. This study sought evidence of apoptotic cell death in retinal ganglion cells from eyes with primary open-angle glaucoma.

Methods.—The study included 18 cadaver eyes from 17 subjects with known primary open-angle glaucoma. A group of 21 eyes matched for age, race, and sex were studied as controls. Histologic evaluation of the optic nerve was performed to stage glaucoma severity. Retinal sections were then prepared and examined for internucleosomal DNA fragmentation—which is characteristic of apoptosis—by the terminal deoxynucleotidyl transferase-mediated deoxyuridine triphosphate-biotin nick end-labeling (TUNEL) technique.

Results.—Ten of 18 glaucomatous eyes showed TUNEL-positive cells. These cells appeared in the ganglion layer with a frequency of 1.15 per 10,000 cells in eyes with mild glaucoma, 1.55 per 10,000 in eyes with moderate glaucoma, and 3.40 per 10,000 in eyes with severe glaucoma. Cells in the outer retinal layers showed no marked TUNEL staining. Of 11 evaluable control eyes from subjects without potentially confounding diseases, only 1 eye showed 1 TUNEL-positive cell. Overall, TUNEL-positive cells were 15-fold more frequent in glaucomatous eyes.

Conclusions.—In eyes with primary open-angle glaucoma, there is evidence that retinal ganglion cells die through apoptosis. The frequency of TUNEL-positive cells varies with the severity of glaucoma; though the cells are relatively rare, this is consistent with previous knowledge of apoptosis and glaucoma. The findings support the hypothesis that blockage of axonal transport at the lamina cribrosa blocks neurotrophic signaling from axon terminals to ganglion cell bodies, thus leading to cell death.

► This is one of the most important studies that have investigated the topic of apoptosis or programmed cell death in the retina. The paper suggests that apoptosis may be the cause of retinal ganglion cell death in glaucoma. Although the number of TUNEL-positive cells found in eyes from patients with glaucoma was small, it was compatible with estimated values. According to the authors' hypothesis, apoptotic death of ganglion cells may be initiated when blockage of axoplasmic flow in the pressure-distorted lamina cribrosa deprives the ganglion cells of a neurotrophic protein made in the brain.

R.C. Eagle, Jr., M.D.

Mutation of the Stargardt Disease Gene (*ABCR*) in Age-related Macular Degeneration

Allikmets R, Shroyer NF, Singh N, et al (NCI-Frederick Cancer Research and Development Ctr, Md; Baylor College of Medicine, Houston; Univ of Utah, Salt Lake City; et al)
Science 277:1805–1807, 1997 11–5

Introduction.—The most common cause of acquired visual impairment in the elderly is age-related macular degeneration, affecting about 11 million individuals in the United States. There are 2 categories of age-related macular degeneration; 20% of the patients have exudative or wet and 80% have dry age-related macular degeneration. The hallmarks of dry age-related macular degeneration are the presence of drusen, irregularities in the pigmentation of retinal pigment epithelium, and geographic atrophy. The hallmarks of wet age-related macular degeneration are serous detachment of the retinal pigment epithelium and choroidal neovascularization. No therapies are available for the dry type, and only about 5% with the wet type are candidates for laser photocoagulation.

Methods.—Screening for alterations in *ABCR*, a gene that encodes a retinal rod photoreceptor protein and is defective is Stargardt disease, a common hereditary form of macular degeneration, was conducted on 167 unrelated patients with age-related macular degeneration. This gene was identified on human chromosome 1p21 and is mutated in Stargardt disease. A member of the ATP-binding cassette transporter superfamily, the ABCR protein corresponds to a previously identified rod outer segment protein called rim protein. In each patient, all 51 exons of *ABCR* were screened for variations.

Results.—In 26 patients (16%), with age-related macular degeneration, 13 different age-related macular degeneration–associated alterations were detected, and most were missense mutations in conserved amino acid positions. Some mutations that cause recessive Stargardt disease may enhance susceptibility to age-related macular degeneration in the heterozygous state, because 3 of the 13 alterations in patients with age-related macular degeneration were also detected in patients with Stargardt disease. Two families were identified in which the parents or grandparents of Stargardt disease probands have age-related macular degeneration.

Conclusion.—Presymptomatic screening of high-risk individuals may be possible with the discovery of specific *ABCR* alterations in patients with age-related macular degeneration. Earlier diagnosis and clinical testing of preventive and therapeutic strategies may be possible.

▶ Heterozygous mutations in the *ABCR* gene that causes the autosomal recessive form of Stargardt disease/fundus flavimaculatus were identified in 16% of elderly patients with the "dry" or atrophic form of age-related macular degeneration. Homozygous mutations cause Stargardt disease in teenagers. Stargardt disease has long been considered a retinal pigment epithelial (RPE) disorder because pathologic examination has shown striking

RPE abnormalities. These include the massive accumulation of abnormal lipofuscin-like material that makes the RPE periodic acid–Schiff (PAS) positive. Surprisingly, the *ABCR* gene is not expressed in the RPE. The gene product appears to be a transport protein that is located principally in the inner segments of rod photoreceptors. What the protein transports, and how defective transport leads to the storage of lipofuscin in the RPE remain to be determined.

R.C. Eagle, Jr., M.D.

Suggested Reading

Pennisi E: Gene found for the fading eyesight of old age. *Science* 277:1765–1766, 1997.

The Clinical and Pathologic Constellation of Wegener Granulomatosis of the Orbit

Perry SR, Rootman J, White VA (Kidderminster Gen Hosp, Worcestershire, England; Univ of British Columbia, Vancouver)

Ophthalmology 104:683–694, 1997 11–6

Objective.—Because Wegener's granulomatosis (WG) is often clinically and pathologically misdiagnosed, patients may experience serious visual or systemic effects. Progress in treatment resulting in improved prognosis has spurred a retrospective review at the University of British Columbia Orbit Unit to identify the clinical, radiologic, and pathologic features that characterize the disease.

Methods.—The records of 13 patients with WG (5 males), aged 9–69 years, were reviewed.

Results.—The most common initial symptoms reported were proptosis with face or eye pain and a red eye with previously diagnosed scleritis. Visual disability was moderate. During the 3 months before ophthalmic examination, 11 patients had experienced plugged ears and nose, epistaxis or clear nasal discharge, pressure in the ears or over paranasal sinuses, draining ears, hearing loss or tinnitus, and throat symptoms. Five patients had systemic symptoms including malaise, weight loss, and arthralgia. Ear, nose, and throat symptoms eventually developed in all patients. Three patterns of orbital symptoms evolved: diffuse orbital involvement, tearing, or midline involvement with increasing vision loss. A nodular mass developed in all patients, including those with scleritis, which was usually described as nodular with necrosis. Eight patients (13 eyes) experienced a decline in visual acuity, and all 11 were given diagnoses of optic neuropathy. Computed tomography showed an orbital mass, usually with infiltrative margins, or a midline change in 12 patients, nasopharyngeal or sinus lesions in 8, and midline bony erosion in 6. Biopsy material showed fat disruption with areas of focal necrosis and giant cells; fibrosis; granulomatous and acute inflammation with eosinophils or polymorphonuclear leukocytes forming granulomatous infiltrates; and smudgy necrosis surrounded by granulomatous or inflammatory infiltrates. Oral steroids were successful in only 1 patient. Cyclophosphamide–corticosteroid treatment allowed the retention of vision and improvement over a period of several months. The patients' conditions were stabilized. Antineutrophil cytoplasmic antibody testing, although initially negative, became positive in 3 patients.

Conclusion.—Diagnosis of WG must be made on a wide variety of clinical, radiologic, and pathologic characteristics. Proptosis, inflammation, and necrosis findings are frequently bilateral. Ear, nose, sinus and throat involvement are common features. Orbital biopsy findings, such as areas of fat necrosis, lipid-containing macrophages, granulomatous or focal abscesses, leukocyte and eosinophilic infiltrates, should be cause for suspicion.

► This excellent clinicopathologic study of Wegener's granulomatosis makes several important clinical points. First, the histopathologic features found in orbital biopsies differ from those of other sites. Orbital biopsy results typically show mixed acute and chronic granulomatous inflammation and necrosis. Active granulomatous vasculitis, a histologic hallmark of Wegener's granulomatosis elsewhere, is usually absent, however. Second, the antineutrophil cytoplasmic antibody test, which has been widely touted as a diagnostic adjunct in Wegener's granulomatosis, was initially negative in 5 of 5 patients. (It eventually became positive in 3). Although the authors agree that the antineutrophil cytoplasmic antibody test is helpful when it is positive, they emphasize that treatment should not be delayed by a negative test result when clinical and pathologic evidence suggest the diagnosis. Finally, a combination of cyclophosphamide and oral corticosteroids appears to be a highly effective therapy for this once fatal disorder.

R.C. Eagle, Jr., M.D.

► This study is an excellent clinical-pathologic correlation of Wegener's granulomatosis of the orbit. The authors indicate that early diagnosis is extremely important because untreated generalized Wegener's is usually fatal within 2 years. From the radiologic perspective, bilateral proptosis and proptosis with scleritis should prompt one to consider Wegener's granulomatosis. Symptoms include nose, ear, and throat features. One interesting aspect of this report is that although 6 of 10 patients had unilateral disease at presentation, ocular features became bilateral in 11 of the 13 patients.

The ocular findings included a diffuse pattern, lacrimal, or midline involvement. Lid swelling was noted in those patients with lacrimal gland involvement. Orbital mass developed in all 13 of these patients. The orbital mass was associated with proptosis and could be located in the lacrimal gland, midline, apex, or inferolateral regions of the orbit. The masses tended to have infiltrating margins obscuring adjacent flat planes. Two patients had the pattern noted in Figure 1 of the original article, which was diffuse bilateral disease. The pattern of onset was generally subacute evolving over weeks with 3 of 10 patients having chronic disease of more than 2 years' duration.

The disease could accelerate after a subacute onset. Midline disease is associated with bone erosion.

Wegener's granulomatosis is characterized by a rapidly progressive multisystem disease involving the upper and lower respiratory tracts, followed by renal failure from necrotizing glomerulonephritis. It can also have limited forms that can spare the kidney. Orbital involvement occurs in approximately 50% of cases and is seen in both typical and limited Wegener's. Respiratory tract or sinus involvement including the mastoids, scleritis associated with classic features of limbal corneal infiltrates, and systemic associations should alert clinicians to a possible occurrence of Wegener's. The disorder affects patients from youth to old age.

Besides the constellation of symptoms, orbital biopsy was felt to be particularly useful in this study, although the mixed inflammatory pattern appears to be more common then necrotizing granulomas with vasculitis. An important feature of the biopsy is the stains for fungi and mycobacteria. The authors claim the mixed orbital inflammation pattern is diagnostic for Wegener's granulomatosis. Other diagnoses include Hodgkin's disease and orbital pseudotumor. Orbital pseudotumor is noted here to have a different course responding promptly to corticosteroids alone with biopsy showing largely lymphocytic infiltration without an acute component, necrosis, or fibrosis, nor is there any evidence of vascular infiltration or destruction. Idiopathic sclerosing inflammation produces fibrosis and is associated with paucicellular inflammatory infiltration.

Clearly this report heightens one's awareness of the diagnostic features of this important disease. Radiology plays a key role, as does the patient's medical history. The bilaterality of the disease limits the differential diagnosis in most cases. In addition to orbital pseudotumor and orbital sclerosing inflammation, I would be concerned about metastatic disease which can be destructive and produce these mass-type lesions. I have seen such patterns in metastatic breast cancer, although the desmoplastic reactions characteristically produce less proptosis. Increased awareness of the orbital manifestations of Wegener's will no doubt improve our diagnostic acumen.

R.I. Grossman, M.D.

Familial Subepithelial Corneal Amyloidosis: A Lactoferrin-related Amyloidosis

Klintworth GK, Valnickova Z, Kielar RA, et al (Duke Univ, Durham, NC; Univ of Kentucky, Lexington; Mayo Clinic and Found, Rochester, Minn)

Invest Ophthalmol Vis Sci 38:2756–2763, 1997 11–7

Introduction.—Familial subepithelial corneal amyloidosis (FSCA) is a rare bilateral corneal disorder that usually begins in the first or second decade of life with severe photophobia, tearing, ocular foreign body sensation, and multiple prominent nodular deposits of amyloid accumulation beneath the epithelium that produce a mulberry-shaped mass. Corneal

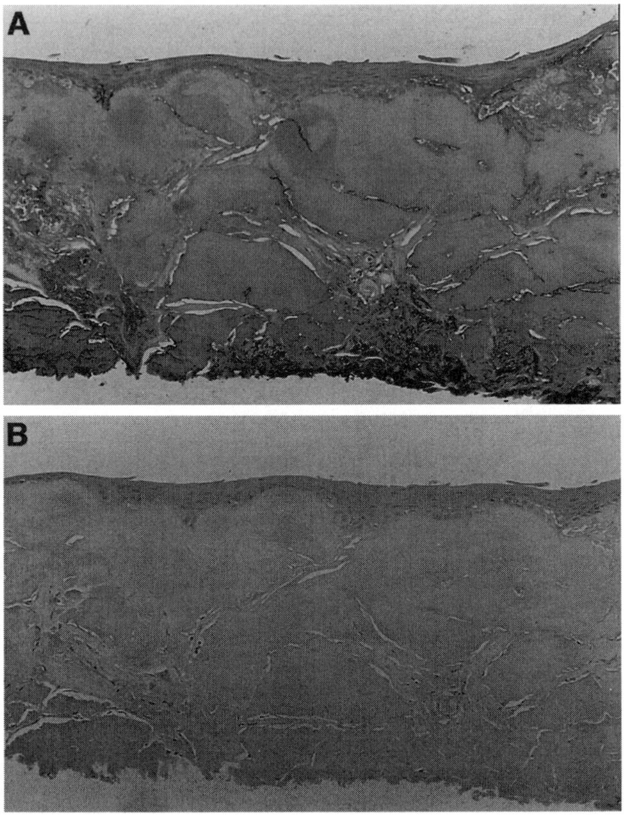

FIGURE 5.—Immunoperoxidase-stained preparations of cornea after treatment with rabbit antihuman lactoferrin antibody (1:3000) (**A**) and normal rabbit serum (**B**). In contrast to the control (**B**), note the brown discolored positive reactivity of corneal amyloid (**A**). The amyloid near the periphery of this formalin-fixed, paraffin-embedded specimen (bottom of **A**) stains more intensely than the amyloid deeper in the tissue. The intense staining in the lower portion of the figure may be an "edge artifact." The epithelium at the top of the figure reacts minimally with the antihuman lactoferrin. In contrast to **A**, the amyloid does not react with normal rabbit serum (**B**). Immunoperoxidase reaction; magnification, ×85. (Reproduced by permission of the Association for Research in Vision and Ophthalmology, from Klintworth GK, Valnickova Z, Kielar RA, et al: Familial subepithelial corneal amyloidosis: A lactoferrin-related amyloidosis. *Invest Ophthalmol Vis Sci* 38:2756–2763, 1997.)

specimens were assessed to isolate the protein that collects in increased quantities under the corneal epithelium in FSCA.

Methods.—Specimens of cornea were taken at the time of lamellar keratoplasty or superficial keratectomy from 2 unrelated patients with clinical and histopathologic features of FSCA. Peptides that result from pepsin digestion of a distinctive protein isolated by sodium dodecyl sulfate-polyacrylamide gel electrophoresis from the frozen corneal tissues with FSCA were purified by high-pressure liquid chromatography, then protein sequence analysis. The protein lactoferrin was identified in the cornea using amino acid sequencing and Western blotting. The reactivity of the amyloid in formalin-fixed, paraplast-embedded corneal tissue sec-

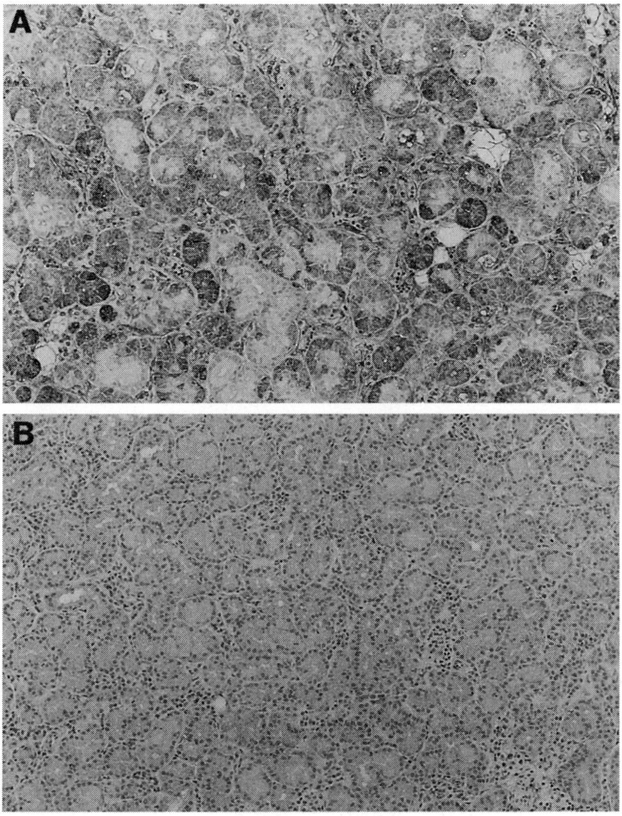

FIGURE 6.—Positive reactivity of normal lacrimal gland with rabbit antihuman lactoferrin antibody (1:3000) (**A**) and negative effect with normal rabbit serum (**B**). Immunoperoxidease reaction; magnification, ×85. (Reproduced by permission of the Association for Research in Vision and Ophthalmology, from Klintworth GK, Valnickova Z, Kielar RA; et al: Familial subepithelial corneal amyloidosis: A lactoferrin-related amyloidosis. *Invest Ophthalmol Vis Sci* 38:2756–2763, 1997.)

tions was evaluated by immunohistochemistry. Lacrimal gland and breast tissues known to express lactoferrin were prepared in the same way as positive controls.

Results.—Light microscopy showed the typical histopathologic features of FSCA, with mounds of amyloid in the subepithelial corneal tissue covered by an epithelium of variable thickness. A protein was detected in the corneas with FSCA that was not seen in normal corneas or in corneas with other disorders. The amino acid sequences of peptides taken from this protein were identical to equivalent portions of lactoferrin. The corneal amyloid (Fig 5) and normal human lacrimal gland tissue reacted with rabbit antihuman lactoferrin antibody (Fig 6).

Conclusion.—Lactoferrin is generated by the lacrimal gland and is responsible for about 25% of the total tear protein. The presence of lactoferrin in corneas with FSCA, combined with positive cross-reactivity of amyloid with lactoferrin antiserum, strongly indicates that lactoferrin is a main component of the corneal accumulations in FSA.

► Amyloidosis is characterized by eosinophilic deposits of amorphous acellular material that is insoluble, stains positively with amyloid stains such as Congo red, and shows "apple green" birefringence under polarized light. A variety of proteins or protein fragments are amyloidogenic. Structurally, these proteins typically contain a segment with beta-pleated sheet conformation, which precipitate in register to form amyloid.

The gelatinous droplike deposits of amyloid that accumulate beneath the corneal epithelium in familial subepithelial corneal amyloidosis appear to be composed of the protein lactoferrin, which is produced by the lacrimal gland and is present in high concentration in tears. Although affected individuals could make too much lactoferrin, the dystrophy probably is caused by a heritable mutant form of the protein, which is prone to form amyloid.

R.C. Eagle, Jr., M.D.

Mutations in Cornea-specific Keratin *K3* or *K12* Genes Cause Meesmann's Corneal Dystrophy

Irvine AD, Corden LD, Swensson O, et al (Belfast City Hosp, Northern Ireland; Jefferson Med College, Philadelphia; Univ of Dundee, Scotland; et al)

Nature Genet 16:184–187, 1997 11–8

Background.—Meesmann's corneal dystrophy (MCD) is a bilateral, autosomal dominant corneal epithelial disorder. During the first year of life, fine round epithelial cysts appear on slit-lamp examination. These cysts may rupture in adulthood, causing erosions and clinical symptoms. Patients with this disorder cannot wear contact lenses, because the lenses traumatize the corneal epithelium. Meesmann's corneal dystrophy meets several of the criteria for a keratin disease. As in other keratin disorders, patients with MCD have fragility of the keratinocytes expressing a particular pair of keratins. Studies in 3 MCD cohorts have shown heterozygous missense mutations in the cornea-specific keratin K3 and K12 polypeptides.

Findings.—Linkage analysis of the German kindred originally studied by Meesmann showed highly significant linkage to the K12 locus. In 2 Northern Irish kindreds, also with typical autosomal dominant inheritances, the phenotype segregated with either the K12 or the K3 locus. Studies demonstrated complete cosegregation of heterozygous missense mutations in K3 and K12 in the MCD families, whereas these mutations were absent in 100 normal unrelated chromosomes. Each of the mutations occurred in the highly conserved keratin helix boundary motifs.

Conclusions.—Mutations in the cornea-specific K3 or K12 gene are identified as the cause of MCD. Such keratin helix boundary motif mutations have been found in other disorders to cause severe compromise of cytoskeletal function, producing keratinocyte fragility phenotypes. The study is the first to illustrate the molecular basis of MCD.

► More than 30 years ago the late Toichiro Kuwabara found deposits of material within the cells of the thickened, irregular corneal epithelium of a patient with Meesmann's corneal dystrophy with transmission electron microscopy. He termed this material "peculiar substance," and thought that it might represent some sort of mucopolysaccharide.[1] In a subsequent EM study, Ben Fine and coworkers emphasized that the abnormal fibrogranular material was associated with the tonofilaments and suggested that its formation probably was related to degeneration of the cytoskeleton.[2] This molecular genetic study confirms Dr. Fine's conclusions. Meesmann's dystrophy appears to be caused by mutations in the specialized keratin molecules that form the cytoskeleton of the corneal epithelium. These mutations compromise intermediate filament assembly leading to cytoplasmic tonofilament clumping and epithelial fragility.

R.C. Eagle, Jr., M.D.

References

1. Kuwabara T, Ciccarelli EC: Meesmann's corneal dystrophy: A pathological study. *Arch Ophthalmol* 71:676, 1964.
2. Fine BS, Yanoff M, Pitts E, et al: Meesmann's epithelial dystrophy of the cornea. *Am J Ophthalmol* 83:633–642, 1997.

Identification of Missense Mutations in the Norrie Disease Gene Associated With Advanced Retinopathy of Prematurity

Shastry BS, Pendergast SD, Hartzer MK, et al (Oakland Univ, Rochester, Mich; Beaumont Eye Inst, Royal Oak, Mich)

Arch Ophthalmol 115:651–655, 1997 11–9

Introduction.—Retinopathy of prematurity (ROP), a leading cause of blindness in children in the United States, is associated with low birth weight and short gestational age. There is also indirect evidence that genetic abnormalities play a role in the disorder. Mutations of Norrie's disease (ND) gene have been found in X-linked familial exudative vitreoretinopathy (FEVR), a vitreoretinal dystrophy with a varied clinical course similar to ROP. To determine whether a genetic component might be involved in the development of stage 4 or 5 ROP similar to FEVR, investigators performed molecular genetic analysis of the ND gene from 16 children.

Methods.—All 16 children had a history of premature birth and low birth weight. There were 3 pairs of twins in the group. Retinal findings were consistent with ROP, and 11 children had stage 4B or 5 ROP in both eyes. Excluded were patients with a family history of FEVR or ND, any ocular findings atypical for ROP, or a history of anemia or blood dyscrasia.

Blood specimens were obtained from the patients, parents, and 50 unrelated healthy controls.

Results.—Molecular genetic analysis of the ND gene demonstrated mutations in exon 3 in 4 (33%) of the 12 children with ROP stage 4B or 5 in at least 1 eye. Sequencing of the amplified product from exon 3 showed a missense mutation at codon 121 in 3 children with advanced ROP: twin 1A, twin 2C, and twin 2D. Twin 1B, the dizygotic twin of 1A, showed a wild-type sequence and did not have ROP. Mutations found in the 4 children were not present in the parents, the unrelated healthy controls, or the 2 patients with regressed stage 3 ROP.

Discussion.—In some premature, low-birth weight infants, ROP regresses spontaneously, whereas in others with similar clinical characteristics ROP progresses to the severe stage. Findings in this group of children suggest that a genetic factor may play a role in the course of ROP. Thus in a subset of predisposed infants, mutations in the ND gene may be responsible for advanced ROP.

▶ Low birth weight, young gestational age, and exposure to supplemental oxygen are the factors that we commonly associate with the development of ROP. This study indicates that genetic factors also may contribute to development of severe blinding ROP in certain premature infants. The authors investigated the Norrie's disease gene because retinal abnormalities that resemble those found in ROP occur in patients who have inherited disorders, such as X-linked familial exudative vitreoretinopathy which are known to be caused by mutations in the ND gene.

R.C. Eagle, Jr., M.D.

Uveal Melanoma: Comparison of the Prognostic Value of Fibrovascular Loops, Mean of the Ten Largest Nucleoli, Cell Type, and Tumor Size

McLean IW, Keefe KS, Burnier MN (Armed Forces Inst of Pathology, Washington, DC)

Ophthalmology 104:777–780, 1997 11–10

Objective.—Patients with uveal melanomas whose periodic acid-Schiff (PAS)–stained vascular patterns exhibited parallel vessels with cross-linking, arcs with branching, loop patterns, or networks had lower survival rates than patients with other patterns. In studies of enucleated eyes, PAS- and hematoxylin-stained sections frequently show loops within uveal melanomas. The relation between the presence of loops in these sections and the predictability of uveal melanomas was investigated.

Methods.—A total of 496 cases of uveal melanomas with PAS- and hematoxylin-stained slides of a center section of the tumor, with data available for the mean diameter of the 10 largest nucleoli (MLN), and with patient follow-up information were evaluated for the presence of loops. Melanomas with epithelioid cells were classified as mixed-cell type 2. Tumors without epithelioid cells were classified as spindle cell type 1. A loop was defined as the presence of at least 1 tumor lobule surrounded by a PAS-stained fibrovascular septum. A blinded observer determined the presence of loops. In instances in which the presence was equivocal, another examiner reviewed the slide. The final classification was determined by consensus. Results were compared statistically using Kaplan-Meier analysis.

Results.—At least 1 loop was present in 119 (24%) slides. Equivocal loops were present in 38 (8%) slides. There was a significant association between the presence of loops and deaths from uveal melanomas. The survival rate at 15 years was 67.5% for patients without complete loops and 33.8% for patients with complete loops. Univariate Cox regression analysis demonstrated that the presence of loops was a better predictor of outcome than age but was a worse predictor than MLN, cell type, or tumor size. Multivariate Cox regression analysis showed that loops and all other predictors but age remained significant. These results confirm the observations of Folberg et al., who showed that the presence of loops was indicative of a poor prognosis in 234 patients with uveal melanomas. This association was independent of MLN, cell type, and tumor size.

Conclusion.—This easy loop assessment method does not require special equipment, as does MLN determination, and is strongly prognostic of outcome in patients with uveal melanomas. The authors recommend that pathologists include the presence and description of loops in their reports.

► This study from the ophthalmic pathology department of the Armed Forces Institute of Pathology (AFIP) confirms that vascular patterns called loops or networks found in uveal melanomas do have prognostic significance. Contrary to earlier reports, however, other features such as cell type, tumor size, and nucleolar parameters were better predictors of outcome. The AFIP's technique for the assessment of vascular patterns uses routine slides stained with PAS and does not require any special equipment, which makes it readily applicable by practicing pathologists. The AFIP recommends that the presence or absence of vascular loops or networks in uveal melanomas should be mentioned in pathology reports along with cell type, tumor dimension, mitotic count, lymphocytic infiltration, and extrascleral extension. This currently is our policy at the Wills Eye Hospital.

R.C. Eagle, Jr., M.D.

Clinicopathologic Study of the Cornea in X-linked Ichthyosis

Kempster RC, Hirst LW, de la Cruz Z, et al (John Hopkins Hosp, Baltimore, Md; Univ of Queensland, Australia)

Arch Ophthalmol 115:409–415, 1997 11–11

Background.—The ichthyosiform dermatoses are classified into 4 groups based on mode of inheritance and clinical characteristics. The second most common form is X-linked ichthyosis, occurring in 1 of 6,190 males in England. Ectropion, superficial corneal changes, nodular swellings and brushlike endings of the corneal nerves, filiform-to-punctate opacities in the deep stroma or the Descemet membrane, and posterior embryotoxon are associated with ichthyosis. The histopathologic and ultrastructural features of a cornea removed from a patient with X-linked ichthyosis and anterior corneal changes clinically were reported.

Methods and Findings.—The corneal button was removed from a 64-year-old man. On examination, a thick amorphous subepithelial material was noted, consisting of proteinaceous material, disorganized collagen fibers, and electron-dense granular material. Many round and ovoid spaces within and between the stromal collagen lamellae were observed, concentrated along the anterior aspect of the Descemet membrane. Some appeared membrane-bound, some had a central dropout appearance, and some contained a laminated electron-dense material, findings similar to those in lecithin-cholesterol acyltransferase disease.

Conclusions.—These data suggest that cholesterol sulfate deposition is responsible for the ultrastructural changes in X-linked ichthyosis. Definitive diagnosis would require assaying for cholesterol sulfate levels in fresh tissue.

▶ This paper from W. Richard Greens laboratory at Johns Hopkins shows that transmission electron microscopy still has a place in this era of molecular biology. The molecular defect in X-linked ichthyosis is known; affected patients are deficient in an enzyme called steroid sulfatase, which is involved in the metabolism of estrogen and cholesterol sulfate. This ultrastructural study shows that the deep stromal opacities that occur just anterior to Descemet's membrane in X-linked ichthyosis correspond to ovoid spaces thought to contain cholesterol sulfate in vivo. Similar corneal vacuoles have been observed in lecithin-cholesterol acyltransferase deficiency.

R.C. Eagle, Jr., M.D.

Kerato-Epithelin Mutations in Four 5q31-linked Corneal Dystrophies

Munier FL, Korvatska E, Djemaï A, et al (CHUV, Lausanne, Switzerland; Hôpital Jules Gonin, Lausanne, Switzerland; Centre d'Etude du Polymorphisme Humain, Paris)

Nature Genet 15:247–251, 1997 11–12

Introduction.—Granular dystrophy Groenouw type I (CDGG1), Reis-Bückler's (CDRB), lattice type I (CDL1), and Avellino (ACD) are 4 human autosomal dominant corneal dystrophy disorders that have been linked to 5q31 in the vicinity of 1L9. The progressive opacification of the cornea associated with these disorders can cause severe visual handicap. A yeast artificial chromosome (YAC) contig of the linked region was created to identify the gene responsible for these corneal dystrophies.

Methods.—A complementary DNA (cDNA) selection was made and the human transforming growth factor (β*ig-h3*) gene was recovered. When aligned with sequences from Genbank, 1 clone was 10% homologous to a portion of *βig-h3*, but was not indexed in the Genome Database. This gene was considered a good candidate because it mapped to 5q31 and showed a distinct expression pattern in the human eye. A systematic search for mutations in *βig-h3* was conducted in patients with CDGG1, CDRB, CDL1, and ACD.

Results.—Mutations were observed in all 4 disorders: R555W in 1 family with CDGG1, R555Q in 1 family with CDRB, R124C in 2 families with CDL1, and R124H in 2 families with ACD. Mutations were detected at the CpG dinucleotide of 2 arginine codons.

Conclusion.—Findings suggest a common molecular origin for 5q31-linked corneal dystrophies.

► Several years ago when the genes for granular, lattice, and Avellino corneal dystrophies were found to be closely linked on the long arm of chromosome 5, it was suggested that all 3 disorders might represent disparate clinical manifestations of a single disease. This important study indicates that all 3 dystrophies, and Reis-Bücklers dystrophy as well, are caused by separate mutations in a single gene called β*ig-h3* that encodes a protein called kerato-epithelin.

The corneal epithelium is a rich source of this protein, which probably is involved in cellular adhesion. The single amino acid substitutions that have been identified appear to affect the structure and folding of the mutant kerato-epithelin in different ways. The protein precipitates as amyloid in patients who have lattice and Avellino dystrophies. In granular corneal dystrophy, the mutation predisposes to the formation of rodlike fibers that aggregate to form the crystalloids that make up the granular deposits.

It is unclear whether the families with Reis-Bückler's dystrophy in whom kerato-epithelin mutations were identified had superficial deposits of granular material or "curly filaments" in their corneas. Curly filaments are associated with Reis-Bückler's dystrophy in the American literature, but Reis and Bückler probably reported a family that had a superficial variant of granular dystrophy.

R.C. Eagle, Jr., M.D.

Homozygous Mutations in the Plasminogen Gene of Two Unrelated Girls With Ligneous Conjunctivitis

Schuster V, Mingers A-M, Seidenspinner S, et al (Univ of Würzburg, Germany; Univ of Bonn, Germany)

Blood 90:958–966, 1997 11–13

Introduction.—An unusual and rare form of chronic conjunctivitis, ligneous conjunctivitis is characterized by chronic tearing and redness of the conjunctivae. The palpebral surfaces have pseudomembranes that form and then become thick nodular masses that replace the normal mucosa. The disease was termed ligneous conjunctivitis because the pseudomembranes have a woodlike consistency. The mucosa of the mouth, tongue, nasopharynx, tracheobronchial tree, and female genital

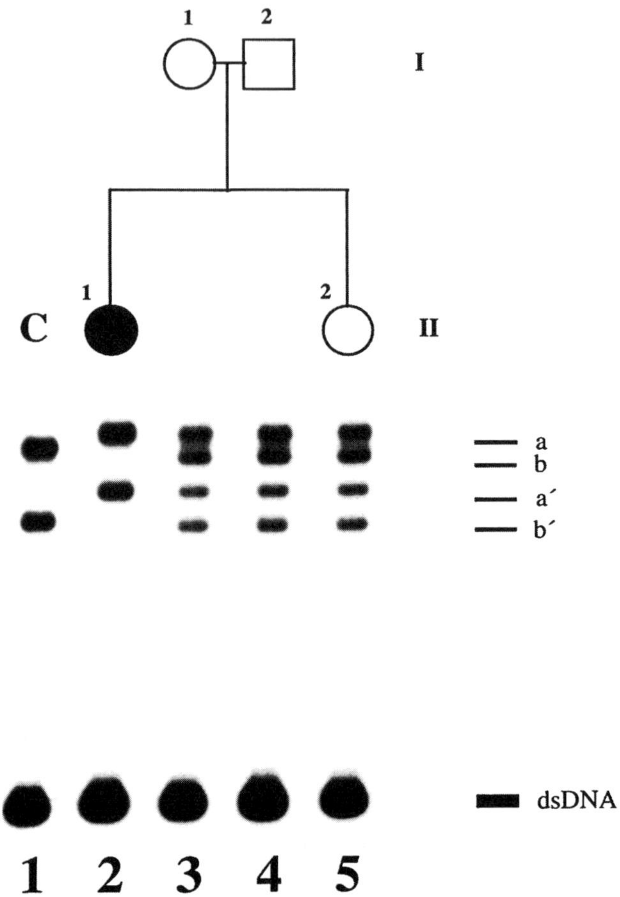

FIGURE 2.—Single-strand conformation polymorphism analysis of plasminogen gene exon 7 in patient 1, her healthy parents, and her healthy sister. Radiolabeled single-stranded polymerase chain reaction products of plasminogen exon 7 were electrophoresed in a nondenaturing 5% polyacrylamide gel. *Lane 1*, healthy control (C); *lane 2*, patient 1 with ligneous conjunctivitis (*II-1*); *lane 3*, healthy mother of patient 1 (*I-1*); *lane 4*, healthy father of patient 1 (*I-2*); *lane 5*, healthy sister of patient 1 (*II-2*). *Abbreviation: dsDNA*, double-stranded DNA. (Courtesy of Schuster V, Mingers A-M, Seidenspinner S, et al: Homozygous mutations in the plasminogen gene of two unrelated girls with ligneous conjunctivitis. *Blood* 90:958–966, 1997.)

tract may have additional similar pseudomembranous lesions. A disrupted epithelium that is replaced by a massive deposition of fibrin and amorphous hyalin-like eosinophilic material and accompanied by an inflammatory cellular infiltration are seen on histologic examination of pseudomembranes from the eyes and from the mucosa of the genital tract. This disease is inherited in an autosomal-recessive manner in some families. Two unrelated Turkish girls with ligneous conjunctivitis and occlusive hydrocephalus were examined.

Methods.—Screenings for mutations in the plasminogen gene by polymerase chain reaction, single-strand conformation polymorphism analysis and DNA sequencing were conducted on genomic DNA from both patients and clinically healthy family members. Peripheral blood samples of both girls and healthy parents and sisters were used to prepare genomic DNA.

Results.—A severe plasminogen deficiency was seen in both children. In plasminogen exon 7 at position 780 leading to an amino acid exchange, a homozygous G→A point mutation was seen in one girl with ligneous conjunctivitis (Fig 2). For this mutation, her healthy parents and sister were heterozygous. In plasminogen exon 15 at position 1924, which leads to a stop-codon, a homozygous G→A point mutation was seen in the other girl with ligneous conjunctivitis. For this mutation, the healthy parents were heterozygous. Another mutation in the same codon was found in the father's second allele.

Conclusions.—Ligneous conjunctivitis may be caused by certain homozygous mutations in the plasminogen gene. In affected patients, it is mainly the extravascular plasmin-mediated fibrinolytic pathway that is impaired, leading to deficient wound healing in mucous membranes.

► In 1986, I reported that fibrin was the major constituent of the mass of "woody" material that is the most striking clinical manifestation of ligneous conjunctivitis.[1] This paper from Germany indicates that this enigmatic form of pseudomembranous conjunctivitis is caused by mutations in the gene for plasminogen, the precursor of the enzyme plasmin which breaks down fibrin. The elucidation of this genetic defect explains why ligneous conjunctivitis is such a therapeutic challenge, and why attacks of the childhood disease are recurrent and frequently persist into adulthood. It is interesting that the plasminogen deficiency only leads to fibrin deposition in injured mucous membranes. Patients do not develop venous thromboses.

R.C. Eagle, Jr., M.D.

Reference

1. Eagle RC Jr, Brooks JSJ, Katowitz JA, et al: Fibrin as a major constituent of ligneous conjunctivitis. *Am J Ophthalmol* 101:493–494, 1986.

Reassessment of the PAS Patterns in Uveal Melanoma

Foss AJE, Alexander RA, Hungerford JL, et al (Inst of Ophthalmology, London; Moorfields Eye Hosp, London; Churchill Hosp, Headington, Oxford)

Br J Ophthalmol 81:240–246, 1997 11–14

Background.—The prognostic importance of patterns of periodic acid Schiff (PAS) staining (the Folberg patterns) in uveal melanoma has been demonstrated. Although these patterns have been attributed to blood vessels, they are different from those occurring with other staining methods for blood vessels. The nature and significance of the PAS patterns were explored further.

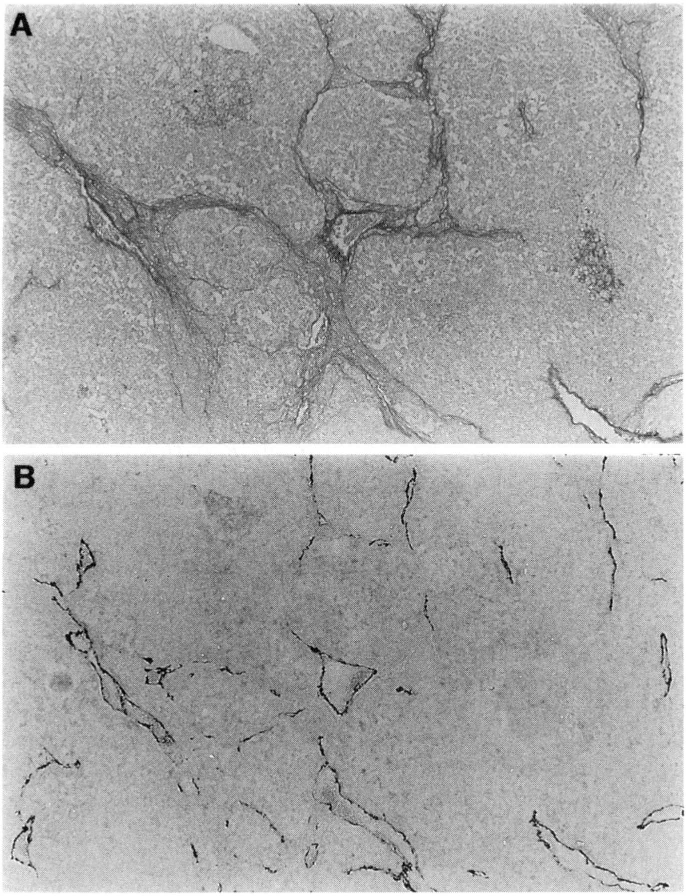

FIGURE 2.—A periodic acid Schiff stained section (**A**) showing the presence of a vascular loop, with a corresponding section (**B**) stained with F8 showing no loops. Original magnification, ×60. (Courtesy of Foss AJE, Alexander RA, Hungerford JL, et al: Reassessment of the PAS patterns in uveal melanoma. *Br J Ophthalmol* 81:240–246, 1997.)

Methods.—Periodic acid Schiff patterns were examined in 117 uveal melanomas. These patterns were compared with those occurring with conventional connective tissue stains and in sections stained for the presence of blood vessels by immunohistochemistry for factor VIII-related antigen.

Findings.—The PAS patterns were based on connective tissue, including fibrovascular tissue. In a principal components analysis, these patterns represented 3 underlying factors, tentatively identified as indicating disordered growth (factor 1), emergence of rapidly growing subclones (factor 2), and section orientation (factor 3) (Fig 2).

Conclusions.—The PAS patterns are formed primarily from connective tissue, including perivascular connective tissue. The patterns appear to be based on 3 underlying factors, the first 2 having prognostic significance, with the first retaining independent prognostic significance in a multivariate Cox model including tumor size and microvessel density.

► In 1992, Folberg and colleagues[1] reported that certain vascular patterns in uveal malignant melanomas, which are evident on histopathologic examination, serve as markers for tumor progression after enucleation. Enclosed vascular loops and networks of loops were the patterns associated with death from metastatic melanoma in Folberg's study. This report suggests that the putative vascular patterns described by Folberg and colleagues are not truly vascular, but actually are composed of fibrovascular connective tissue. The authors believe that microvascular density is a better prognostic factor.

At the present time, both of these prognostic techniques are basically research tools. The current emphasis on cost-containment makes it unlikely that either technique will become a standard procedure in most anatomical pathology laboratories.

R.C. Eagle, Jr., M.D.

Reference

1. Folberg R, Pe'er J, Gruman LM, et al: The morphologic characteristics of tumor blood vessels as a marker of tumor progression in primary human uveal melanoma: A matched case-control study. *Hum Pathol* 23:1298–1305, 1992.

Melanogenic Neuroectodermal Tumor of the Retina (Primary Malignant Melanoma of the Retina)

Freitag SK, Eagle RC Jr, Shields JA, et al (Thomas Jefferson Univ, Philadelphia; Tufts Univ, Boston; Baylor College of Medicine, Houston)
Arch Ophthalmol 115:1581–1584, 1997 11–15

Introduction.—Many primary intraocular tumors of early childhood are neuroectodermal neoplasms, including retinoblastoma and medulloepithelioma. In a young child with leukokoria, an erroneous clinical diagnosis of retinoblastoma was initially made.

Case Report.—Girl, 35 months, was born prematurely and weighed 0.9 kg at birth. A white pupil was detected; ophthalmoscopic examination showed a white retinal tumor with inherent vessels that filled most of the eye. Macroscopic examination revealed a white tumor consistent with a retinoblastoma in the posterior portion of the eye. A diagnosis of unilateral sporadic retinoblastoma was made and the eye was enucleated. Light microscopy showed an unremarkable anterior segment and a malignant neoplasm that seemed continuous with the neurosensory retina posteriorly. On cytologic examination, the tumor did not resemble a retinoblastoma and was composed of 3 distinct populations of cells: sheets of relatively undifferentiated neuroblastic cells; a population of large spindle-shaped cells with vesicular nuclei and prominent nucleoli; and epithelioid cells with abundant granular eosinophilic cytoplasm. No neuroepithelial bands, cords, rosettes, or heteroplastic elements were observed and the tumor was negative for synaptophysin and neurofilaments. Patchy moderate staining for S100 protein was observed in small and large tumor cells. The Fontana-Masson stain revealed scattered intracytoplasmic granules of melanin in some tumor cells. Parts of the tumor demonstrated convincing moderately heavy immunoreactivity for melanoma-specific antigen HMB-45. Transmission electron microscopy confirmed the presence of premelanosomes in tumor cells.

Conclusion.—Described is a child with an unusual retinal tumor with an uncertain prognosis. The most appropriate name for this never-described neoplasm is melanogenic neuroectodermal tumor of the retina.

▶ This unique pediatric intraocular tumor initially was thought to be a retinoblastoma on ophthalmosopic examination and during gross pathologic examination by experienced clinicians. Light microscopy revealed a retinal tumor that was a "melanoma" in the generic sense. The tumor contained spindle and epithelioid cells that contained melanin pigment and expressed melanoma-specific antigen HMB 45. Whether this unusual pediatric neoplasm will behave like a retinoblastoma or a melanoma is uncertain.

R.C. Eagle, Jr., M.D.

12 Social Economics

1997—The Year in Review

by Elisabeth J. Cohen, M.D.

The major shifts in managed care this year are more evident in the newspapers than in the scientific literature. The power of the HMOs is being questioned by the government and the public. Physicians' efforts continue to be weak, despite attempts to shape their own future.

Laws were passed in various states to halt drive-through deliveries and out-patient mastectomies. Egregious limitations on patient care mandated by HMOs were met with public outcry, followed by these legislative responses. In the face of the outrageous HMO policies, the public, through elected representatives, responded on a limited case-by-case basis. There was recognition that doctors should have some say in determining the medically appropriate length of hospitalization. When quality of care was obviously threatened, the government responded incrementally, not globally. In 1998 a patient's Bill of Rights may become law.

The HMOs have also been the subject of a number of unfavorable newspaper headlines. Columbia/HCA has been the target of a major ongoing federal investigation throughout the year and is trying to redefine itself rather than expand. Oxford Health Plan reported financial losses attributed to "computer problems" and then lost more than half its stock value in a day. It is not surprising that this "high end" HMO, which promised to be quality-oriented, had higher than expected expenses. Payers and patients are more concerned about getting good health care for their money than about the returns to stockholders and HMO executives. How could one possibly think enormous profits for the HMO could continue to grow without reducing the medical care provided to a level that would cause patients to demand better?

The year ended with an announcement in the newspaper that a Medicare HMO was ending prescription coverage. This may sound like a small item. However, cost of medication is a major concern for Medicare patients, especially those with medical problems. Coverage of prescriptions has encouraged many Medicare patients to enroll in HMOs, and loss of this coverage will certainly encourage people with a choice to leave HMOs. What sounds like a cost containment measure is actually another way to select healthy patients for Medicare HMOs and thereby improve their profitability.

The upshot of these developments in 1997 is that the power of the HMOs is under attack, albeit a limited one. From the physicians' point of view, the payers maintain control. However, at the end of 1997 there appeared to be increased interest among HMOs to interact with physician organizations. Physicians are trying to regain control by forming their own insurance organizations and running for public office. As always, it is impossible to predict the future, but I think the HMOs may weaken as the public resists restrictions on care it deserves.

The Value of Routine Dilated Pupil Screening Examination

Batchelder TJ, Fireman B, Friedman GD, et al (Kaiser Permanente Med Ctr, Richmond, Calif; Kaiser Permanente Med Care Program, Oakland, Calif; Kaiser Permanente Med Ctr, San Rafael, Calif; et al)

Arch Ophthalmol 115:1179–1184, 1997 12–1

Objective.—Although routine dilated examination (RDE) is recommended because of frequent findings of retinal anomalies, most of these do not reveal harmful conditions. The value of routine screening RDE for detecting uncommon conditions has not been evaluated. The cost effectiveness of RDE in improving visual outcomes was tested.

Methods.—Routine dilated fundus examination was performed in 1.75 million patients who had not undergone a dilated examination within 2 years for patients aged 65 or older, within 4 years for patients age 40–64, and within 5 years for patients age 20–39. The purpose was to detect rhegmatogenous retinal detachment, exudative retinal detachment resulting in loss of visual acuity, uveal melanoma, or tumor metastasized to the choroid. All were diseases that might have improved clinical outcome if detected early. American Optometric Association guidelines calling for a dilated examination within 1 year for patients aged 61 years or older, within 2 years for patients age 41–60, and within 3 years for patients age 20–40 were also tested. The cost of a dilated examination to the provider was based on the cost of an undilated examination plus an estimate of the cost of 5 minutes of extra time for an ophthalmologist ($10.40) and 10 minutes of extra time for an optometrist ($8.25).

Results.—Vision-threatening peripheral retinal disease, primarily rhegmatogenous retinal detachment (greater than 90%), was detected in 207 patients, 127 of whom were excluded because of a pre-existing diagnosis. Five patients had uveal melanoma, and 4 patients had tumors that had metastasized to the choroid, 2 from the lung and 2 from breast and colon. In 42 patients, the condition could not have been prevented by performing RDE rather than undilated examination. Of the 38 patients whose conditions may have been preventable, 36 had retinal detachment, 1 had choroid melanoma, and 1 had a tumor metastatic to the choroid. In 3 patients, the retinal detachment appears to have been a chronic and unpreventable problem. Earlier detection by RDE may have been beneficial for the patient with choroidal melanoma but not for the patient with a tumor metastatic to the choroid who died of lung cancer 6 months later. If prevention were 10% effective (1:50,000 patients), the provider cost per prevented case is estimated at $433,000.

Conclusion.—Although the RDE screening test is inexpensive, a screening program is not cost effective because conditions detected by RDE are rare and/or unpreventable.

► This study provides evidence that RDE of the fundus is not cost effective in preventing vision threatening peripheral retinal diseases. It is interesting that coding was not used to determine the cost difference as comprehensive ophthalmic codes (92004, 92014) are often used for RDEs.

I think that RDEs facilitate the examination of the posterior pole as well as the peripheral retina and that their value is underestimated in this study, which considers only the diagnosis of asymptomatic peripheral retinal disease. The study does not question the indication of RDEs for patients with symptoms or risk factors for posterior segment pathology.

E.J. Cohen, M.D.

Variations in Cataract Extraction Rates in Medicare Prepaid and Fee-for-Service Settings

Goldzweig CL, Mittman BS, Carter GM, et al (Veterans Affairs Med Ctr, West Los Angeles; Univ of California Los Angeles; RAND, Santa Monica, Calif; et al)

JAMA 277:1765–1768, 1997 12–2

Background.—The movement toward managed care continues to grow, but little is known about variations in elective surgery for elderly patients enrolled in prepaid vs. traditional fee-for-service (FFS) Medicare plans. Because of utilization review and prior approval, rates of cataract extraction (which accounts for Medicare's single largest expenditure) are likely to be lower in prepaid settings. A cross-sectional analysis using 1993 Medicare beneficiaries aged 65 years and older examined rates of cataract extraction in 3 health care models: the staff-model HMO, the independent practice association (IPA), and and traditional FFS plan.

Methods.—All Medicare beneficiaries lived in Southern California and had self-selected into a prepaid or traditional plan. The study population included all 43,387 staff-model HMO enrollees, all 19,050 IPA enrollees, and a 5% sample (47,150) of FFS beneficiaries. Sources of data included 1993 HMO Medicare claims and encounter files, the Health Care Financing Administration (HCFA) 5% Medicare Part B provider/supplier file, and the HCFA October 1992 100% Medicare population file. Cataract extraction rates were obtained by dividing the total number of surgical procedures by the total number of beneficiary-years in a given setting.

Results.—When prepaid and FFS settings were compared, the unadjusted rates of cataract extraction per 1,000 beneficiary-years varied significantly. The FFS rates were more than twice as high as HMO rates (35 vs. 17 extractions/1,000 beneficiary-years); IPA rates were 22 extractions/1,000 beneficiary-years. These differences persisted even after adjusting for age, sex, and diabetes status. In all settings, the probability of having a cataract extraction was significantly greater for older patients (aged 75 to 84 years) and for those with diabetes. In the FFS group, women were twice as likely as men to undergo cataract extraction; rates were similar for men and women in staff and IPA settings.

Conclusion.—Elderly Medicare beneficiaries enrolled in FFS settings are twice as likely as similar patients in prepaid settings to undergo cataract extraction. Although the financial incentive to perform more surgery exists in the IPA setting, this group and the staff-model HMO had similar extraction rates. The quality implications of these rate differences need to be explored.

► It is impressive that in a Southern California Medicare population, patients with FFS insurance were twice as likely to have cataract surgery as patients enrolled in HMOs. This was true for both staff-model HMOs, in which the primary care gatekeepers were salaried, and IPA HMOs, in which the primary gatekeepers were capitated and the ophthalmologists were reimbursed by discounted FFSs. It is noteworthy that women—who are known to have a 50% increased risk for cataracts—were twice as likely as men to have cataract surgery in FFS settings but not in prepaid settings.

Although assessment of visual disability was not undertaken to determine whether there was overuse of cataract surgery in the FFS setting or underutilization in the prepaid setting, it is more likely that the latter is the case. It would also appear that women, in particular, are bearing the brunt of reduced/managed care. Functional evaluations are needed to test these suspicions and should become a routine part of preoperative and postoperative ophthalmic care. It is very difficult, however, to evaluate the need for surgery in patients who are not even referred for it.

E.J. Cohen, M.D.

Outcomes of Stroke Patients in Medicare Fee for Service and Managed Care

Retchin SM, Brown RS, Yeh S-CJ, et al (Virginia Commonwealth Univ, Richmond; Mathematica Policy Research Inc, Princeton, NJ)

JAMA 278:119–124, 1997 12–3

Background.—Although most studies of Medicare beneficiaries enrolled in HMOs have found patient care to be similar to that provided in fee-for-service (FFS) settings, there is evidence that HMOs reduce selected services as a cost-cutting measure. Stroke patients often need expensive resources for posthospital care, and such services appear to be performed less often or less intensively for HMO patients. An observational study of 402 HMO patients and 408 FFS patients compared discharge destinations and survival rates after stroke.

Methods.—Patients eligible for the study were hospitalized during 1989 with the diagnosis of cerebrovascular accident, stroke, or cerebral thrombosis. The HMO sample was selected from 19 HMOs in 12 states; FFS patients were drawn from the same geographic areas. Data abstracted from medical records included demographic and clinical characteristics, co-morbid illnesses, and discharge destinations. The February 1992 Health Insurance Printout file from Medicare provided follow-up data on death.

Results.—The HMO and FFS patients were similar in most of the analyzed personal and clinical characteristics. Compared with FFS patients, HMO patients were slightly younger and more likely to be married; FFS patients had a higher prevalence of recent myocardial infarction and a significantly higher prevalence of history of dementia. Forty-nine HMO (12.2%) and 60 FFS (14.7%) patients died during hospitalization. After controlling for age, marital status, and dependency level at discharge, HMO patients were more likely than FFS patients to be sent to nursing homes (41.8% vs. 27.9%). The rate of discharge to rehabilitation hospitals or units was 23.4% for FFS patients vs. 16.2% for HMO patients. Survival rates after discharge were similar for the 2 groups. By the end of follow-up (25 to 37 months), 191 HMO (47.5%) and 219 FFS (53.7%) patients had died.

Conclusion.—Medicare beneficiaries hospitalized for stroke are more likely to be discharged to nursing homes and less likely to be sent to rehabilitation facilities when they are enrolled in an HMO vs. an FFS setting. Survival rates, however, were similar for the 2 groups after adjusting for selected factors. A question raised by HMO practices is whether the functional level of stroke survivors is compromised.

▶ It is not surprising that this study shows that stroke patients are more likely to be discharged to nursing homes than rehabilitation centers when covered by HMO compared with FFS insurance. This result needs to be combined with previous studies showing that rehabilitation improves functional outcome and reduces long-term nursing home institutionalization among stroke patients. It is not enough that survival is similar. Quality of life is the critical issue when considering the care of stroke victims. It is obvious that HMOs reduce their costs by limiting rehabilitation. Medicare patients should have access to this kind of information when selecting their insurance if they have a choice.

Is this what our elected representatives want when they support policies encouraging Medicare enrollment in HMOs? What are the politicians going to do about the situation? Although the majority of people are healthy, eventually most families will be touched by debilitating chronic disease and would prefer rehabilitation to long-term nursing care. Long-term institutionalization in nursing homes is costly relative to short-term rehabilitation and improved independent living.

E.J. Cohen, M.D.

The Medicare-HMO Revolving Door: The Healthy Go In and the Sick Go Out

Morgan RO, Virnig BA, DeVito CA, et al (Univ of Miami, Fla; Washington Univ, Washington, DC)

N Engl J Med 337:169–175, 1997 12–4

Introduction.—Reduction in the length of stay and the number of bed-days associated with the traditional fee-for-service system has been credited to HMOs serving Medicare beneficiaries. The growth in the costs of health care for the elderly is assumed to go slower with HMOs; however, recently, this assumption has been questioned. There is a theory that selective enrollment of healthier Medicare recipients benefits HMOs and that sicker patients are more likely to disenroll from Medicare HMOs, which would raise the average fee-for-service costs.

Methods.—To examine differences in the use of inpatient medical services by 375,406 beneficiaries in the Medicare fee-for-service system,

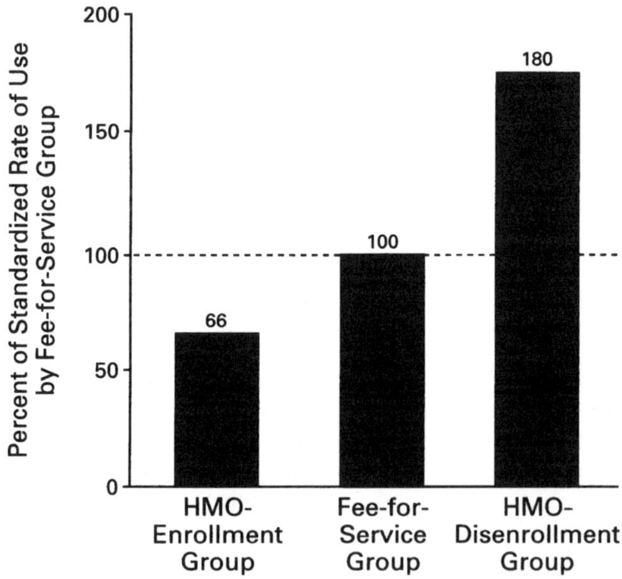

FIGURE 1.—Use of inpatient services by Medicare beneficiaries who switched from the fee-for-service system to HMOs (*HMO-Enrollment Group*), those who remained in the fee-for-service system (*Fee-for-Service Group*), and those who switched from HMOs to the fee-for service system (*HMO-Disenrollment Group*). Rates of use are shown as percentages of the standardized rate of use by the fee-for-service group (100%). (Reprinted by permission of *The New England Journal of Medicine*, from Morgan RO, Virnig BA, DeVito CA, et al: The Medicare-HMO revolving door: The healthy go in and the sick go out. *N Engl J Med* 337:169–175. Copyright 1997, Massachusetts Medical Society. All rights reserved.)

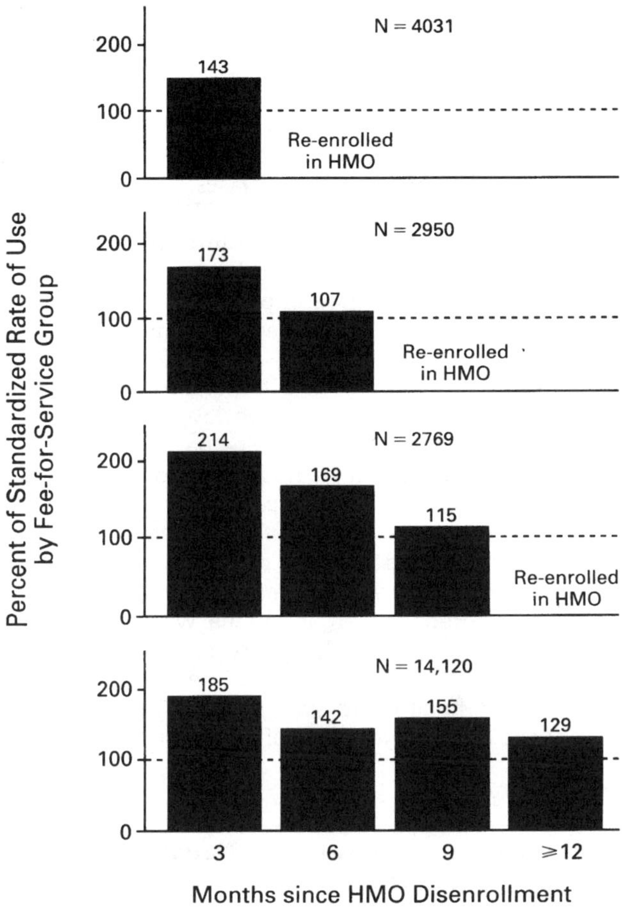

FIGURE 2.—Use of inpatient services by Medicare beneficiaries who switched from HMOs to the fee-for-service system, according to the length of time since disenrollment. Rates of use are shown as percentages of the standardized rate of use by beneficiaries continuously in the fee-for-service system (100%). (Reprinted by permission of *The New England Journal of Medicine*, from Morgan RO, Virnig BA, DeVito CA, et al: The Medicare-HMO revolving door: The healthy go in and the sick go out. *N Engl J Med* 337:169–175. Copyright 1997, Massachusetts Medical Society. All rights reserved.)

48,380 HMO enrollees before enrollment, and 23,870 HMO enrollees after disenrollment, Medicare enrollment and inpatient billing records were used from a 3-year period. Whether the pattern of use after disenrollment persisted over time and whether these differences were related to demographic characteristics were also determined.

Results.—During the year before enrollment, the rate of use of inpatient services in the HMO-enrollment group was 66% of the rate of the fee-for-service group. After disenrollment, the rate in the HMO-disenrollment group was 180% of that in the fee-for-service group (Figs 1 and 2). Those who disenrolled from HMOs and re-enrolled had a higher rate of admissions than the fee-for-service beneficiaries. At least 1 inpatient stay was found in twice as many beneficiaries in the HMO-disenrollment group and they had twice as many inpatient days and twice the inpatient hospital payments when compared to those who remained in the fee-for-service system.

Conclusion.—With respect to HMO enrollment and disenrollment, there are marked selection biases. The effectiveness of the Medicare managed-care system is undermined by these biases. The need for longitudinal and population-based studies is highlighted. There is a strong suggestion that those who disenroll from HMOs move into the fee-for-service system to obtain needed services and then return back to Medicare HMOs after they are healthier. There is also a greater proportion of younger individuals using Medicare HMOs who are low-use beneficiaries.

▶ This study provides impressive data demonstrating that Medicare patients who choose to enroll in HMOs have lower rates of hospitalization before enrollment compared to fee-for-service patients. In addition, patients who choose to disenroll have higher hospitalization rates and tend to re-enroll when this rate levels off. The bottom line is that healthy patients enter HMOs and sick patients choose to leave if they have the choice. This works to the advantage of the HMOs who are paid 95% of fee-for-service rates; however, it means that Medicare HMOs make money, but do not save health care costs. Health maintenance organizations will be popular among the majority who are healthy, but clearly do not best serve the needs of the acutely or chronically ill. Preventive care is important, but many illnesses cannot be prevented. A health care system that does not care well for the sick clearly is not the solution to our health care crisis.

E.J. Cohen, M.D.

The Oregon Health Plan: Lessons for the Nation. First of Two Parts

Bodenheimer T (Univ of California at San Francisco)

N Engl J Med 337:651–655, 1997 12–5

Introduction.—In 1989, the state of Oregon added more than 100,000 uninsured individuals to its Medicaid program and funded it by reducing the number of services available to all by ranking more than 700 diagnoses in order of importance and rationing treatments. The program is popular and has no more serious problems than do other health care programs throughout the country.

History.—In 1987, John Kitzhaber, an emergency room physician, approached the problem of covering the medical expenses of low-income individuals by reducing Medicaid expenditures using 1 of the 3 legislative options: removing people from the Medicaid, lowering the reimbursement rate to providers, or reducing the benefit package. Deciding on the last, Kitzhaber introduced legislation that would extend Medicaid coverage to individuals with incomes below the federal poverty level according to a ranked list of diagnoses and treatments with a cutoff point below which no

TABLE 1.—The Oregon Health Plan's Prioritized List of Health Services, 1995.

The five top items
Line 1. Diagnosis: severe or moderate head injury, hematoma or edema with loss of consciousness. Treatment: medical and surgical treatment.
Line 2. Diagnosis: insulin-dependent diabetes mellitus. Treatment: medical therapy.
Line 3. Diagnosis: peritonitis. Treatment: medical and surgical treatment.
Line 4. Diagnosis: acute glomerulonephritis, with lesion of rapidly progressive glomerulonephritis. Treatment: medical therapy, including dialysis.
Line 5. Diagnosis: pneumothorax and hemothorax. Treatment: tube thoracostomy or thoracotomy, medical therapy.
The five bottom items
Line 741. Diagnosis: mental disorders with no effective treatments. Treatment: evaluation.
Line 742. Diagnosis: tubal dysfunction and other causes of infertility. Treatment: in vitro fertilization, gamete intrafallopian transfer.
Line 743. Diagnosis: hepatorenal syndrome. Treatment: medical therapy.
Line 744. Diagnosis: spastic dysphoria. Treatment: medical therapy.
Line 745. Diagnosis: disorders of refraction and accommodation. Treatment: radial keratotomy.
Six items near the 1997 cutoff line
Line 576. Diagnosis: internal derangement of the knee and ligamentous disruptions of the knee, grade III or IV. Treatment: repair, medical therapy.
Line 577. Diagnosis: keratoconjunctivitis sicca, not specified as Sjogren's syndrome. Treatment: punctal occlusion, tarsorrhaphy.
Line 578. Diagnosis: noncervical warts, including condyloma acuminatum and venereal warts. Treatment: medical therapy.
Line 579. Diagnosis: anal fistula. Treatment: fistulectomy.
Line 580. Diagnosis: relaxed anal sphincter. Treatment: medical and surgical treatment.
Line 581. Diagnosis: dental conditions (e.g., broken appliances), Treatment: repairs.

Note: Data were adapted from Oregon Health Plan Administrative Rules (Oregon Health Plan Administrative Rules. Salem: Oregon Office of Medical Assistance Programs, 1995).

(Reprinted by permission of *The New England Journal of Medicine*, from Bodenheimer T: The Oregon Health Plan: Lessons for the nation. First of two parts. *N Engl J Med* 337:651–655.

reimbursement would be provided. Above the cutoff point, unreduced reimbursements would be made to providers, Medicaid services would be available through managed care plans and employers would insure employees. The Oregon Health Services Commission ranked 17 categories of health problems according to 13 criteria. Treatments preventing death and leading to complete recovery were ranked first, maternity care second, and treatments preventing death but not resulting in full recovery third. In 1991, the plan was rejected by the Bush administration. When each diagnosis/treatment pair was re-ranked according to probability of death or disability with and without treatment, the plan was approved by the Clinton administration in 1993 and implemented in 1994, with 85% of the items ranked almost the same as on the original list. Kitzhaber was elected governor of Oregon that year.

Accomplishments.—States can mandate managed care. Any qualified Oregonians not enrolled can enroll when they become sick and be covered that day. According to the Census Bureau, the percent of uninsured Oregonians dropped from 14% to 12% (state data suggest a drop from 18% to 11%). Minnesota, Tennessee, Massachusetts, New York, and Arizona have since implemented similar programs. Nationwide, the uninsured population is growing. Coverage has expanded 11%, and Medicaid expenditure have increased 30%. Oregon increased its Medicare population by 39% and their expenditures by 36%.

Managed Care.—Managed care has been part of Oregon's health care system for decades. Capitation payments (about 30% above former Medicaid fee-for-service payments) have been kept high to support funding for the program and to attract physicians. Capitation payments in other states have declined as much as 40%. Oregon physicians are not dissatisfied with the arrangement and 88% of patients are satisfied.

The List.—There are few complaints about the ranked list (Table 1). Diagnoses below the cutoff of 578 can be managed by selecting a treatment above the line. The Oregon plant has expanded coverage. Denied services are low on the list. A diagnosis is required before a treatment can be denied, and physicians occasionally choose a diagnosis above the line even though the illness falls below the line; adherence to the list is required only for 13% of patients. For the 87% of Medicaid enrollees in capitated health plans, the state deducts 10% of all expenditures for items below the line from capitation payments. The plans decide what treatments are medically necessary.

Conclusion.—The Oregon Health Plan incorporates a common sense ranked list of diagnostic and treatment categories. Its benefits package design is a new approach to the effective rationing of health care.

The Oregon Health Plan: Lessons for the Nation. Second of Two Parts

Bodenheimer T (Univ of California at San Francisco)

N Engl J Med 337:720–723, 1997 12–6

Introduction.—The part of the Oregon Health Plan that required employers to provide insurance was defeated in the legislature. A 1996, 30-cent increase in the tobacco tax funded the addition to the plan of 25,000 children and provision of state subsidies for private health insurance to 21,000 individuals.

Problems.—Oregon's safety net includes Oregon Health Sciences University, public health clinics, urban and rural health centers, and county hospitals. Many clinics get federal grants. Increasing Medicaid growth threatens this safety net. Whereas ample Medicaid reimbursement rates to community centers have been used in the past to subsidize care of the uninsured, section 1115 waivers may eliminate reimbursement on a cost basis, leaving the uninsured worse off than before the Oregon plan went into effect. Section 1115 waivers also allow Medicaid disproportionate-share funds to be added to the general Medicaid funds rather disseminated to hospitals serving a disproportionate share of uninsured patients. The effort to shift Medicaid patients to private managed care plans is causing the plans to try to attract healthy individuals and leave high-risk and uninsured patients to public providers. Because the federal government requires high reimbursement rates for safety net HMOs, the state prefers to contract with private HMOs that are reimbursed at lower rates. Care-

Oregon, a safety net provider, has asked the legislature to base its capitation payments on risk. The downside is that physicians can overreport expensive diagnoses and inflate reimbursements. Oregon instituted sliding-scale premiums in 1995. Oregon's mental health benefits are generous but may suffer with the switch to managed care. A similar system in Tennessee is unravelling. Capitated mental health services do not always provide the best outcomes for individuals with severe or chronic mental illnesses. Whereas the elderly and disabled use 59% of Medicaid expenditures, section 1115 waivers allow the state to require them to join managed care plans. A national survey found that 26% of Medicare-HMO enrollees would not recommend their plan. Another study found that elderly HMO enrollees with chronic illnesses had worse outcomes over a 4-year period than did similar elderly persons in fee-for-service plans.

Fiscal Uncertainty.—Oregon is a fiscally conservative state. The health plan does not allow large reductions in numbers of enrollees or cuts in provider reimbursements. The Health Care Finance Administration will not permit a substantial reduction in the number of covered treatments. In 1991, property taxes were reduced; the state has no sales tax, and federal Medicaid funds may be reduced. Oregon has a strong economy and a low rate of inflation in medical costs. If the business cycle takes a downturn, health care funding will be problematic, and the line on the priority list may be moved upward.

► This 2-part article (Abstract 12–5 and 12–6) nicely reviews the history, early (2-year) results, and remaining issues of the Oregon Health Plan. The plan uses a prioritized list of diagnoses to determine services covered by Medicaid. A physician, John Kitzhaber, now governor, developed the plan to increase insurance for low income people and provide coverage for life-saving treatment. Effective, expensive therapies are ranked high. The plan has expanded benefits more than it has reduced them. The original requirement that employers provide insurance based on this list of minimum benefits has been repealed and with it hope of universal health insurance.

Use of managed care to provide Medicaid services is associated with a number of problems discussed in Part 2 of the report, including financial losses for academic centers providing care to the sickest and poorest patients. Adjustment of the capitation rate on the basis of risk remains a challenge. Although the Oregon plan has worked relatively well so far, increased inflation or a weaker economy would make it less viable. One plan administrator has a sign on the wall that reads "Cost, access, quality—pick any two."

It is important to assess the outcome of rational attempts at health care reform to learn how to make further improvements. It was naive to think health care in the United States could be reformed in 90 days. Different approaches should be tried and studied on a relatively small scale so that mistakes are not too devastating. Universal access must remain a goal. Quality should not be sacrificed. Cost is what has to give sooner or later.

Patients, employers, and insurers need to recognize that quality health care is worth paying for.

E.J. Cohen, M.D.

Is Gatekeeping Better Than Traditional Care?: A Survey of Physicians' Attitudes

Halm EA, Causino N, Blumenthal D (Harvard Med School, Boston)

JAMA 278:1677–1681, 1997 12–7

Introduction.—In the restructuring of the health care system, nearly all managed care plans rely on primary care physicians as gatekeepers to orchestrate and control the health care of its enrollees, including referrals to specialists, hospitalizations, and other expensive services. The expectations of managed care plans is that gatekeepers can increase the quality of care by increasing coordination and reduce costs. Previous studies have not separated the effects of gatekeeping as an administrative arrangement from the confounding effects of different payment mechanisms such as capitation.

Methods.—There were 330 physicians who served as primary care gatekeepers and traditional providers and who were surveyed to assess their attitudes about the effects of gatekeeping compared with traditional care on quality of patient care, administrative work, appropriateness of resource use, and cost.

Results.—Control of costs, frequency, and appropriateness of preventive services and knowledge of patient's overall care were considered to be the positive effects of gatekeeping compared with traditional care by physicians. The negative effects of gatekeeping, according to the physicians, were that they increased paperwork and telephone calls, and negatively affected access to specialists, ability to order expensive tests and procedures, overall quality of care, freedom in clinical decisions, physician-patient relationships, time spent with patients, and appropriate use of hospitalizations and laboratory tests. The survey revealed that 7% of physicians were of mixed opinion, 21% said gatekeeping was worse, 40% said gatekeeping was the same as traditional care, and 32% rated gatekeeping as better than traditional care. Fewer years in clinical practice, generalist training, and experience with gatekeeping and HMO plans were associated with positive ratings of gatekeeping.

Conclusions.—Positive and negative effects of gatekeeping were identified by physicians. Gatekeeping was considered to be better than or comparable to traditional care arrangements by 72% of physicians overall.

▶ This is an interesting, well-designed, controlled scientific study of physician perceptions of the impact of gatekeeping on patient care. The price of good science can be controls that limit generalizability. In this case, there were no financial incentives for gatekeepers, which is different from their usual situation in risk contracts. Nonetheless, gatekeeping was perceived to have a significantly positive effect only on costs, knowledge of patient's overall care, and preventive care. Unfortunately, cost data were not gathered to compare perceptions to realities about reduced costs. Not surprisingly, gatekeeping was perceived to have a significant negative impact on many aspects of patient care, appropriate use of resources, administrative work, and overall quality.

The conclusion that the majority of physicians thought gatekeeping was better than or equal to traditional care is somewhat misleading because the data were calculated from mean differences rather than directly from questionnaire responses, and cost benefits balanced quality issues. Younger doctors were more favorable about gatekeeping, so perhaps perceptions will improve with time as older physicians retire.

E.J. Cohen, M.D.

Physicians' Views on Capitated Payment for Medical Care: Does Familiarity Foster Acceptance?

Wynia MK, Picken HA, Selker HP (AMA, Chicago; New England Med Ctr, Boston; Tufts Univ, Boston)

Am J Managed Care 3:1497–1502, 1997 12–8

Introduction.—Although ethical concerns are voiced about capitated payments for medical care among third-party payers, little is known about what practicing physicians think about capitated payment for medical care. The inherent financial conflict of interest between patients and physicians has been the focus of ethical concerns with capitated payment because there is a strong incentive to reduce expenditures at the expense of quality patient care, whereas fee-for-service payment encourages physicians to provide more services, perhaps even some that are marginal or unnecessary. Some believe that once physicians become familiar in working within a capitated payment system, they will begin to see these plans as ethically acceptable and financially attractive and will become more comfortable with capitated payment.

Methods.—There were 200 physicians who were given a written survey, of which 41% responded. Of these respondents, 26% were primary care physicians, 22% were medical subspecialists, and 22% were surgeons. Forty-three percent participated in capitated payment arrangements, and 71% were providers for managed care plans.

Results.—A conflict of interest in capitated payment was cited by 100% of those physicians who did not participate in capitated care, and 77% of these physicians believed that participation in plans that reduce physician income in proportion to medical expenditures is not acceptable (Table 2). Of those who did participate in capitated plans, 95% said that there was a conflict of interest, and 72% believed this was not acceptable. Those who received capitated payment were 50% more likely to have never discussed capitated payment with any patient than those who were not receiving capitated payment. Those who received capitated payment were 70%

TABLE 2.—Percentage of Respondents Who Answered "Yes" to Questions About Capitated Payment for Medical Care

Question	Physicians Who Do Not Receive Capitated Payments [%(n)]	Physicians Who Receive Capitated Payments [%(n)]	Total [%(n)]	*P* Value for Difference
■ Is there some or very clear conflict of interest in capitated payment for medical care?	100 (31)	95 (41)	96 (79)	0.40
■ Is physician participation in payment arrangements that discourage expenditures by reducing physician income in proportion to expenditures for care *not* acceptable?	77 (23)	72 (31)	74 (57)	0.66
■ Would you be willing to give up more than 10% of your income to avoid capitated payment?	26 (7)	42 (17)	38 (27)	0.19
■ Is it impossible to avoid capitated payments and stay in the practice of medicine?	65 (20)	84 (36)	76 (60)	0.06

(Reprinted by permission of *The American Journal of Managed Care*, from Wynia MK, Picken HA, Selker HP: Physicians' view on capitated payment for medical care: Does familiarity foster acceptance? *Am J Managed Care* 3:1497–1502.)

more likely to very strongly oppose the use of capitation to pay their own family's physicians than those who were not receiving capitated payment (Table 4). Those who received capitated payment were 30% more likely to believe it is impossible to stay in the practice of medicine without participating in capitated payment, compared with those physicians who were not receiving capitated payment.

TABLE 4.—Percentage of Respondents Who Answered "Yes" to Questions or Statements About Preferences for Physician Payment

Statement	Physicians Who Do Not Receive Capitated Payments [%(n)]	Physicians Who Receive Capitated Payments [%(n)]	Total [%(n)]	*P* Value for Difference
■ Is there some or very clear conflict of interest in fee-for-service payment for medical care?	48 (15)	58 (25)	54 (44)	0.70
■ I very strongly do not prefer capitated payment for the physicians of my own family members.	29 (9)	50 (21)	43 (34)	0.07
■ My own healthcare is through a managed care plan.	61 (19)	67 (28)	64 (48)	0.76
■ My own physician is paid a capitated rate.	3 (1)	5 (2)	4 (3)	N/A*

**N/A* = not applicable. Cell with fewer than 5 individuals, so statistical testing was not performed.

(Reprinted by permission of *The American Journal of Managed Care*, from Wynia MK, Picken HA, Selker HP: Physicians' view on capitated payment for medical care: Does familiarity foster acceptance? *Am J Managed Care* 3:1497–1502.)

Conclusions.—Greater levels of experience with capitated plans did not cause physicians to believe that capitated payment arrangements are acceptable. Views were as negative or more negative on the acceptability of capitated payment by those who participated in existing capitated payment managed care plans as those who did not participate. In spite of these negative views, many were participating because they feared that if they didn't they would be forced out of medical practice.

► This paper discusses a nonrandomized study with a relatively low response rate (41% vs. 61% of Abstract 12–7) providing compelling evidence that both physicians who do and do not participate in capitated contracts think capitation involves an unacceptable conflict of interest. Not surprisingly, physicians participate in capitated contracts because they think they don't have a choice. The most telling result is that physicians do not want their own families' physicians to be capitated. All this adds up to a terrible report card for capitation from the physicians' point of view. Hopefully, capitation will be an experiment in delivery of medical care that is not the wave of the future in the United States.

E.J. Cohen, M.D.

Listening In on the Duke University Private Sector Conference
Iglehart JK (Health Affairs, Bethesda, Md)
N Engl J Med 336:1827–1831, 1997 12–9

Introduction.—The Private Sector Conferences held at Duke University Medical Center bring together a group of physicians who direct academic health centers, professional associations, and medical journals, together with managed-care executives and health policy analysts. The 1997 conference, entitled "Beyond Managed Health Care: The Role of the Academic Health Center," concluded that the market-driven system has only started to implement its goals. Depending upon ones point of view, the best—or worst—is yet to come. Several topics discussed at the conference were reviewed.

The Insurance Pool.—Medical savings accounts were promoted by some conference participants, whereas others see this development as socially irresponsible because healthy individuals are removed from the insurance pool. One solution proposed had payers increasingly shifting from offering their beneficiaries defined packages of benefits to making defined financial contributions, as the preferred way to limit their liability. Some payers are already moving in this direction.

A Large Corporate Purchaser.—General Motors, with 1.5 million employees, retirees, and dependents, is seeking to moderate the cost of health care through market mechanisms. The corporation's close to \$5 billion annual health care expenditures, almost half spent on retirees, account for about \$1,200 of every vehicle General Motors produces in the United States. General Motors ranks the plans it offers and gives workers financial incentives to join 1 of the 15 plans with the highest rankings. All 15 plans operate on a not-for-profit basis and are characterized by General Motors as being "highly integrated . . . with great medical leadership." The for-profits are losing their credibility, a development that may enable academic medical centers to work actively to improve quality of care.

The Academic Response.—Several themes appeared in presentations by the academic medical centers. Because health care is a locally based phenomenon, tailored responses are needed. All medical centers are seeking to affiliate with primary care physicians to obtain new referrals. Reducing expenses is an important concern, and department-based structures are being replaced by multidisciplinary teams. Many centers are seeking to exploit the commercial potential of the laboratories.

The Physician Work Force.—Marketplace pressure has led more doctors to train as generalists, but the geographic maldistribution of physicians continues, as does the underrepresentation of ethnic and racial minorities in medical schools. A solution proposed for the current problem of an oversupply of physicians is a reduction in the number of residency training positions.

Conclusion.—The health care system in the United States can be characterized as pluralistic and uncoordinated. Academic medicine needs to identify and aggressively pursue a strategy to protect its missions of education, research, and patient care.

▶ This is a rather depressing summary of a meeting of leaders including physicians, managed care executives, and health care policy makers. There was agreement that the worst is yet to come for academic medicine, that there will be a war on health care costs, and that health care is not a profession but a business. There has been a shift toward training more general physicians but no progress regarding maldistribution of physicians or underrepresentation of minorities. The only somewhat optimistic prediction was that there would be a shift from primary care gatekeepers toward greater access to specialists. The prognosis for academic medicine is grim.

How will physician educators maintain their morale so that new physicians in training do not lose their enthusiasm and idealism? Academic medicine in the United States has set the gold standard for medical care and research for the world, but in the current climate in which cost is the only issue, that standard appears to be in danger. If high quality academic medicine is sacrificed, the future of medicine in the United States is in jeopardy.

E.J. Cohen, M.D.

To Tell the Truth: Disclosing the Incentives and Limits of Managed Care

Morreim EH (Univ of Tennessee, Memphis)

Am J Man Care 3:35–43, 1997 12–10

Purpose.—With the rise of managed care have come increasing concerns about the way managed care companies do business. One controversial issue is whether patients should be told about the financial incentives and treatment limitations of their health care plan. Although it is clear that patients should be provided with this information, difficult questions remain regarding who should tell them and what they should be told. Key issues related to informing patients of the financial incentives and limits of managed care were reviewed.

Why Disclosure Is Necessary.—Recent years have seen the rise of new and aggressive means of cost control in managed care. These include gatekeeper systems, financial incentives rewarding physicians for withholding resources, and utilization controls or "micromanagement." Such methods raise troublesome ethical questions in that they bring the physician's obligations to the patient in conflict with their own financial interests and their obligations to the managed care organization. Most patients probably do not know about their physician's financial incentives to "earn more by doing less." For moral, medical, legal, and practical reasons, patients must receive explicit information on their managed care organization's cost-containment program.

The primary responsibility to provide this information rests with the managed care organization. This obligation stems from the contracts between managed care organizations, their patients, and physicians; the fiduciary relationship between managed care organizations and patients; and certain federal requirements, including stop-loss protection for physicians at financial risk and annual beneficiary surveys. Physicians also have an obligation to disclose their financial incentives, in that they are implementing responsibility on the part of the managed care organization; they are responsible for providing information "material" to making informed consent decisions; they have a fiduciary relationship with their patients; and they face possible legal consequences stemming from denial of care. "Gag rules" prohibiting disclosure by physicians may violate the physician's fiduciary duty to the patient.

How Incentives Should Be Disclosed.—Once the decision is made to disclose, the challenge becomes how to do so. The organization should prepare a sample disclosure document that informs patients of the potentially competing obligations and interests of providers and health plans. This document must explain why these conflicts are often unavoidable, and why cost controls are actually in the patient's best interests. The disclosure should not be too detailed but should encourage patients who desire more information to ask for it. A sample disclosure document, written in intentionally "upbeat" language, is presented in the article. The managed care organization is honest and direct about its cost-containment program, without portraying itself in a negative light. The document includes 3 areas of disclosure: utilization controls and treatment limits, explaining the need for and benefits of fair enforcement of those limits; common types of incentive arrangements, namely fee-for-service and capitation; and some patient incentives.

Even if every patient does not understand every point of the disclosure, it can still have beneficial effects. Such "sunshine" effects can include a clear look at the acceptability of the incentive scheme. An incentive plan that cannot be clearly described and justified is probably not an acceptable one. Thus, the act of putting the plan into plain English offers insight into its acceptability from a moral standpoint.

Discussion.—The physician must disclose any incentive that interferes with his or her ability to make a particular patient care decision. The managed care organization must develop an incentive system that facilitates prudent resource utilization while allowing physicians to provide the care their patients need.

► This article argues that incentives to limit care under managed care policies should be disclosed to patients and suggests how this can be done by HMOs in an upbeat and positive way. Incentives that can be openly discussed are probably less bad than those that cannot be revealed. The argument that incentives should be disclosed is more convincing than how it can be done in such a rosy way.

The accompanying editorial[1] takes the interesting, ethical position that incentives should not be disclosed because a balanced disclosure would confuse and scare patients. Patients are concerned about quality but the authors think that there is no evidence that capitation affects quality.

I think there is accumulating evidence that incentives to reduce care impact quality. The most egregious examples are taken to one court or the legislatures for redress. Outcomes research is important, but until the information from them is available, disclosure of financial incentives is indicated when it is in the interest of the patient.

E.J. Cohen, M.D.

Reference

1. Noone GC, Ubel PA: Managed care organizations should not disclose their physicians' financial incentives (editorial). *Am J Man Care* 3:159–160, 1997.

Putting Patients First: A 100-Year Tradition

Lichter PR (Ann Arbor, Mich)

Ophthalmology 104:347–354, 1997 12–11

Objective.—Recent advances in medical knowledge and technology have been beneficial to millions of people. These same advances are leading to difficult changes in the health care delivery system. On the occasion of the centennial annual meeting of the American Academy of Ophthalmology, academy president Paul Lichter discusses the need to protect patient's interests during this time of change.

Primacy of the Patient in a Time of Change.—Physicians and patients find themselves torn between medicine's enormous capabilities and powerful cost inhibitions. Dr. Lichter maintains that the present "epidemic of discovery" sometimes feels like an "epidemic of despair." A great deal of insight into the history of medicine over the last 100 years can be gleaned by reading the speeches of the presidents of the Academy. In doing so, Dr.

Lichter found more similarities than differences. Throughout the years, the presidents have sought to impart new concepts to help patients, maintained a focus on what is now called "quality of life," and emphasized the need to care for patients as human beings. Although these objectives are shared today, now, as in the past, there are economic forces that threaten the shared goals of patients and physicians. Although the dilemma is not new, physicians are increasingly asked to meet the medical needs of more patients while using fewer resources. High-quality care is expensive, but physicians know that "cut-rate care" has its own costs, especially in terms of unsatisfactory patient outcomes. More so than in the past, America is investing not in the health of its citizens but in the "bottom line."

Ophthalmologists know the value of specialty care. However, in the managed care environment, the primary care physician is expected to grasp an ever-widening base of knowledge, to the detriment of patients who should be seen by a specialist. For fear of economic reprisals, patients may be kept ignorant of what kind of care they need. These "gag rules" are insulting for physicians and dangerous for patients. "Managed cost" is perverting the benefits of managed care. Dr. Lichter maintains that physicians must tell patients what care they should receive when their health plan will not cover it. They should advocate patients' rights to specialty care and to fair consideration. Physicians must participate in the debate over patient care, rather than simply saying no to change. Physicians and nonphysicians must work together to make positive changes in the health care system. Physicians must listen to their patients.

Summary.—Throughout the 20th century, ophthalmologists have held the best interests of patients as their primary concern. Now, as in the past, these physicians strive to meet high ideals, to be the best they can, to teach and learn from one another, and to bring that knowledge back to serve patients. At a time of unremitting change in health care, that initial vision of the primacy of the patient must remain paramount.

▶ The address of the president of the American Academy of Ophthalmology, Paul Lichter, M.D., at the opening ceremonies of the centennial annual meeting in 1996 put the current state of ophthalmology in its historical context. He discussed how the "current health care climate" threatens the doctor-patient relationship. He unequivocally concluded that we must tell patients when their insurance will not allow care we think is indicated. He hopes that the "primacy of the patient" will remain the vision for the American Academy of Ophthalmology. All this seems rather straightforward. However, disclosure of insurance policy incentives and limits is actually a controversial subject! (See Abstract 12–10 for more information.)

E.J. Cohen, M.D.

The Two Cultures and the Health Care Revolution: Commerce and Professionalism in Medical Care

McArthur JH, Moore FD (Harvard Business School, Boston; Harvard Med School, Boston)

JAMA 277:985–989, 1997 12–12

Introduction.—The commercial and professional traditions are in sharp contrast to each other. Described are the threats to the quality and scope of medical care if medical professionalism is overtaken by the commercial ethic and corporations seeking profit.

The Two Cultures.—The primary priority in the medical profession is the patient. For commerce, it is providing dividends to investors. The cost containment goals of commerce are not always in keeping with quality of care in medicine. Control of medicine by commerce may cause several potential hazards and problems, including: diversion of funds, raising costs, risk avoidance, increased load on public providers, downgrading of personnel, loss of free speech, distortions of clinical care and ethical dilemmas, monopolies with loss of free choice, and neglect of community responsibility and teaching and research. Minimal standards may be needed to abate hazards to society and abuses of patient care arising from commercial pressures on commercial behavior.

New National Agency.—A new agency is needed to set standards and provide surveillance for medical commerce. A national agency could be the basis for state enforcement through licensing. Two models have been proposed—one based on the National Academy of Sciences as the initiating force and the other an initiative provided by a consortium of national charitable foundations with an interest in health policy. Wide support from these national foundations would be needed.

Conclusion.—In this time of needed cost containment, corporate-commercial medicine could work with appropriate agencies for surveillance, reporting, and local assessment of the adequacy of health practices.

▶ This paper and its accompanying editorial[1] describe the tension between business and professionalism in medicine. The conflict is well outlined, but solutions are less obvious. The authors suggest various approaches for private agencies to set standards to safeguard professionalism from commercialism. It will be a challenge for bureaucratic organizations to protect patient care.

E.J. Cohen, M.D.

Reference

1. Emanuel L: Bringing market medicine to professional account (editorial). *JAMA* 277:1004–1005, 1997.

The Impending Physician Surplus: Is it Time to Quit?
Reinhardt U (Princeton Univ, NJ)
JAMA 277:69–70, 1997 12–13

Introduction.—Over the last 2 decades, the number of physicians whose major activity is patient care has been steadily rising without depressing the average physician income. This trend may not be able to continue because of revolutionary changes in insurance reimbursement. There may be a physician surplus.

Impact of Changes.—The restructuring of the health care system to meet the demands of the insurance sector has reduced the typical American physician to that of employee. Self-employed physicians will at some point in the future find their livelihood dependent on a handful of contracts with a powerful employer. If 60% of Americans are enrolled in managed health care plans by the year 2000, there may be a surplus of 140,000 specialists and 29,000 generalists (about 30% of patient care physicians).

Prospective Physicians.—Medical students need to consider what they want to do if a physician glut occurs. It may be that well educated surplus physicians will become administrators in the upper echelons of health care administration or in other sectors of the economy. They may become entrepreneurs within the health care sector or other sectors. To argue that an M.D. degree is not necessary for these pursuits is no greater argument than to assert that a liberal arts education is not necessary to become an investment banker or engineer.

Unionization.—Unionization has been contemplated by organized medicine, but the issue of supply and demand could catch up to medicine, just as it did to car manufacturers.

Conclusion.—A surplus of physicians is possible in the present health care environment. Even so, physicians can still attempt to be among the excellent few who will always be in short supply.

▶ This is one of the most appalling articles I have read on this subject. The author, one of the architects of the Clinton Health Care Reform Proposal, suggests that M.D. degrees will be useful for pursuits outside of medical practice, just as liberal arts degrees are necessary for investment bankers. He predicts surplus M.D.s will be health care administrators and entrepreneurs. How many administrators do we need? It seems to me it is a waste of time, money, and effort for individuals to become doctors and not have the opportunity to practice medicine. I remain unconvinced that there will be such a surplus of doctors if we value quality care for our growing aging population.

E.J. Cohen, M.D.

Suggested Reading

Asch DA, Ubel PA: Rationing by any other name. *N Engl J Med* 336:1668–1671, 1997.

▶ This is a very interesting and relevant discussion of rationing or compromise in the selection of less expensive and less effective treatment options. The term *compromise* has a much more positive connotation than *rationing*. The authors believe compromise is inevitable, and that the best way to analyze the choices is by considering how big the compromise is.

The accompanying editorial (by J.P. Kassier) describes three types of physicians: the first refuse to compromise and are tireless advocates for their patients, the second are also patient advocates but they become frustrated and retire, and the third convince themselves that low-cost care is quality care. The third group probably have promising careers ahead for them in medicine or in working directly for managed care organizations. Doctors who can only put the patient first may graduate from the first to second group. They hope they will last in medicine long enough to see quality valued over cost.

E.J. Cohen, M.D

Kassier JP: Our endangered integrity: It can only get worse (editorial). *N Engl J Med* 336:1666–1667, 1997.

13 Office Management

Practice Management

by Patricia M. Salmon

Many articles suggest that the key to increasing practice profitability is to decrease costs while still maintaining, or better yet, improving the quality of the services provided by the practice. While there is wisdom in that advice, all too many practices respond by arbitrarily reducing overhead without considering how such reductions affect productivity. Others respond by signing up with every insurance carrier in their area without considering the impact that any given contract has on the bottom line or the operation as a whole.

The challenges for medical practices increase daily. Non-traditional health care partners change community dynamics overnight. Legislative issues, such as Fraud and Abuse and Stark II, quickly become a mine field for the unprepared practice.

Practices succeed only if they have a solid foundation on which to build. Successful practices have the data and talent needed to respond quickly to change. Those practices understand Private Practice Management 101. They build a structure that encourages creativity, growth, and accountability. Do you belong to one of those practices?

Let us take a few minutes to review my version of Practice Management 101.

1. *Set goals regularly*. It is difficult to know if sacrifices are worth it if you (and your staff) do not have a clear understanding of the goals toward which you are working. Short-term goals may be the only goals you can develop in this environment. The process of developing those goals is key, however. Successful goal setting requires good communication, accurate data, and group buy-in. Even if the goal towards which you are working does not come to fruition, the process itself separates struggling, reactive practices from successful, proactive leaders.
2. *Develop an understanding of your costs*. This goes beyond reviewing individual expense items on your Income and Expense Statement. Cost analysis forces you to focus on the costs of providing each individual service and running each satellite office. In the process, you may find that while you like having refractive surgery as part of your practice (as

an example), the cost associated with marketing it, etc. is offset by the dollars, time, and energy it takes. This is particularly true if it diverts resources away from more viable areas of the practice. Allocation of resources becomes easier once you understand the return you receive on your investment.

3. *To help understand costs, evaluate the processes involved in implementing practice systems and routines.* Out of date equipment, duplication of effort, inefficient business office layout, and the like affect staffing levels and operating costs (supplies, etc.). Streamlining processes may not cut down on the number of existing employees in the practice; it will, however, help control future hires.
4. *Invest in your staff.* Offer competitive salaries for quality employees. Develop job descriptions that use resources appropriately. In a managed care environment, billing begins at the front desk. All too many practices are not staffed appropriately in that key area. As a result, one or two employees are responsible for answering phones, scheduling appointments, collecting insurance information, etc. Their attention is so diverted by those tasks that patients sign in to record their arrival rather than being greeted by someone whose primary goal is to make the patient feel as if he or she is the most important person who has come in all day. Help cultivate your investment through a well-defined training program for new and existing employees. Many delayed or denied insurance claims can be avoided if employees know the intricacies of the plans with which you participate and the impact poor information has on the entire practice.
5. *Evaluate line-item expenses yearly.* Involve the staff in the process by asking them for ideas on how to decrease supply costs, etc. You will be surprised at the feedback you get when employees feel ownership in the process.
6. *Do not rely exclusively on your staff to code for your service (CPT and ICD-9).* In today's fraud and abuse environment, you must develop an understanding of the codes that apply to your practice and the rules that govern them.
7. *Conduct regular patient and referring doctor satisfaction surveys at least quarterly.* Review the results with everyone in the practice (as appropriate). Involve the staff in solving controllable problems. Compare your progress from one quarter to the next.
8. *Establish good systems of communication—physician to physician, physicians to management, etc.* Most practices are amazed at what can be done if the team takes the time to discuss problems and solve them together.
9. *Review your scheduling plan every 6 months.* Your goal should be to maximize the use of your and your patients' time without either group feeling rushed or compromised.
10. *Last but not least, pick a week each year and designate it "Practice Health Week."* Encourage everyone to see that as a time for reevalu-

ation. Have your manager review the distribution of job duties, flow-chart processes, etc. Then meet (perhaps on a Saturday so as not to interfere with office hours) and discuss the goals for the year ahead. Develop a "change plan" as needed. Adhering to these basic principles can help you reach desired goals time. Equally as important, they also help you respond to surprise.

Quality: Your New Pay Yardstick
Grandinetti D
Med Economics 74:73–77, 1997 13–1

Objective.—The issue of quality has not accounted for a significant percentage of a physician's compensation in the past. Some businesses have found a way to provide significant rewards to physicians for quality performance.

Gallatin Medical.—This organization developed a system that provides physicians with merit bonuses of up to 30% of their salaries. Half of the bonus depends on their patient-satisfaction scores, 20% on organizational performance, and 30% on the physician's performance on HEDIS (Health Plan Employer Data and Information Set) measures. These quality-based measures are the first step in a process that ultimately will grade physicians' quality in regard to patient outcomes.

Prairie Medical Group.—Bonuses as high as 25% to 30% of their salaries are paid to physicians who score well on patient satisfaction results, HEDIS compliance, utilization review, group participation, and group management responsibilities. Those who score below 85 on a 100-point scale must pass an audit in the next quarter or go before the board of directors. Physicians get report cards.

Sentara Medical Group.—Twenty percent of a physician's salary is at risk if quality goals (patient-satisfaction and involvement in clinical quality improvement projects) are not met, admissions and pharmacy utilization comparisons are sub par, and there is poor compliance with HEDIS criteria. The group wants to increase physician awareness of good practice methods and to hold physicians accountable for their work in the clinic.

Conclusion.—Quality-based pay systems are on the rise. Such systems will provide incentives to medical groups to improve their competitive profile in the health care marketplace.

► Quality is a term with elusive meanings. Now, more than ever before, physicians are asked to indicate the quality of medical service that is delivered from a variety of sources. Physician acceptance of this new evaluation system varies. Many do not fully understand the impact of quality in today's market place and how it can affect patient volume. Managed care companies such as Aetna U.S. Healthcare are linking physician pay to quality. Some medical practices are now allocating a percentage of annual compensation to performance scores on quality measures such as patient satisfaction surveys and the Health Plan Employer Data and Information Set. If your medical practice currently uses methods to monitor the quality of service delivery, it may well be at the cutting edge of the medical service delivery system.

This article does not provide an in-depth analysis of the functional aspects of quality measures. It does, however, provide an entry level presentation of the concept and gives examples of how quality measures are being used in the United States in 3 medical practices.

P.M. Salmon

How to Increase Your Staff's Productivity: Start With a Vision for Your Practice's Success

Yerkes LA (Catalyst Consulting Group, Cleveland, Ohio)
Physician's Manage 37:53–58, 1997 13–2

Objective.—Productivity depends on how well a physician and the physician's staff can meet the needs of the patient. It begins with a vision of what constitutes a successful practice.

Productivity Killers.—Doing anything twice, including rescheduling patients because you don't have what you need to treat them; inadequate billing systems that don't send out timely bills; and having patient "no shows" because the office doesn't have a confirmation system are productivity killers.

How to Get Productive Personnel.—Hire right the first time, know what skills and experience are necessary to get the job done, select those with a "can-do" attitude, clearly define the individual's role and responsibilities and your expectations, provide support and clear and specific instructions, learn "how-to" from physicians whose practices are working the way you'd like yours to work, and pay competitive wages. Most importantly, don't hire someone just like you; surround yourself with a diverse staff. If you are always hiring and training, you may want to hire an expert to diagnose your business problems. Provide your staff with the technology they need to do their jobs effectively and efficiently.

Track Performance.—Set benchmarks and compare them regularly with previous standards, give your staff feedback, provide formal and informal performance appraisals. Provide monetary and other incentives such as formal and informal recognition and sincere praise.

Final Points.—Trust your staff to do their jobs. Do not try to control everything. Stay in touch with your staff. Don't have a double standard; perform as well as you expect your staff to perform.

► More and more, physicians are called upon to make administrative decisions that affect staff productivity and, consequently, the profitability of the practice. In hiring staff, it is important to hire the right complement of individuals who will work effectively together in performing their separate functions. Even small practices need to follow concepts used by corporate management to assure that their staffs are able to produce a high quality of work while exhibiting a team approach. After hiring the appropriate staff, it is important to find performance evaluation methods that are motivational. It is also important to provide all employees with the proper tools for performing their jobs, from a scheduling system to the medical supplies used by the physician. Participation of staff in the decision-making processes and fair performance appraisals are being used within medical practices to empower employees in their daily activities. This article discusses the steps toward having a productive and efficient medical office.

P.M. Salmon

How to Spot the Unscrupulous Employee

Valancy J (Jack Valency Consulting, Cleveland Heights, Ohio)
Physician's Manage 37:34–39, 1997 13–3

Purpose.—About one fourth of physicians will have an employee steal from them sometime during their career. Such criminal behavior most often happens because the physician does not adequately check out new hires or fails to respond to the signs of trouble. Some important steps for preventing theft by employees in medical practices were reviewed.

Before the Hire.—Checking references is the most important step in detecting potentially unscrupulous employees. Candidates for jobs should provide written references and a statement authorizing release of information to you. Special attention is needed to gaps in employment. The physician should check dates of employment and type of work performed. The physician should call former and, if possible, current employers and ask to speak to the applicant's immediate supervisor. A key question to ask this person is whether they would hire the employee again. For fear of lawsuits, employers may be reluctant to provide any more information than the former employee's dates of employment. In interviews, the physician should take a positive approach to the issue of potential wrongdoing. No more than a brief mention of office policy regarding employee theft is needed.

After the Hire.—By adding fidelity bonds to their insurance coverage, business owners can be reimbursed for losses to employee theft. Bonding employees provides a good preventive measure at low cost. System controls are needed to remove any opportunity for embezzlement. Such controls include balancing the practice daysheets every day and checking the total charges, payments, and adjustments against source documents. Bank deposits should be reconciled with daysheets and deposit receipts checked. The physician should examine each bill before signing checks and should sign checks personally. The physician should resist pressure from employees not to balance daysheets every day. In very large practices, accounts should be balanced twice a day.

As much as possible, the physician should separate office functions and make sure staff are cross-trained. Having only 1 employee know how to do a certain job not only creates the opportunity for malfeasance, it means that that job doesn't get done when the employee is out. One person should open the mail and add up the checks, while another employee does the posting. To ensure proper checks and balances, the practice accountant should perform a regular operational audit of the books. When a problem does arise, the physician should deal with it firmly; ignoring wrongdoing invites repetition.

Discussion.—Several steps can help prevent employee theft, both in detecting potentially unscrupulous behavior before the hire and in ensuring proper controls afterward. Prospective and current staff should understand that the purpose of these measures is not to place them under suspicion but rather to detect and correct errors.

► As managed care penetrates the marketplace, affecting the revenues of a practice, it is increasingly important to hire and retain quality employees. How can you spot the best applicant to minimize any criminal or immoral actions within your practice? It is important to follow the steps used by human resources personnel within larger companies when hiring employees. For example, verify credentials and references; ask for a previous supervisor's reference to verify past performance. During the interview, listen to the applicant's verbal and nonverbal communication. Once the applicant is hired, be sure the environment minimizes any risk for dubious behavior.

Having job descriptions provides a clear definition of the employer's expectations within the job as well as a base for evaluating performance. Institute a system of checks and balances to minimize any temptation for dishonesty. Provide a working environment that empowers employees and motivates them to excel. This article provides the reader with a sound checklist of considerations in hiring and retaining employees. It is presented in an easily comprehensible manner.

P.M. Salmon

How Fast Can Things Change?

Chesanow N

Med Economics 74:42–67, 1997 13–4

Objective.—As the trend toward managed care grows, local health care markets can change very quickly. Recent developments in the Philadelphia market were reviewed to illustrate this point.

The Philadelphia Experience.—At the beginning of 1994, HMO penetration in the Philadelphia market was only 27%. However, physicians felt the impact of managed care very shortly thereafter, whether or not they did managed care business. The many academic medical centers in the area were unable to keep up with the trend toward ambulatory care and hoped to receive global capitation by managing care for large numbers of enrolled patients. As a result, they quickly developed large, integrated health care delivery systems. They began linking up with high-quality, high-volume primary care practices, whether by affiliation or purchase. Although physicians in many smaller practices remain unconcerned, by the end of 1995, HMO penetration had risen to 43%. Estimates suggest that it will reach 60% by the year 2000. Practice sales and defensive mergers are the order of the day.

The options for smaller practices are limited. Selling directly to a hospital network may not be possible for specialty practices, but the market is booming for primary care practices. Systems will pay market value for practices to keep their competitors from getting them. Physicians are eager to get the money for their practices but may not understand the consequences of becoming hospital employees. Signing a contract is no guarantee of renewal once the contract is up. Merging offers another option, with the reasoning that "bigger is better." However, it can be difficult to arrange mergers and to make them work. Independent practice associations may offer a way for physicians to take part in managed care and retain some control over what is done. However, there are questions about the difficulty of setting up such associations and their ability to compete in the health care market. They gain leverage in markets where managed care organizations realize that choice is the basis for competition. Other practices are trying to wait out the managed care trend. By making their operations run more efficiently, these practices make themselves even more attractive to managed care. Quality reports and computerized records are important in keeping up with managed care entities, and as the basis on which hospital networks decide their offers when buying practices.

Discussion.—The Philadelphia market has seen a particularly sharp trend in the growth of managed care. Physicians are urged to take a more active role in the changes taking place in health care delivery.

► Health economists flaunt the financial advantages of managed care in delivering a more streamlined package of medical care. The impact of managed care has been felt in every metropolitan area of the United States. It is the popular answer to today's rising health costs. With carefully selected data from health care markets saturated with managed care, marketers promote reduction of costs through utilization control and capitation agreements while demonstrating a high quality of care. Market penetration of managed care insurance companies has accelerated faster than expected because of the financial savings that have been presented.

In Philadelphia, from 1994 to 1995, managed care coverage increased from 27% of the market to 43% by year end. Physicians have frenetically gathered together to combat this growth by joining larger networks. Major health care systems are replacing the solo practitioner. This article presents the effects that managed care has in today's health care environment in a way that is empathetic to physicians and administrators.

P.M. Salmon

A Tool to Help Doctors Review Each Other

Wiley MJ (Health Care Management and Consulting Services Inc, Bay Shore, NY)

Med Economics 74:86–93, 1997 13–5

Introduction.—Having doctors review each other is a useful management tool. Although the concept may be upsetting to some, such reviews may solve problems and settle differences that have remained unresolved in the past.

Methods.—Systematic and objective performance tools can provide an objective process by which doctors can review each other in a nonconfrontational way (Figure). For example, these reviews can highlight a difference in 1 doctor's style that does not fit a group's practice style, identify excessive coding documentation, pinpoint where a doctor is ignoring a practice's rules, point out when a new doctor does not know what the group expects, reveal scheduling misadventures, and disclose when the group is not keeping up with changes in the market. For some groups, an outside facilitator may be preferred to supervise and referee the process.

Conclusion.—Performance reviews that are sensitively prepared and flexible and concentrate on what can be fixed minimize the resentment and negative outcomes of criticism.

► Forces in the health care marketplace, such as managed care and its emphasis on cost containment and quality, have impacted the formation of physician groups. Because the performance of the individual practitioner can

Physician Performance Review

Dr.__________________

Date____/____/____

	Below average	Average	Above average
Time and effort spent—patients			
Time and effort spent—business			
Patients per hour or per day			
Communication with partners			
Communication with referral sources			
Communication with patients			
Communication with staff			
Helpful and cooperative attitude with partners			
Consideration shown toward partners (rooms, equipment, etc.)			
Completes business projects in timely manner			
Adheres to decisions made by group			
Promotes practice in daily contacts			
Chart documentation			
Patient satisfaction			
Unjustified negative outcomes			

FIGURE.—A tool to help doctors review one another. Source: Healthcare Management and Consulting Services. (Courtesy of Wiley MJ: A tool to help doctors review one another. Med Economics 74:86–93. Copyright 1997 by Medical Economics Company. Reproduced with permission from *Medical Economics* magazine.)

influence the total practice, it is important that physicians have a tool to evaluate each other's performance. This article presents 1 physician performance tool designed by a practice management consultant in Bay Shore, New York. One of the major advantages it provides is a peer evaluation. It can stimulate a healthy discussion for resolving personnel differences as well as making administrative decisions.

The cohesiveness and mental health of the individual physicians will certainly be reflected in their service delivery. By evaluating each other's performance, physicians can objectify a colleague's weak points, thus improving the service delivery and overall health of the practice.

P.M. Salmon

Getting Patients to Pay

Dolan KP

Med Economics 74:48–62, 1997 13–6

Introduction.—The first step to increasing collections is to evaluate your current collections system. Policy should be clearly established and all staff members should understand their role in the collections process. You should know your collection ratio and how old the accounts receivable are (See "Test Your Collections IQ").

TABLE.—Test Your Collections IQ

If you have the right answers to these 20 questions, your collections policy is likely to be a winner.

1. Is your collections policy in writing?
2. Is your collections policy clearly defined?
3. Does everyone who needs a copy of your policy have one?
4. Do you fully explain your collections policy to all new staff members?
5. Do you fully inform your patients of your financial policies before treatment?
6. Is your staff able and willing to answer all patient questions about your financial policies?
7. Do you update patient-registration information regularly?
8. Do you track collections success at the time of service?
9. Do you inform staff about the insurance plans in which your practice participates?
10. Do you update your staff immediately on new plan requirements and developments?
11. Do you monitor collections schedules?
12. Do you document collections follow-ups?
13. Do you train collections personnel in insurance coding?
14. Do you advise all relevant personnel immediately of coding-rule changes?
15. Do physicians, staff, and administrators regularly review collections developments?
16. Do you regularly monitor vital financial statistics, such as net collection ratio and average age of accounts receivable?
17. Do you provide training tools and workshops for collections personnel?
18. If you use an outside collection agency, do you evaluate its performance?
19. Does one individual have ultimate responsibility for your collections system?
20. Have you enlisted professional help to develop the best system for your practice?

Score 1 for each Yes answer.

20 points: Keep up the good work!

15 points: Not bad, but some fine tuning could result in better collections.

10 points or fewer: You need help. Review this article carefully.

(From Dolan KP: Getting patients to pay. *Med Economics* 74:48–62. Copyright 1997 by Medical Economics Company. Reproduced with permission of *Medical Economics* magazine.)

TABLE.—A Seven-Step Collections Timetable

Here's what to do if a patient doesn't pay in full at the time of service.

30 days. Send a statement of the account in an envelope marked "address correction requested."

45 days. Call the patient and try to get a commitment to pay, either in full or on an installment schedule.

60 days. Send a second statement. Use an envelope without your practice's name in the return address.

75 days. Call the patient again and send a statement with a letter pointing out that the account is two-and-a-half months past due. Try to set up a schedule for payment if you haven't already done so.

90 days. Send a letter stating that you'll have to take further action on the account. Review the account with your office manager to decide whether to write it off or give it to a collection agency.

105 days. Call the patient and tell him you're turning his account over to a collection agency. Then wait 15 days.

120 days. Send the account to the agency, and send the patient a letter telling him you've done so.

(Courtesy of Dolan KP: Getting patients to pay. *Med Economics* 74:48–62. Copyright 1977 by Medical Economics Company. Reproduced with permission of *Medical Economics* magazine.)

Set Policy.—Do some soul-searching and decide what you will allow the staff to do to collect on an account. The policy should be in writing and should be distributed and explained to all employees. Your staff may need a pep talk with a reminder that the health of the practice depends on how collections procedures are followed through. Also, remind staff that the practice has a right to the money and that patients know of their finanicial responsibility when they accept treatment.

Common Sense.—Encourage your employees to use common sense and some heart when whey approach patients with overdue accounts. Also, make sure that every employee understands federal and state regulations regarding communicating information about debts to an outside person

TABLE.—Collections "Dos" and "Don'ts" for You and Your Staff

Remember that it's illegal to communicate the fact of a debt to an outside person. Make sure your staff knows, too. The best-intentioned employees may inadvertently break this and other laws. Make sure you— and they—know the applicable federal and state rules.

Don't: Put collection notices on postcards, mark envelopes "past due," or try to make your letters look like court documents or communications from attorneys.

Don't: Call the patient at home before 8 a.m. or after 9 p.m. *Don't* call him at work if his employer prohibits it or if the patient has asked you not to.

Don't: Leave messages that identify the practice or the purpose of the call; give only your first name and phone number.

Don't: Tell other people why you want information about the patient's current address, phone number, or employment when you're trying to track him down.

Don't: Threaten, lie to, or harass patients.

Do: Approach collections with kindness and professionalism. If at any point the patient refuses in writing to pay, or asks in writing that your office cease contact, or your office learns that the patient is represented by an attorney, halt collection efforts until your lawyer says it's okay to proceed.

Do: Create templates for your past-due and collection notices. This makes letters ready at a moment's notice. Write scripts for employees to use when making collection calls. Occasionally turn staff meetings into training sessions and have employees practice collections by role-playing.

Do: Document all calls made and letters sent in connection with an overdue account.

(Courtesy of Dolan KP: Getting patients to pay. *Med Economics* 74:48–62. Copyright 1997 by Medical Economics Company. Reproduced with permission of *Medical Economics* magazine.)

(See "A Seven-Step Collections Timetable"). Assign collections duties to the right person—someone who is comfortable asking for money, is assertive but not aggressive, and who will not let patients push them around. Do not get personally involved; it is not a physician's place to be involved in collections.

More Tips.—Keep patient records up to date and keep a copy of insurance cards. Post a sign that payment is expected at the time of service. The receptionist should ask, "How will you be paying today?" Have the office file insurance claims. Make it easy for patients to pay by accepting credit cards. Allow patients with financial difficulties to pay in installments, but with ground rules. Regularly contact patients with overdue accounts by mail or phone.

Discussion.—Do not let accounts go that are more than 90 days overdue. Get into a regular routine and review overdue accounts every month (See "Collections 'Dos' and 'Don'ts'"). Write off everything under $10 and first concentrate on accounts over $100. Maintaining the attitude that nearly every patient contact is a chance to reinforce your payment policy will help keep your collection ratio at 95% or more.

► With the number of uninsured persons growing each year, more patients have to pay out of pocket for their medical care. In addition, managed care insurance and self-insured insurance plans have many different levels of copayment. It is important to develop a policy for your medical practice that assists you in collecting these patient obligations. The other confounding factor is that medical care has been viewed primarily as a social good and not perceived as a product to be purchased (this is psychological).

Before developing a policy, it is important to evaluate the collection system. The collection policy that is subsequently developed must be supported throughout the practice from the physician to the receptionist. Roles should be defined which permit the physician to focus on clinical treatment with administrative staff focusing on billing and collection. This article presents many good suggestions that can be used in establishing a documented collection policy which encourages patient payment.

P.M. Salmon

Use Your HMO Profile to Your Advantage

Grandinetti D

Med Economics 74:165–171, 1997 13–7

Introduction.—Your bargaining power with health plans can be strengthened with profiling information from managed-care organizations. Concessions from the sponsoring health plan may be achieved even from a profile that paints you as an outlier. An assertive response may be necessary among physicians with their profiling information, particularly by understanding what the numbers mean and responding appropriately to prevent deselection. You can also use reports by managed care companies to add to your information systems.

Marketing.—Profiles generally include overall per-member-per-month capitation and costs for specialist referrals, inpatient charges, prescriptions, outpatient surgery, laboratory and imaging tests, and emergency department use. If your numbers look good, take the opportunity to meet with the director to ask for more tips on how to be better. Your marketing material can highlight your patient satisfaction scores, for example, if they are well above average. If many of your patients go to a particular specialist, you may have the bargaining power to request that the specialist see your patients more quickly.

Meeting.—Get any mistakes rectified in the profile quickly by calling the medical director and insisting on a meeting. If the medical director won't respond, ask the medical society to provide you with additional data to help you understand why your numbers are skewed. The medical association may even agree to send a representative to intervene.

Conclusions.—A performance profile should be looked at with a critical eye. A favorable performance assessment should be used as a marketing tool for your practice, and a poor assessment should not be left unchallenged. The parameters of performance will be determined by the statisticians if you ignore your performance profile.

► Statistical analysis courses may have seemed of minor importance in the pursuit of one's clinical education. In today's managed care environment, wherein physicians receive profile information rating their performance to their peers, the tenets learned in statistics can be used. Profile data is only as sound as the algorithm used to calculate the desired outcome measure. Examine the database, the independent and dependent variables' validity and reliability, and look for confounding variables. Concepts that may have been shelved in the recesses of our cognitive processing have a new meaning!

Interpreting your practice's profile can assist you in obtaining a different level of reimbursement, or it can be used in marketing materials to increase your patient base. Using profile data in a constructive process can only assist you in maintaining a high quality of medical service delivery. Of primary importance is not to simply ignore an insurer's rating of your performance. Develop a relationship with the medical director of the major insurers represented by your patients so that there is a forum to discuss your profile results. This article encourages physicians to be their own advocates and statisticians. It provides the physician and administrator with many positive outlets for what has been a little appreciated statistical analysis of practice patterns.

P.M. Salmon

Activity-based Costing Management in a Private Practice Setting

Carlomagno M, Draper V (Knoxville, Tenn; Knoxville Orthopedic Clinic PA, Tenn)

MGM J 45:68–78, 1997 13–8

Introduction.—Activity-based costing (ABC), a management tool for valuing services, focuses on the cost of patients' visits. An ABC project must be clearly defined, a timeframe determined, a working model created, operational and financial data entered into the model, and calculations prepared and checked. Resources, processes, and services must be identified. Resource consumption must be apportioned according to the activities provided. Cost information data can then be used to make necessary operational changes, generate data that can be used when negotiating for managed care, and provide physician income guidelines. The resulting model can be used to create scenarios for studying the effect of adjusting patient volume, staff, capacity utilization, and revenues. Commitment of upper management and of financial systems, accounting, and management information systems personnel is crucial.

Developing the Model.—The model uses financial, volume, and operational data to tally the cost of moving a patient through the system, regardless of why the patient is in the system or the resources—including type of physician—required for the visit. Resources used will be specialty specific and charges are apportioned on the basis of payer mix.

Conclusion.—The ABC plan does not replace a financial report. It provides a model for change that relies on management commitment and is based on cost reduction and process improvement.

► Calculating the costs associated with your medical practice is crucial to its financial success. Activity-based costing is a management tool used to determine the cost of a practice based on its operational components. By identifying resources, processes, and demands (services) that are specific to your practice, information is obtained to assist the practice manager in making informed cost-benefit decisions. Specifically, ABC can be used in your practice to make appropriate operational changes, as well as provide a basis for physician income.

An additional benefit is in the area of managed care contracting. Because managed care has infiltrated the health care environment, knowing your practice's cost can be an invaluable tool in negotiating reimbursement within managed care contracts. This article focuses on the components used in the ABC process. The principles of ABC can be applied to any medical practice. This approach allows qualitative practice components to be quantified, thus helping the practice administrator in financial and personnel decisions.

P.M. Salmon

Guarding Patient Confidentiality Under Managed Care

Walker LM
Med Economics 74:155–173, 1997 13–9

Introduction.—Managed care poses a new threat to patient privacy. Usually without knowing they are doing so, patients sign away their right to confidentiality in exchange for managed care coverage. In addition, the concept of managed care itself implies further scrutiny for such measures as quality assurance and utilization review. Once patient information is entered into the managed care company's computer system, it poses new risks to confidentiality. In this article, key issues concerning patient confidentiality in managed care were discussed.

Deciding What to Record.—The best way to make sure sensitive information does not get into the wrong hands is not to write it down in the first place. Language should be neutral and precise, including only what another clinician might need to know. Although sensitive information is protected under various state laws, there are limits to how well patient information can be shielded from insurers. The best way to protect the patient's privacy may be to ask what information he or she considers sensitive.

Patient Consent.—It is a good idea to obtain patients' informed consent regarding who has access to their records. The amount of information patients want to share may be affected by how ill they are and may change over time. Even when patients have given permission for something to be recorded, it is a good idea to warn them when sensitive information is released, such as information regarding substance abuse or an HIV test.

Respect for Privacy.—In their practices, physicians should strive to develop an organizational commitment to patient privacy. Staff should realize the importance of privacy and the consequences of breaking it. Privacy should be both a personnel and a technical issue. Problems are most likely to arise when staff do not question a request for information.

Technical Security.—The practice computer system should have security measures built in, with different levels of access for different types of information. This makes the system more complex, but it limits access to sensitive information while maintaining the value of computerized medical records. Additional protection—such as firewalls and data encryption—are needed if the system interacts with the Internet in any way. A computer security consultant can provide useful input for practices that are part of a larger network. Staff must understand that there are clear penalties for breaches of confidentiality.

Rules for Other Users.—When other users have access to patient records, there must be clear policies on confidentiality. The physician can set limits on the reasons for which records will be released and the length of time of the release, but the physician cannot always control what the recipient does with the records. If an HMO is requesting information, the physician should find out its policies on record keeping. When records are audited, the physician should ask to select the records and screen out possible patient identifiers. Although it is not always possible to challenge reviews, the physician can let patients know how the payer may use their information. Even though insurers have broad permission to examine records, there are still specific rules as to what kind of information can be shared and when.

Summary.—Key considerations in patient confidentiality in the managed care era include what to record, obtaining patient consent to release records, respect for patient privacy, and technical measures. Although physicians can no longer offer absolute confidentiality, they can still do much to protect patient privacy.

► Patient confidentiality is of primary concern to the physician. It is the fundamental basis for the physician-patient relationship. With the penetration of managed care and computerization of the medical record, physicians must secure the confidentiality of the patient record as much as possible. By establishing procedures and policies regarding the release of patient information, the physician can control the type of information released. If clinical information is entered into a computerized milieu, designing different levels of security access to clinical information is recommended. The physician must also reflect upon the pertinence of the recorded information to the patient's current condition and medical treatment.

It is best to remain clinically sterile when choosing language to be used in record keeping. Involving patients in deciding what is to be recorded (if there is some delicacy to the information) as well as informing them of the possible outcome of signing specific medical release forms promotes a healthy physician-patient relationship. The article provides the physician and practice administrator with sound suggestions for insuring that patient confidentiality is maintained.

P.M. Salmon

Success Factors of Risk Based Specialty Networks

Krohn RW (Med Alliances, Alexandria, Va)

MGM J 45:28–34, 1997 13–10

Introduction.—Specialty physicians are feeling the heat of managed care with shrinking reimbursement, selective paneling, and clinical reengineering. Specialists have begun to form groups and networks, and their success lies in their response to payer demands for business and clinical efficiency and geographic diversity.

Planning.—A mission is necessary to impart a clear sense of the true purpose or intended capabilities. The network must establish itself as the premier provider network within a geographic region and align itself with other groups. The true costs of launching a functional network should not be underestimated. A comprehensive business plan with 5-year projections should be developed. Equity in the organization must be obtained. To attract quality physicians, physician equity participation in the network is effective.

Strategies.—More risk should not be accepted than can be absorbed. Member volume must be captured because profitability in a risk-contracting environment relies on managing patient care provided to a defined membership. There is a greater actuarial probability that the contract can be managed successfully with a larger volume of patients assigned to each physician through a network contract. Payer diversity must be established and maintained. Practice management services should support network efficiencies. Alliances should be formed with noncompeting physician organizations. The panel should not be overloaded with specialists, otherwise the network will become inefficient.

Conclusions.—Physicians must be educated about the emergence of managed care, the impact on their future lives, and the need to position their practices in a shrinking specialty service environment. Careful planning and execution are necessary for successful specialty networks.

► When speaking to physicians regarding practice patterns, one realizes that the majority of physicians want to maintain the control in medically treating patients. Inherent to the formation of risk-based specialty networks is the maintenance of physician control in the clinical and financial decision making of their practice. It empowers the physician in deciding the direction of his clinical future. Designed to minimize financial loss in this era of shrinking reimbursement, selective paneling, and clinical reengineering, the formation of specialty networks has made the physician more accountable for his clinical decisions, which ultimately affect the bottom line on the financial statement. The author does an excellent job of presenting the advantages of forming your own physician network. He explains the philosophies behind the mentality of the managed care insurance companies and provides the steps to succeed financially in the current health care market while maintaining operational control. This article provides a *ray of hope* for physicians who may be reluctantly faced with the prospect of using a physician practice management company to administer their practice.

P.M. Salmon

Making Risk Contracting Work in Specialty Networks

Krohn RW (Med Alliances, Alexandria, Va)

MGM J 45:13–20, 1997 13–11

Introduction.—Contracting arrangements will be increasingly influenced by capitation of specialties. Amid a shrinking market for their services, specialists and networks must position themselves to operate in this environment. Before accepting capitation, a self-appraisal of the specialist network should be conducted to understand its capability to succeed in this milieu.

Questions.—Can the network manage capitation? Capitation is a numbers game, and the physicians must determine whether the number of covered lives is sufficient to make the actuarial estimate of cost and patient population behavior work. Networking and risk contracting are best done by specialties that do not experience wide variations in patterns of patient treatment. Should the network have specific specialty services or subcapitate with a primary care network for full medical risk? To determine how much is too much, don't accept risk over which you have no control.

Strategies.—To gain market share, build alliances. A strategic plan should be crafted by the specialty network that is supported by alliance. Efficiencies must be established throughout the entire network before rival provider groups do. Network physicians must firmly understand the specific risk-bearing provisions of the contract, including accountabilities. The pool of payers comprising the network's contracting base should be evaluated. To provide a minimum actuarial probability of profitability, the capitation rates must be supported by a sufficient patient panel size. To comply with unique clinical and administrative requirements of each capitation agreement, additional training and education must be anticipated.

Conclusions.—Physician leaders and members must be well informed about the quality and financial issues associated with capitation. Practice guidelines, clinical protocols, peer review, outcomes measurement, and patient satisfaction surveys are used to promote clinical efficiencies. As the network gains experience and establishes the tools and techniques of successful risk management, the risk component of contracting can be expanded.

► Specialty physicians have traditionally been reimbursed by all insurance carriers including managed care companies on a fee-for-service basis. Cost-containment efforts at controlling specialty physician usage has focused on the primary care physician. Primary care physicians are expected to control utilization because their capitation agreement places them at risk for issuing specialty referrals. Managed care companies are beginning to formulate capitation arrangements with specialty groups. To prepare for this eventuality, specialty physicians must begin to quantify the quality of their service, to investigate their practice patterns as well as utilization patterns, to determine the cost of delivering care, to evaluate their use of information systems, and to examine the staffing used to deliver their medical care. The economic concept of *economy of scale* becomes ever more important. Developing internal standards and measures for the aforementioned areas will improve the negotiating position of the specialty physician engaged in capitation contracting. This article is excellent in orienting the practice administrator and physician to the methodology required to successfully negotiate a capitated contract that minimizes their risk while maximizing reimbursement.

P.M. Salmon

Evaluation of the Business Side of the Group Practice

Fulmer JG Jr, Weekly KJ (Univ of Tennessee, Chattanooga)
MGM J 45:37–50, 1997 13–12

Introduction.—As capitation continues to spread and complicate finances, the business side of a group practice has become even more important. Physicians can create their own internal management team, or a professional management firm can be hired for managing the business side.

Evaluating a Firm.—The firm's track record should be evaluated by contacting at least 3 clients for references. To see how the firm makes decisions, the firm should be asked how to solve a particular problem (one that has already been solved by the group practice). Evaluate the firm's personality to see whether it fits in with the group practice. Audited financial statements should be reviewed, particularly balance sheets, income statements, and statements of cash flows. Three years of historical and projected statements should be obtained.

Evaluating Internal Management.—An internal management team must be well versed in accounting and finance, and statistical, managerial, and strategic planning. The internal team should assist with such managerial issues as communication, understanding the economics of plans, and assisting in changing habits of physicians who are not cost-effective. Decide whether the team will have a bookkeeper or an accountant or an individual with an MBA degree. The group also needs to decide whether to retain a legal firm.

Conclusions.—Strategic planning is necessary for the success of a group practice. Change must be built into the management strategy and organizational structure. Contract negotiation, quality assessment, utilization management, claims administration, financial performance reporting, and member eligibility are required in managed care. Business expertise is necessary to obtain data and use it in the design of practice systems to succeed in the managed care environment.

► Traditionally, physicians have been able to focus on the clinical aspects of their business. Today, as the solo practitioner becomes an anomaly and physician groups become the mode, the business side of running a medical practice has become a higher priority in the delivery of medical care. Physicians can either choose to manage the administrative components of their practice through using a practice management firm, or internally designing a management structure. This article seems a bit redundant in its presentation of the 2 choices. The presented concepts are covered in most entry-level management courses. It would have helped if some real-life examples were provided that demonstrate the differences between the 2 management options. The article makes it seem simplistic. If physicians hire a practice management firm, they are purchasing at a *one stop shopping mall.* If they decide to design an internal management structure, they may need *to shop* at several malls until all required management expertise is purchased. Even though the article has some pertinent points, the adage, *less is best,* could be applied.

P.M. Salmon

Physician Practice-Management Company Buyouts: Is Taking the Leap Worth the Risk?
Finger AL
Med Economics 74:106–118, 1997 13–13

Introduction.—Depending on the company, physician practice management companies may be a good deal for physicians, but caution is still necessary. Generally, buyouts occur with one-third cash, one-third stock, and one-third a combination of debentures, options, or compensation plans, and the purchase price is usually 5 times the estimated annual profit figure. Generally, however, the stock prices of physician practice management companies lag behind the stock market as a whole.

How to Practice.—Physicians may practice differently because of their concerns about the bottom line. Physicians are lured by the promise that these companies will take care of management, so that they are free to practice medicine. Arrangements can vary from paying a management fee and having the physicians continuing to practice as before, or from physicians being employed by the corporation with the company keeping up to 50% of practice revenues for management. About 5% of physicians belong to 1 of 25 physician practice management companies.

Going It Alone.—More doctors are getting together and forming their own companies. They merge together and approach a bank for capital. This effort can eliminate out-of-pocket costs that doctors have for legal, accounting, or investment-banking fees. The doctors can control the stock and the board. Doctor-controlled physician practice companies can own facilities, ancillary services, surgicenters, and birthing centers.

Conclusions.—Small groups of doctors working together may be the future of medicine. There is some debate about how well doctors work together, but the Mayo Clinic is one example of a diverse group of physicians coming together to form a successful entity. Whatever manner the doctors decide, the patients must come first, and the doctors must come second.

► Physicians focused their education toward clinical development. In today's medical environment, the physician is faced with an ever increasing amount of managerial, especially financially based, decisions. Some physicians have turned to physician practice management companies for their administrative management. Others have chosen to develop their own internal management company or infrastructure for this function.

One of the major factors to be considered in deciding how your practice will address its current administrative dilemma is the amount of financial and managerial control you want when the decision has been actualized. In forming physician practice management relationships, some physician practices have met with financial success, whereas others have regretted their loss of input in the daily operations. Regardless of the chosen option, it is best to understand your current costs and operation including your insurance-related contracts. This article hits the major features to consider through the examples provided.

P.M. Salmon

14 Medicolegal Issues in an Era of Health Care Reform

Legal Issues for Ophthalmologists: The More Things Change the More They Stay the Same

by Alice G. Gosfield, Esq.

The last year has seen a continuing intensification in the legal context which defines the ophthalmologist's environment. While some salutary developments can be observed, the law continues to act as both a goad and a barrier to physician business and clinical interests. The three articles that are included in this YEAR BOOK manifest the dynamism of the ophthalmologist's reality.

Managed care continues to exercise a major force in the health care world. One of the principal concerns of physicians in relating to managed care entities (MCOs) is the extent to which the physicians are likely to be held liable for their actions in reliance on and compliance with their contractual obligations to the MCO. While it is apparent that the courts increasingly impose liability on MCOs for the bad clinical outcomes of their patients, the strange impact of the Employee Retirement Income Security Act (ERISA) has distorted much which has developed in this arena. In the *AGG Note* "Managed care and liability: As the world turns," the issues of the forms of managed care entities to which ophthalmologists may relate and the types of liability such entities can incur are addressed. The impact of ERISA in affording broad protection to managed care entities and its significance to physicians cannot be overstated. However, as the *Note* points out, as a result of a 1995 case it will be important to keep an eye on developments because cases which used to be dismissed as falling under the ERISA laws now are being sent to state court to be tried as traditional malpractice cases. This *Note* also considers the new forms of payment arrangements that may increase liability for physicians and points out specific contract terms which define the parameters of the ophthalmologist–MCO relationship. Seven explicit practical tips are offered.

As the reimbursement world has narrowed for physicians, they are considering a range of options in dealing with their patients. One of the obstacles to an ordinary business relationship has been Medicare's insistence on controlling physician fees even when the patient would choose to enter into a private contract with the physician. As part of the Balanced Budget Act passed at the end of 1997, a provision was enacted to permit patients to engage in private contracts with their physicians should they choose to do so. Originally it was intended that this law would permit physicians on a case-by-case basis to enter into private relationships. As a result of last minute legislative negotiations the law was substantially changed. In "Private contracting by Medicare physicians: The pit and the pendulum," the historical development of Congressional control over physician fees is presented along with an explanation of the new law. Already the subject of some further Congressional maneuvering, this is a piece of legislation which has evoked intense interest despite its very narrow potential impact. It is an interesting symbol of the role of legislative policy in the private financial lives of all physicians.

In potentially the most confusing and detailed manifestation of regulatory implementation of congressional policy, the Stark II regulations have been published in proposed form. Although the law became effective on January 1, 1995, regulations dealing with services other than clinical laboratory services were only published in January of 1998, and then only in proposed form. The vagaries and confusions in these regulations have been generated in part by bad legislative drafting and distorted Congressional policy. Nonetheless, the regulators have spoken on issues that drive directly to the heart of physician practices. In a proposed provision that would affect ophthalmologists directly, they have taken the positive position that an optical shop within a physician practice is a legitimate exercise of the physician's business rights provided that the general rules pertaining to in-office ancillary services are taken into account. In addition, matters dealing with bona fide employment arrangements and the definition of a group will affect those subspecialists, such as retina specialists, who relate to general ophthalmology practices in a variety of ways. In "Stark II proposed regulations: Down the rabbit hole," the salutary developments as well as the major confusions are addressed. However, since the regulatory material submitted to the Federal Register to provide these explanations exceeded 400 pages in length, the article can only highlight those matters of general applicability. Again, ophthalmologists would be well advised to carefully monitor developments in this context. In the meantime, decisions will have to be made as to whether to conform with regulations that do not yet have the force of law.

Taken as a whole, the physician practice environment is one which cannot function without taking into account the impact of the law. These three articles are only part of what will continue to define the ophthalmologist's world.

Managed Care and Liability: As the World Turns*

In managed care, traditional liabilities for malpractice and bad outcomes to patients are triangulated among the patient, managed care organizations (MCOs) and physician. Because continuing developments in the marketplace create ever more complex relationships, the courts will face novel arrangements when lawsuits are filed. The context is volatile. The stakes are high. The answers are not yet clear. We do know, however, that there is a burgeoning consideration of the influential role played by MCOs which is changing traditional theories of liability, while new ones emerge. This *AGG Note* (1) presents now standard views of managed care liability based on traditional organizational forms and caselaw, (2) considers liability issues in new managed care arrangements, (3) discusses contract terms which are especially relevant, and (4) provides practical guidance.

Tradition and Managed Care Liability

The earliest forms of managed care were *group model* HMOs with Kaiser as the premier example. The Kaiser Health Plan obtains its physicians through a contract with the Permanente-Medical Group which provides its employees exclusively to Kaiser. This model has frequently been described as a true staff model, but that is inaccurate. In a true *staff model* HMO, the comprehensive benefits which the plan agrees to provide are offered by physicians directly employed by the plan. Caselaw has long held that in the staff model, the HMO is liable for the acts of its employed physicians.

Similarly, in the group model HMO, courts have often found that the HMO can be held liable for the acts of the physicians working for the group which staffs it. But the group model is not particularly prevalent on the east coast. There, other styles predominate. In the *IPA* (*Independent Practice Association*) form the HMO contracts with a corporation which arranges for care to be provided by its own network of contracted, but otherwise independent physicians. From there—the prototype originally used by US Healthcare—many HMOs moved to *network model* arrangements, where they would contract directly with individual physicians who were otherwise independent, adding groups or IPAs into the mix, too. The advent of *Physician Hospital Organizations* (*PHOs*) evolved these early formats still further into one in which the HMO would contract with a single entity representing the hospital and selected members of its medical staff (whether participating as individuals or through their own IPA) to provide both physician and facility services. Some of these entities have joined with other PHOs or multiple hospitals to create super-PHOs which contract with payors, including employers. Now, even more complex entities calling themselves *IDSs* (*or integrated delivery systems*) are participating directly with payors on behalf of their affiliated hospitals, group practices, IPAs, PHOs and other institutional providers. To understand the

---

*From *AGG Notes,* published by Alice G. Gosfield, Esq. Copyright 1997 Alice G. Gosfield, Esq.

liability implications to these various players, a familiarity with the state of liability caselaw in managed care is useful.

Caselaw

Managed care liability caselaw has focused on three essential aspects of managed care archetypes: (1) whether a business entity which is not licensed to practice medicine can be held liable for the medical outcomes experienced by its beneficiaries; (2) the legal effect of the entity's selection of a limited network of providers from whom the beneficiaries obtain the services covered under the insurance contract; and (3) the significance of the medical management programs through which managed care produces both cost savings and a style of practice different from fee-for-service medicine. However, in considering the implications of caselaw, it is important to note the very long time period between a bad outcome to a patient and a decision from an appellate court. Those decisions create precedent. Jury trials do not. In addition, frequently in managed care cases, because the law has been unsettled, precedent is made on decisions involving preliminary motions to dismiss (motion for summary judgment). This means that market developments far outstrip judicial guidance on the allocation of liability among the relevant actors.

Entity Liability

Using theories of ostensible agency (the patient perceives the physician as the representative of the plan), corporate negligence (because of the activity the entity engages in, it can be held liable for its negligent business behavior) and vicarious liability (even though the entity itself did not directly create the harm, it can be held liable because of the special relationships involved), most of the caselaw has found that HMOs can be held liable for bad outcomes to their subscribers. There is decidedly less guidance available when you move from the HMO to an IPA or network which has contracted with the HMO. In fact, there are a few cases that have held that where an HMO contracts with an IPA which itself then contracts with the professional corporation which employs the physicians which caused the problem, the HMO really cannot be held liable since it does not control the actions of the physician. These cases are decidedly in the minority.

Negligent Selection

In cases which have found HMOs can be held liable, the plan's negligent selection of the provider who caused the harm has been the primary basis for liability. The fact that the patient is limited to obtaining covered services from the HMO's pre-selected physicians is the key to this analysis. While this notion seems logical as applied to participating physicians, in *Decker v. Saini*, a 1991 Michigan case, it was extended to include liability for out of network providers too. There the court found that an HMO should not be able to avoid liability simply by referring patients out-of-network when the HMO has agreed to provide comprehensive benefits.

Utilization Management

A number of cases have sought to impose liability for HMO utilization decisions, whether in denying access to a service in the first place, or in limiting hospitalization in others. Some courts have held that as a matter of law any party dealing with the patient can be held liable when its decisions harm a patient because either no appeal was taken by the attending physicians, no appeal opportunity was made available, appeal requests were arbitrarily ignored or denied, or where the standard of care was not followed. In the few cases which have so held, though, at trial the plan was not actually held liable. In addition, although in a few instances the courts have said liability could exist, in far more cases the ERISA laws have thwarted attempts to impose liability. This now appears to be changing.

ERISA

The Employee Retirement Income Security Act (ERISA) was Congress' effort in 1974 to assure that pension dollars promised to employees were there when they retired. The law imposed a federal scheme which would preempt any state laws on the same subject. Since the major focus was on preserving bank accounts, the primary remedy provided for the aggrieved beneficiary was to grant him the value of the benefit denied. This approach made good sense when the benefit was money. However, because health benefits are made available as part of the same employee welfare programs that provide for retirement benefits, ERISA turned out to apply to health care. In health care cases then, certain issues which would appear to be traditional malpractice cases to be decided in state court under long-standing tort principles end up as ERISA cases in federal court where the courts are restricted in what they can do for the plaintiff. The results have been quite startling. Two cases with dramatic results frame this issue well.

In *Corcoran v. Blue Cross of Louisiana*, when a high risk pre-term mother was admitted to the hospital for fetal monitoring, the insurer and utilization review (UR) company found that she would be fine at home with a home monitor and a nurse. The patient was discharged. One night when the nurse was off duty, the baby went into fetal distress and died. The family sued both the insurer and UR company for wrongful death. In response, however, they removed the case to federal court where ERISA would preempt. The federal court judge wrote an anguished opinion in which she said, essentially, I am compelled to find that in this case the UR decision was a benefit decision with a medical component. Because ERISA preempts challenges to benefit decisions, there is no remedy for this family in either state court or federal court.

Similarly, in *Kuhl v. Lincoln National*, when Buddy Kuhl made arrangements to have heart surgery performed out of network, his physicians and the consulting physicians thought the surgery necessary. Just before the surgery was to occur, the HMO discovered the case had not gone through the proper prior authorization. The surgery was canceled until authorization could be obtained. By the time it was, Kuhl's condition had deteriorated so only a heart transplant would help him. He died awaiting a heart.

The family sued with the same result as in Corcoran—no remedy available. Some will raise the issue of cases like *Fox v. HealthNet* where Nellie Fox's family won an $89 million verdict against her plan when she was denied an autologous bone marrow transplant for breast cancer. Although liability was assessed against the HMO, ERISA did not pertain there, because Ms. Fox worked for the school district which was exempt from ERISA. About 85% of health benefits made available in this country arise under plans affected by ERISA. Its reach has been extensive and the protection it offered plans significant. This appears to be changing now.

Dukes and After

In 1995, in *Dukes v. US Healthcare*, the plaintiffs brought their action differently. Instead of arguing that the test the patient didn't get was the basis for plan liability, the plaintiff argued that the HMO had an on-going obligation to monitor the quality of the care provided by its network of physicians. Its negligence in performing this responsibility led to the harm. The HMO defended by arguing ERISA preempted; but the court did not buy that. Holding that the quality of the network had nothing to do with benefit decisions, the case was remanded to state court where traditional malpractice principles will apply. As we write this, the trial was pending. Cases around the country have now started to move in the same direction. State legislatures are also leaping into the fray. Texas has enacted a statute which makes HMOs liable for malpractice. In the future, more managed care liability cases will be litigated in state court under traditional principles than during the last half-dozen years. Consider, then, the shifting sands of liability in light of new developments in the marketplace, some of which providers are seeking at all cost.

Trends in the Marketplace

With the new organizational structures discussed in the opening of this *AGG Note* have come new payment techniques, too. Traditional managed care gives capitation payments to primary care gatekeeping physicians to motivate them to provide only those physician services which are truly necessary to the patients' immediate needs. Over time some plans moved to pay primary care physician groups increased capitation rates to include ancillary services—laboratory, radiology, physical therapy. This evolution itself expanded. Set forth below are some new models which we have seen in our practice.

Global Risk Contracting

Through this technique, the entity with the insurance license (the HMO) gives a significant portion of the premium dollar to another organization to manage a full continuum of care—physician services, external ancillary services, prescription drugs, hospital services and even long term care. While in California much global contracting has found a home in large medical groups, in the east the principal seekers of this payment technique are IDSs still in their formative stages. Frequently, although enthusiastically negotiating these contracts, these putative integrated entities have had little experience with managed care generally and now have created a maze of relationships among providers with little infrastructure to manage yet in place.

Global risk contracting has produced striking data. In a 1995 study of the large California medical groups taking global risk, hospital admissions were 40% below California managed care rates! The basic strategy of capitation and global risk arrangements rests on the basic theory of insurance—namely that there are enough healthy people on whom premiums are paid but who will never use the service to balance the sicker patients. Based as they are on an insurance model, these payment mechanisms contain two fundamental risks for those who accept them: (1) the risk that the actuarial assumptions pertaining to the incidence of disease in the assigned population and the anticipated utilization of services upon which the premiums were calculated were accurate; and (2) the risk that the insurance product will be sold to groups whose incidence of disease conforms with the actuarial assumptions. Whether clinically valid standards for the health care needs of the projected population are taken into account in the construction of premium rates or rates of payment in global risk arrangements is a critical issue often overlooked in the rush to assume financial risk.

A new "global risk" opportunity has emerged for some provider entities in the recognition in the Medicare Balanced Budget Act of "*Provider Sponsored Organizations*" (PSOs). Who will qualify as these organizations is, so far, unclear. The idea is that provider entities would be able to contract directly with HCFA, like an HMO, to provide a full range of services to Medicare beneficiaries under the Medicare+ Choice program. One of the major points of contention for policy-makers has been what protection against insolvency will be imposed on these organizations.

Managed care organizations have been concerned about "leveling the playing field", meaning that provider sponsored entities should not be permitted to avoid the financial reserves required of licensed HMOs. Financial reserves are a critical aspect of insurance regulation. They protect against bad actuarial assumptions, among other things. In the HMO context financial reserves are especially important since, if the plan goes bankrupt, as some have, not only are the providers left holding the bag, the beneficiaries have paid premium dollars and cannot receive health care for their payments.

Because of the arguments over this issue, Congress mandated that the Secretary of DHHS enter into a negotiated rule-making process—a technique newly applied to two major issues under federal law—this solvency issue and safe harbor protection under the anti-kickback statute for physician incentive plans. In this process, representatives of the affected interests sit at the table with government and literally negotiate the terms of the regulations. It will be awhile until we know what the landscape of the PSO option will incorporate.

From a liability perspective, though, where an entity takes global risk it becomes a managed care organization. It cannot survive if it does not truly manage delivery of care, responding to the financial incentives to safeguard premium dollars. While the caselaw on liability for HMOs—which do not even provide services directly—is still evolving, for provider entities the duality of managing and delivering all of the care, makes for very short steps to large jury awards. The link between payment and underservice is far clearer in this type of payment system. Disappointed patients will draw the connection easily. By way of analogy, data today show that although family physicians and internists have traditionally experienced very low rates of malpractice suits, with the introduction of gatekeeping the number of suits filed against them has gone up significantly.

Specialty Carve-Outs

While global contracting heads toward a highly consolidated model, a contradictory phenomenon is also developing with other payors. Some are increasingly *carving out* of the primary care payment arrangement certain specialty care services. Traditional carve-outs have been focused around behavioral health. Many MCOs take a portion of the premium dollar and dedicate it to behavioral health entities to manage those services. A major lawsuit was filed against an HMO in Philadelphia recently involving alleged negligent credentialing by a carve-out behavioral health company. Other liability cases around the country have involved denial of or foreshortening of psychiatric benefits. Carve-outs are now spreading to other specialty services including vision care, oncology and cardiology, where a portion of the capitated per member per month payment is assigned to the specialty arrangement. Here, the fundamental questions turn on where the utilization controls exist. Do patients have direct access to the specialist? Must care still funnel through a primary care gatekeeper? Is that gatekeeper still at risk for referrals for specialty services? Whether the amounts paid will be sufficient to cover medically necessary patient care services depends on these factors in addition to the fundamental actuarial assumptions as well. But, as we have seen, financial risk relates directly to the extent of liability risk. Compare the implications from still another variant of carve-outs.

Case Rate

In case rate payments, instead of capitation, the provider contracts to provide, for a single fixed rate which extends over a defined timeframe, a full spectrum of services associated with a specific procedure or patient condition. Case rates are often associated with specific surgical procedures or defined disease processes. "We agree to provide a hip replacement for $X over a year regardless of how many times the patient needs to be readmitted" or "We will treat a Stage II breast cancer patient for a year for $X." Sometimes the payment is not restricted either to physician or hospital services alone, but encompasses all relevant services including physical therapy, durable medical equipment, home nursing or more. Certain high cost cases like bone marrow transplants are also paid for on this model.

In case rates, the financial assumptions rest on an understanding of what the typical patient will need medically and what it costs to provide those services. Case rates cannot be undertaken safely without clearly articulated clinical practice guidelines or algorithms which define the typical process of care. The incidence risk disappears because the payor agrees to pay for each patient who manifests the triggering condition. The case rate does create an incentive to efficient utilization which in an atypical patient can be financially problematic. Consequently one of the major challenges in case rate payments is to avoid including patients with co-morbid conditions that would undermine the validity of the clinical algorithm which is the basis for the payment calculation. Depending on the scope of the rate, the provider may have to select other individuals or entities to render services within the case payment. The case rate contracted provider, then, is at risk for selection of those providers, careful determination of how to pay them as well as for those providers' capacity to treat in accordance with the algorithmic protocol. Case rates also generally are constructed with the assumption that some patients will need somewhat more than the full scope of the payment whereas others will need less. It is beyond those marginal differences that trouble lurks.

To work, case rates must be predicated upon a specifically articulated algorithm of care; so these cases provide clear points of evaluation for liability purposes. The choice of the algorithm, its applicability to the patient, and adherence to the applicable guideline or carefully explicated deviation from it will be the critical issues in a liability case focused around a case rate. Since this approach is founded upon clinical judgments, it shifts the nature of the debate somewhat away from the under-service potential inherent in capitated models. Of course, a rigidly defined algorithm which does not reflect good clinical judgment can create just as much of an incentive to under-serve, and because of its explicit nature would likely be easier to criticize in a malpractice case.

EPISODE OF CARE (EOC)

A different version of the case rate which has emerged in some markets is an episode of care payment system. Here, the payor establishes a budget for services provided by a specific specialty—say cardiology or gastroenterology. All physicians to be paid under the system are guaranteed to be paid a fixed rate for a defined period of time to cover all those services included in the EOC. The payment amount fluctuates, however, with the number of episodes initiated. If the performance of a simple EKG triggers the same payment over 90 days as a cardiac angioplasty then two essential issues emerge: (1) which types of services, identified by CPT code, fall within the payment; and (2) what system controls utilization which determines how many episodes are initiated. Assumptions in this payment methodology are that all physicians will pare back their utilization since the more services that are rendered and the more episodes which are triggered the less money will be available to pay each of them. The financial incentive in this type of system, however, is so diffuse as to be essentially meaningless. If physicians with absolutely no relationship to each other are at risk financially they have no ability to influence their colleagues' behavior. If there are no controls on the primary physicians referring patients to the specialists, then episode volume increases while payment amounts decrease. The physicians are incentivized to limit services but not only do they have no control over the payment that will be available to them, there is no clarity whatever regarding the amount of that payment.

Here the liability will likely be allocated between the HMO and the provider. To the extent the calculation of the budget is so strict as to contradict reasonable actuarial projections for necessary services, the plan likely would be liable for its breach of the duty to provide contractually mandated benefits. But the physicians have some exposure as well, particularly as the budgets become more aggressive, since high volume lowers payment to all which can further reduce service provided to individuals.

Contract Terms

Against this background a number of typical managed care contract provisions take on new meaning. The most problematic clauses in managed care contracts have been *indemnifications*—here one party, typically the HMO, wants the other (the provider) to step in and pay any damages levied on the HMO but caused by the provider. Where multiple layers exist, (HMO to PHO to IPA to physician) there are often indemnifications throughout. Most malpractice policies exclude coverage for contracted-for-liability, so agreeing to an indemnification clause can mean there is no insurance to pay that contractual obligation. Some carriers will cover for negligence in the provision of medical services if they would have been required to pay in the absence of the clause. Indemnification clauses can be so problematic, though, that they have been outlawed both in California and in provider contracts under the new federal Medicare+ Choice program. There is a real question as to whether they are necessary at all, since contracting parties have a common law right of contribution from the party which causes their economic damages. This theory has already been applied in managed care.

In *Dunn v. Praiss*, a 1995 New Jersey case, although the court had held that the HMO could be liable for the capitated urologist's late diagnosis of the patient's testicular cancer, when the physician settled his case, he turned around and sued the HMO for contribution. The court held that as a matter of law the right existed, but the demand should have been made in the original response to the lawsuit and not after it was settled.

Related to indemnifications are the almost ubiquitous provisions that the physician exercises independent medical judgment. While not problematic on their face, some of these clauses, however, go on to say that the provider "acknowledges" that the plan's medical management programs do not influence clinical decision-making. Given the purpose of managed care, this is disingenuous at best. We do not, yet, however, have caselaw which either confronts plan responsibility for the effects of their medical management programs nor clear guidance to offer physicians regarding their exposure when the plan has said it will not pay for the service the physician thinks is necessary. As managed care becomes more prevalent, however, we may see a shift in the fundamental standard of care. If the point of managed care has been to change provider behavior, then where most care is no longer provided in an unfettered fee for service setting, the standard of care itself may change to a managed care model. If challenged, in defense a physician might well argue he acted exactly as other physicians in a managed care setting might. These issues have not been squarely addressed by the courts either.

Related contract provisions sometimes say that the providers recognize and acknowledge that they are not the plan's agents. As indicated above, however, the courts seem to be headed in a different direction. These contract clauses, then, seem to ask providers to assume by their acknowledgment the HMO's potential liability as established in ostensible agency cases.

Some clauses state specifically that each party is liable for his own acts. Although relatively straightforward, these provisions could undercut common law contribution rights where they exist. Some indemnification clauses attempt to parse out carefully who does what—the physician is responsible for medical care and the plan is responsible for coverage and benefit determinations. These characterizations often beg the question of the utilization review programs and other medical management techniques.

Some contracts actually try to limit any damages which might be obtained under an indemnification to only the amount paid by the plan in benefits, and even then to during the previous twelve months only. This approach could render the plan's indemnification essentially meaningless.

Practical Tips

There is virtually no caselaw looking at the more complex relationships in IDS, PHO, PSO and global risk arrangements. Still some practical steps can be taken, given what we know today.

1. In negotiating the provider contract, it is extremely important to focus exquisite attention on the specific roles played by the various parties. Broadly drafted provisions can only lead to major battles later. A PHO, for example, makes available its providers, so it should have risk for negligent credentialing and selection, but not for the malpractice of its physicians, for which they themselves should be responsible.
2. **Read your liability policy** to determine if it is appropriate to the risks assumed. Where provider entities accept new forms of payment which entail expanded management responsibility or changed financial incentives, they should carefully disclose all of their activities to their liability carrier and assure that appropriate expansions in coverage are obtained.
3. Where provider entities take on delegated credentialing and utilization management, accreditation may be beneficial for both parties. Judicial judgment of the standard of care for these functions has not yet been

enunciated. MCOs can be accredited by a range of organizations—NCQA, JCAHO, URAC, TMQC, AAAHC. To establish whether the parties behaved as similarly situated entities would under the circumstances, accreditation may demonstrate adherence to a standard of the industry.

4. Using accredited or certified entities to assist in delegated functions is also worth considering. NCQA now accredits managed behavioral health entities and certifies credentials verification organizations as well as physician organizations taking delegation of certain functions from an HMO. An HMO carving out to an NCQA - accredited behavioral health entity, or an IDS using a credentials verification organization to provide some of the basic information needed, can help forestall a claim of negligence in performing those functions.
5. Physicians should always appeal UR judgments with which they disagree medically. Although the fundamental question of how far the physician must go in providing uncompensated care has not been squarely addressed by the courts, failure to appeal would certainly arise in a malpractice case.
6. Those seeking some of the newer forms of payment should seek out good clinical practice guidelines and make sure that the payment reflects the clinical assumptions there. (See *AGG Note,* June, 1995).
7. Given the burgeoning caselaw on network quality, MCOs should engage in aggressive credentialing and on-going monitoring of physician performance. Physicians should expect more intrusive inquiries from MCOs and more focused profiling of behavior, with termination of participation for those who cannot conform with quality mandates.

As risk assumption moves around the developing labyrinth of entities and relationships, it can be assumed that fingers will be pointed when things go wrong. Smart players will seek to manage their risk by focusing on potential operational pitfalls. With increasing competitive emphasis on quality performance, HEDIS measures and scorecards (see *AGG Note,* June 1995) risk management merges with strategic planning. Both in managed care liability and competition, good quality care and properly implemented medical management are the keys to managed care success for all players.

For more information on legal issues in managed care quality see, Gosfield, ***GUIDE TO KEY LEGAL ISSUES IN MANAGED CARE QUALITY,*** *253pp, available from Faulkner and Gray, www.faulknergray.com, or 1–800–535–8403, described in the enclosed review from* Healthplan *magazine.*

Private Contracting by Medicare Physicians: The Pit and the Pendulum*

Throughout the history of Medicare physician payment, potential government intrusion in private financial relationships between physicians and patients has been at issue. Congressional action on this subject has gone from an affirmative avoidance policy to one of increasing involvement in private activity, and now back in the other direction. The Balanced Budget Act of 1997[1] ("BBA") enacted a provision[2] to liberalize the restrictions imposed by Medicare law on private financial arrangements between physicians and their Medicare patients, by lifting the imposition of limiting charges in some situations. However, as a result of a controversial Conference Committee modification, the statute is confusing at best, internally inconsistent, and, in the last analysis eviscerates the whole point of the provision in the first place. This article considers the problems in the law as enacted, evaluated against the historical Medicare context on this issue.

I. Historical Background[3]

When Medicare was first introduced in 1966, it was sold to physicians as a program that was voluntary and would not interfere in the practice of medicine, clinically or administratively. This position was even incorporated into the statute and remains in effect.

> Nothing in this title shall be construed to authorize any Federal officer or employee to exercise any supervision or control over the practice of medicine or the manner in which medical services are provided, or over the selection, tenure or compensation of any officer or employee of any institution, agency or person providing health services, or to exercise any supervision or control over *the administration or operation* of any such institution, agency or person.[4]

This freedom from interference was further bolstered by a provision guaranteeing free choice by patients in their selection of providers. "Any individual entitled to insurance benefits under this title may obtain health services from any institution, agency, or person qualified to participate under this title if such institution, agency or person undertakes to provide him such services."[5] For many years, the hands-off approach in these two sections remained the underlying social policy on the fundamental relationship between physicians who would treat Medicare patients and the program itself. Over time, however, the bonds between the Part B program and all physicians would become tighter; and Medicare would reach directly into the wallets even of physicians with whom the program was not in privity.

A. Assignment and Participation

From the beginning of the program, the right to receive Part B payment for physician services has belonged to the patient alone. The patient can assign that right to the physician, who has the freedom to decide whether to accept assignment or not. Carriers who administer the Part B program are statutorily required to pay claims to physicians where payment will be made on the basis of an assignment under which the Medicare allowable amount ("reasonable charge") is the full charge for the service; the physician agrees not to charge for services denied by a peer review organization ("PRO") and agrees not to charge the patient where waiver of liability would pertain.[6] Through this system, the physician steps into the shoes of the beneficiary for purposes of Medicare payment, accepting the Medicare amount as payment in full on the basis of the contractual assignment by the beneficiary, acknowledged in writing by the physician when he submits the claim for the service. Where the physician does not accept assignment, Medicare pays the patient the allowable amount. For some time, physicians who chose not to accept assignment had unfettered discretion to charge the Medicare patient what they chose ("balance billing"); but as physicians increased their fees, Congress began to consider other ways of influencing physicians to accept assignment more often.

Effective July 18, 1984, Congress created the participating physician and supplier program—an approach to assignment that, for the first time, contained incentives to physicians to accept assignment all of the time. Through this mechanism, a physician signs an agreement prior to the beginning of the next year, in which he agrees to "participate" with Medicare, meaning he agrees to accept assignment 100% of the time and not to balance bill for a year. Reenrollment is automatic unless affirmatively terminated before the beginning of the next year.[7] The names of these physicians are published in a directory to be made available by each carrier; preference for electronic claims submission is given to these physicians; and annual notices are sent to beneficiaries informing them of who these physicians are. Where services are provided by a nonparticipating physician, the Secretary places a notice on the Explanation of Benefits indicating the advantages of assignment to the beneficiaries and notifying them of the existence of the directories so they can identify participating physicians. When this "buyer beware" approach failed to yield significant results, Congress went further.

B. Charge Limits and Balance Billing

In 1986, Congress linked non-participation status to financial limitations when physicians did not accept assignment. The law created "Maximum Actual Allowable Charges" ("MAACs"), an individually calculated physician-specific limit on what the non-participating physician could charge the Medicare beneficiary on an unassigned claim.[8] The amount of the limit was based on 1984 historical data. Violations were punishable by civil money penalties or exclusion from Medicare.

The American Medical Association ("AMA") sought an injunction to delay implementation of MAACs on the grounds that the carriers had not provided each physician with information about their own applicable limits. The case was dismissed not only as moot on the injunction and lacking ripeness on the overcharging penalties but also because the plaintiffs lacked standing.[9] MAACs were also challenged in another case as unconstitutional, regulating purely intrastate private physician patient contracts. That case was also dismissed.[10] MAACs were only in place for six years.

In 1989, OBRA replaced MAACs for services after 1991 with the "limiting charge."[11] Limiting charges are keyed to the "recognized payment amount," the most that a non-participating physician can get on an assigned claim—which is itself limited to 95% of what the participating physician would receive. The limiting charge was then set at a rate 115% above the recognized payment amount. Like the MAAC system, the carriers reviewing the limiting charge monitor actual charges and violators are subject to civil money penalties. As additional inducements to participate, expedited payment for electronically billed claims and direct deposit of Medicare payments were made available to participating physicians. In *Garelick v. Sullivan,*[12] a group of anesthesiologists argued that the limiting charge was a taking of property in violation of the Fifth Amendment of the Constitution. They too were unsuccessful.

These absolute charging limits were combined with a number of other features to discourage non-participation. By the time the limiting charges were in place, non-participating physicians were prohibited from billing a patient for unassigned fees where services were deemed not medically necessary by the carrier or PRO. All claims, for all services, whether assigned or unassigned, must be submitted by the physician in accordance with Medicare requirements. Non-participating physicians were subject to special rules for dealing with elective surgeries for which they did not accept assignment. For elective surgical procedures for which the actual charge is more than $500, the physician who does not accept assignment must disclose to the patient in writing: the estimated actual charge; the estimated approved charge; the difference; and the applicable co-insurance. Violations of any of these rules can result in civil money penalties.

Following this federal approach, some states enacted prohibitions on balance billing linked to the Medicare rates. In some ways, these states extended the limits further. In at least four states, litigation challenged the constitutionality of such state controls. None was successful. In Massachusetts, all physicians were required as a condition of licensure to agree not to bill in excess of the Medicare reasonable charge.[13] Pennsylvania's Health Care Practitioners Medicare Fee Control Act—colloquially called the Medicare Overpayment Measure or the "MOM Law"—prohibited billing more than the Medicare allowable amount regardless of participation status.[14] A New York law capped the allowable amount a physician could balance bill at 115% of Medicare allowable charges.[15] Finally, Ohio's law preventing physicians from charging a Medicare beneficiary an amount in excess of the Medicare reimbursement rate was also upheld.[16]

Taken together, by 1996, at both the state and federal levels, the right of the government to insert itself into the business relationships of physicians who treated Medicare patients but had no contractual relationship with the federal government was well established. The swing of the pendulum in the other direction has now come with the Balanced Budget Act.

II. The Original Proposal

The initial theory on private contracts was that some affluent Medicare patients are happy to pay their physicians' full charges. Other patients do not want to be compelled to use their Medicare benefits for certain covered services. Senator Kyl (R-AZ) introduced the legislative remedy, which he characterized as necessary because of HCFA's overreaching interpretation of 1994 Medicare legislative technical corrections. His proposal was intended to overcome HCFA's then-proposed prohibition on physicians accepting any private payments for their services to Medicare patients. "Surely a law that made it illegal to supplement with private funds the amount received from Social Security would be met with disbelief and derision," he argued.[17] Apparently, he was wrong.

The Senate version was relatively straightforward as described in the Conference Committee Report.

> [N]othing in Medicare law shall prohibit a physician or another health care professional who does not provide items and services under Medicare from entering into a private contract with a Medicare beneficiary for health services for which no Medicare claim is to be submitted. Medicare's limiting charge provisions would not apply to services provided to a beneficiary under such a contract. . . .[18]

After four years of the program, the HCFA Administrator was to prepare a report on the effect of these private contracts.

The controversies over the Senate proposal, which had no analogue in the House, turned on the references to services "for which no Medicare claim is to be submitted." Senator Kyl reportedly described the original language to have permitted the private contracting only for physicians who did not provide items or services under the Medicare program, which Kyl had said was only 9% of doctors.[19] With changes agreed to late in the evening before the budget deal was finally struck, Kyl reported that there was panic at the prospect of a Clinton veto if the original private contracting provision remained in the bill. It seems that some lawmakers were concerned that the Senate's provision could have been interpreted by HCFA to require a lifetime opt out from Medicare for physicians who privately contracted.[20]

Although lifetime exclusion was not enacted, the language that became law defeats the original concept, which was to permit physicians on a case-by-case basis to enter into private arrangements with patients who choose to pay the full amount and can afford to do so. The statute does not allow this case-by-case approach, requiring that if a physician wants any private charging relationship with a single patient that would exceed the limiting charge, he must remove himself from the Medicare program, on any level, whether fee-for-service or capitated, for two years.

III. The Law

The basic provision amends the provision in the law allowing freedom of choice of provider by patients (SSA § 1802), which dates to the inception of Medicare.[21] The statute now expressly permits any physician or practitioner to enter into a private contract with a beneficiary for which no claim for payment will be submitted to Medicare, and for which the physician will not receive any Medicare reimbursement directly on a fee for service basis or indirectly on a capitated basis. The provision by its language would permit even the participating physician to break his agreement to accept assignment 100% of the time for a year.

To protect beneficiaries from pressure by physicians to forgo their Medicare benefits, a series of protections were adopted. The arrangement must be documented in a written contract signed by the beneficiary before any item or service is provided pursuant to the arrangement and the contract may not be entered into when the beneficiary is facing an emergency or urgent healthcare situation.[22] The provision specifies the required contents of the contract with the beneficiary. By signing the contract, the beneficiary agrees not to submit or to request the physician to submit a claim for any Medicare covered services; agrees to be responsible, "whether through insurance or otherwise," for payment for the services and understands that no reimbursement will be available from Medicare; acknowledges that no limits will apply to the amount the physician may charge; acknowledges that Medigap plans do not and other supplemental insurers may not make payments because no Medicare payment will be made; and acknowledges that the Medicare beneficiary has the right to have the items or services provided by other physicians or practitioners for whom payment would be made.[23]

These provisions go well beyond a buyer beware policy to an affirmative red flag approach. Given the legislatively imposed constraints, the circumstances under which any beneficiary would choose a private and unlimited relationship would be rare indeed. That, in and of itself, is not particularly problematic. Within the context of Medicare, the long-standing policy justification for limiting charges has been to protect from outright gouging those Medicare beneficiaries who will receive only limited payments from Medicare for unassigned services. Of far more troublesome significance are the enacted requirements for physicians.

A private contract cannot be considered effective unless the physician has filed with the Secretary a formal affidavit providing that the physician or practitioner will not submit *any* claim under Medicare for *any* beneficiary—not just the ones who have chosen the private contract path—during a two-year period extending from the date of filing of the affidavit.

The affidavit itself must be filed with the Secretary no later than ten days after the first contract to which the affidavit applies.[24]

Now for the internal inconsistency. The enforcement provision establishes that if a physician or practitioner who has signed an affidavit knowingly and willfully submits a Medicare claim during the two-year preclusion period (or receives any reimbursement during that time), then the permission to privately contract does not exist on and after the date of the submission, *and* no payment shall be made by Medicare for *any* item or service furnished by the physician during the two-year period. However, the statute already establishes that no payment may be made for *any* Medicare item or service for *any* Medicare beneficiary during the two-year period anyway. So what kind of enforcement is this? It looks as if the original intent was that if the physician entered into an individual private contract and submitted claims in breach of that contract, then the punishment would be preclusion for all Medicare patients for two years, but with the change so that the preclusion existed for two years for all beneficiaries even if one contract was entered into, the enforcement provision makes no sense.

The opacity in drafting is noteworthy.[25] An additional potential consequence of a knowing and willful submission of a claim or receipt of payment in breach of the affidavit rests on the following brilliant construction: "(I) this subsection shall not apply with respect to any items and services provided by the physician or practitioner pursuant to any contract on and after the date of such submission and before the end of such period."[26] This language opens the door to the reimposition of the limiting charges (and requirement to file all claims) for all services rendered by the physician and the outright nullification of the private contract. In that instance, the civil money penalties applicable to limiting charge violations would be triggered. It was apparent that clarifications would be necessary. HCFA has stepped in, although it has not addressed enforcement.

IV. HCFA Clarifications

HCFA issued in November 1997 a six-page question and answer document attempting to clarify the practical implications of the law.[27] The substance of its answers is largely but not entirely incorporated into a Program Memorandum for Carriers that itself provides the camera ready version of the *1998 Fact Sheet,* which carriers must provide to physicians to assist them in determining whether to participate. Because of the understandable confusion over the practical import of this law, HCFA has extended the participation decision deadline for physicians until February 2, 1998.

A. To Whom the Law Pertains

The statute defines the "physicians" and "practitioners" to whom the law pertains.[28] HCFA explains that this includes doctors of medicine and osteopathy, physician assistants ("PAs"), nurse practitioners ("NPs"), clinical nurse specialists ("CNSs"), certified registered nurse anesthetists

("CRNAs"), certified nurse midwives, clinical social workers ("CSWs") and clinical psychologists ("CPs"). Because of the law's reference to SSA § 1861(r)(1) for the definition of "physician," HCFA has clarified that optometrists, podiatrists, dentists, doctors of oral surgery, physical therapists in independent practice and occupational therapists in independent practice may not privately contract or opt out of Medicare.

The ability of some non-physician practitioners to opt out is especially interesting because other provisions in the Medicare program establish that PAs, nurse midwives, NPs, CNSs, CRNAs, CSWs, and CPs services may only be paid on an assigned basis, in essence statutorily making them "participate" in the program. In addition, HCFA obliquely confirms that the statute would allow a participating physician to opt out, but it sees potential administrative issues. In discussing the standard requirement for termination of the participation agreement at the end of the preceding year for the subsequent year, HCFA states that it will not allow a participating physician whose agreement to participate has automatically renewed or been entered into for 1998 to enter into any private contracts in 1998. "HCFA is exploring whether it would be administratively possible to permit physicians and practitioners to exercise the private contracting option at times other than the annual participating physician enrollment period."[29] HCFA's decision on opt out during the term of participation would be made prior to February 2, 1998, the extended deadline for physicians to decide whether to participate for 1998. Physicians who reassign their rights to benefits to an entity that participates in the Medicare program—such as a hospital, an integrated delivery system or a clinic—may not use the private contract mechanism unless the entity that receives payment for them terminates its own participation. In contrast, however, HCFA further confirms that a single member of a group may opt out without affecting the other members of the group, but the corporation itself may not opt out. This is a physician-by-physician decision.

B. Scope of the Private Contract

HCFA clarifies that the opt out does not extend to services *ordered* but not provided by the physician, so long as the physician or practitioner has acquired a unique personal identifying number ("UPIN") from Medicare. But once a physician opts out of the program, all services provided by that physician—including durable medical equipment, independent diagnostic testing facilities or clinical laboratories—are considered out of the program. The private contract is also applicable even where Medicare is a secondary payor.

The "clarifying" questions and answers speak to the complete sweeping effect of a single private contract.

> 8. *Can a physician or practitioner have "private contracts" with some beneficiaries but not others?*
>
> No. The physician or practitioner who chooses to opt out of Medicare may provide covered care to beneficiaries only through private agreements, regardless of who bills and is paid for the

> services. . . . Once the physician or practitioner has opted out, such physician or practitioner must enter into a private contract with each Medicare beneficiary to whom he or she furnishes covered services (even where Medicare payment would be on a capitated basis or where Medicare would pay an organization for the physician's or practitioner's services to the Medicare beneficiary), with the exception of a Medicare beneficiary needing emergency or urgent care.[30]

There is an exception to provide Medicare services in an emergency or urgent care situation to a beneficiary with whom the physician has not entered into a private contract, in which case the physician is limited to the limiting charge in what he may charge the patient. Medicare pays to the beneficiary for covered services provided.

C. Non-Covered Services

When the Conference language was first released, many believed that the opt out pertained only to non-covered services, based on the language that said "for which no claim will be submitted." If services are non-covered services, there is no limiting charge that pertains to them, and no need to opt out of the program. HCFA has confirmed that the usual rules for advance notice to beneficiaries of their financial obligation to pay for services which are non-covered or will likely be deemed not reasonable and medically necessary (e.g., screening studies not specifically covered, extra nursing home visits, specific therapies for conditions which Medicare does not consider covered) are unaffected by the private contract option. In other words, physicians do not need to have a private contract to charge beneficiaries for these services, because they were never covered in the first place. Even those services that are conditionally non-covered do not require a formal private contract arrangement for the physician to charge the beneficiary directly without the limiting charge caps.

Still further, HCFA addresses yet another aspect of the physician relationship with Medicare that seems to have a very broad effect. HCFA states unequivocally, "A physician who has not opted out of Medicare must submit a claim to Medicare for services that may be covered by Medicare unless the beneficiary, for reasons of his or her own, declines to authorize the physician or practitioner to submit a claim or furnish confidential medical information to Medicare that is needed to execute a proper claim."[31] Here, HCFA asserts that the limiting charges still apply, even though no claim will ever be submitted. If neither the physician nor the beneficiary submits a claim for payment, how will HCFA ever know if the limiting charge was used?

D. Physician Issues

Although the statute says the affidavit must be filed with the Secretary, HCFA says that when a physician files the affidavit, he or she must file with each carrier that has jurisdiction over any claims of that physician. On the other hand, a physician must opt out for all carriers in all jurisdictions. The preclusion is complete and absolute for the two-year period. After the two-year period, the physician could elect to return to Medicare or to opt out again. Patients who are not enrolled in Part B are not affected by the opt out and "Medicare does not preclude physicians from treating Medicare beneficiaries if they treat private pay patients, whether they are persons age 65 or seniors who choose not to enroll in Part B."[32]

V. The Future

Senator Kyl, who sponsored the original Senate Bill, introduced legislation himself (S. 1194) and with Congressman Bill Archer (R-TX) (H.R. 2497) to eliminate the two-year preclusion for all Medicare patients. House Democrats reportedly stated that the new bills would alter the basic intent of Medicare "by allowing doctors to charge what they wish for services, thus creating a two-tiered program in which the wealthy would be able to pay for more extensive and expensive care, while other beneficiaries would not have that option."[33] Congressman Pete Stark (D-CA) has characterized the proposal as a "stealth amendment that would destroy the Medicare program."[34] The AMA considers restoration of the case-by-case, patient-by-patient approach a top priority. The American Association of Retired Persons is dead set against the private contracting provision. Confirmation of the HCFA Administrator's appointment was initially delayed by Senator Kyl over this issue, but he eventually relented, stating that rectifying the problems with the enacted language was a congressional leadership decision. The Administrator has stated that she expects the issue to be revisited by Congress because both Democrats and Republicans are dissatisfied. Against this background, the likelihood of reformation is speculative at best.

The policy behind private contract options turns primarily on the argument that physicians and patients ought be able to enter into private relationships without government interference. In 1996, a national poll cited by Senator Kyl found that 60% of Americans believe that Medicare patients should be able to add their own money to government payments in order to get unrationed health services.[35] Senator Kyl has made some arguments that go further, asserting that prohibitions on private contracting not only impair patient free choice, but the imposition of penalties for private contract relationships "would also end the practice of cost shifting, whereby doctors have an incentive to treat more Medicare patients who can't afford to supplement Medicare's low reimbursement rate with funds from those who choose to pay out of pocket."[36] How much cost shifting actually occurs is questionable, especially given the penalties associated with limiting charge violations. Moreover, the real cost shifting is likely not among Medicare patients, but between Medicare patients who need and use more services and healthier younger patients. Whatever the speculative economic impact of private contracting opportunities, the pendulum's swing in the legislation in effect today is only one of a few degrees and not to the status quo ante.

For physicians and other practitioners, the total preclusion of any Medicare payments for any Medicare beneficiaries for two years guts the real value of the provision for the occasional patient who might choose to use it. On the other hand, there are some physicians who have been fiercely opposed to Medicare's ability to govern their interactions with their patients when they have no contractual relationship with Medicare and do not accept Medicare dollars. One can assume that in a very few instances, those physicians will choose to take the extremely limited path the Balanced Budget Act has offered. At the same time, although the likelihood of change in the law may not be great, at least the inevitable rhetoric and positioning regarding private contracting as demonstrated in Congressman Stark's most recent proposal assures health lawyers of some modicum of entertainment in the coming Congressional session.

Alice G. Gosfield, Esq.

1. Pub. L. No. 105–33 (signed Aug. 5, 1997).
2. BBA § 4507.
3. For general background on the development of Part B physician reimbursement law until 1989, *see* Gosfield, "Part B Physician Reimbursement: Developments, Limits and Pitfalls," in Gosfield ed. *1990 Health Law Handbook,* Clark Boardman Co., Ltd., New York, 1990, pp. 275–310.
4. Emphasis added, § 1801 of the Social Security Act ("SSA"); 42 U.S.C. § 1395.
5. SSA § 1802; 42 U.S.C. § 1395a.
6. *See* SSA § 1842(b)(3)(ii); 42 U.S.C. § 1395u(b)(3). Waiver of liability is keyed to whether the patient or the physician knew or should have known that services later deemed not medically necessary and so non-covered and would not be paid for. *See also* SSA § 1879; 42 U.S.C. § 1395pp, and Gosfield, *supra* note 3, at 283–4.
7. SSA § 1842(h); 42 U.S.C. § 1395u(h).
8. SSA § 1842(j)(l); 42 U.S.C. § 1395u(j).
9. *American Med. Ass'n v. Bowen,* 659 F. Supp. 1143 (N.D. Tex. 1987); *vacated, appeal denied,* 857 F.2d 267 (5th Cir. 1988).
10. *Isaacs v. United States.* No. CIV 87–64 PHX RGS (D. Ariz. Oct. 14, 1987), Medicare & Medicaid Guide (CCH) ¶37,235. In *Metrolina Family Practice Group v. Sullivan,* 767 F. Supp 1314 (W.D.N.C. 1989), the plaintiffs also lost their challenge to the MAAC provisions, along with the restriction on billing for services deemed not medically necessary.
11. SSA § 1848(g); 42 U.S.C. § 1395w-4(g).
12. 987 F.2d 913 (2d Cir. 1993), *aff'g* 74 F. Supp 108 (S.D.N.Y. 1992), *cert. denied,* 510 U.S. 821 (1992).
13. *Massachusetts Med. Soc'y v. Dukakis,* 815 F.2d 790 (1st Cir. 1987), *aff'g* 637 F. Supp. 684 (D. Mass. 1986), *cert. denied,* 484 U.S. 896 (1987).
14. *Pennsylvania Med. Soc'y v. Marconis,* 942 F.2d 842 (3d Cir. 1991), *aff'g* 755 F. Supp. 1305 (W.D. Pa. 1991).
15. *Medical Soc'y of N.Y. v. Cuomo,* 976 F.2d 812 (2d Cir. 1992), *aff'g* 777 F. Supp. 1157 (S.D.N.Y. 1991).
16. *Downhour v. Somani,* 85 F.3d 261 (6th Cir. 1996), *cert. denied,* 117 S. Ct. 389 (1996).
17. Remarks of Sen. Kyl, 143 Cong. Rec. S. 6383 (June 25, 1997).

18. Explanation of the Conference Committee Affecting the Medicare and Medicaid Programs, "Balanced Budget Act of 1997 H.R. 2015, As Cleared by Congress for the President July 31, 1997," H. Rep. No. 105–217 at 90B.
19. Martin, "Private Contracts—at a Price," 40 *American Med. News* 1, at p. 32 (Oct. 6, 1997). Today, more than 80% of physicians nationally "participate" in Medicare. The range is from a low of 62.8% in New Jersey to a high of 93.5% in Alabama. *Part B News,* at p. 7, (May 26, 1997).
20. Martin, *supra* note 19, at p. 32.
21. Gosfield, *supra* note 3, at pp. 275–310.
22. BBA § 4507(a)(1); 42 U.S.C. § 1395(b)(1)(A).
23. BBA § 4507(a)(1); 42 U.S.C. § 1395(b)(1)(B).
24. BBA § 4507(b)(3).
25. For another example of late-night Conference Committee drafting, *see* SSA § 1877; 42 U.S.C. 1395nn—the Stark II law.
26. BBA § 4507(b)(3)(C)(i).
27. *Qs and As on Private Contracts* (HCFA Nov. 1997).
28. SSA § 1842(b)(18)(C); 42 U.S.C. § 1395u.
29. HCFA Fact Sheet, published with Program Memorandum Carriers Transmittal B-97–9 (Nov. 1997).
30. This statement is *not* included in the Fact Sheet, but is part of the *Qs and As* document.
31. *Qs and As,* Q. no. 21, *supra* note 27 at p. 6.
32. *Qs and As,* Q. no. 14, *supra* note 27 at p. 5.
33. "Democrats Charge Contracting Bill Would Dismantle Medicare Program," *Medicare Report,* (BNA) (Oct. 10, 1997 at 964).
34. *Id.* This observation should, perhaps, be evaluated in light of Congressman Stark's proposed legislation, the No Private Contracts To Be Negotiated When the Patient is Buck Naked Act of 1997, H.R. 2784, 105th Cong., 1st Sess., a related bill which this author recommends highly for its literary merit, if nothing else.
35. 143 Cong. Rec. S. 6383 at 6384, *supra* note 17.
36. *Id.*

Stark II Proposed Regulations: Down the Rabbit Hole*

> "But I don't want to go among mad people" Alice remarked. "Oh, you can't help that", said the Cat: "we're all mad here. I'm mad. You're mad." "How do you know I'm mad?", said Alice. "You must be," said the Cat, "or you wouldn't have come here."
>
> —Lewis Carroll

The Stark II proposed regulations have been published. These are *not* final regulations. They offer nothing more than a glimpse into HCFA's thinking at this moment in time. Join us in a trip down the rabbit hole to learn more about HCFA's views of life as we know it here on planet earth—today. How long their positions will remain viable only the Caterpillar knows.

Background and Context

On January 9, 1998, Stark II proposed regulations were published. Although the law they interpret became effective on January 1, 1995, until now, the only guidance available for those providing designated services other than clinical laboratory services was the final Stark I regulations published in August, 1995. (See *AGG Note*, Sept. 1995, "Stark I Regs: The Good, The Bad and the Incomprehensible".)

Because these are only proposed regulations, issues pertaining to referrals by physicians for clinical laboratory services will continue to be determined under the August, 1995 final regulations. For all of the other designated health services, the proposed regulations demonstrate HCFA's current thinking on many points, but they are not law.

In addition, given the major confusions these proposed regulations will generate, it is especially comforting to know that HCFA published simultaneously its interim final regulations (meaning having the force of law, but requesting comments anyway) for advisory opinions which HCFA will offer on Stark law issues. (The advisory opinion regulations will not be addressed here.)

The Essence of Stark II

The Stark statute prohibits a physician or an immediate family member from referring a Medicare or Medicaid patient for a "designated health service" to an entity with which the physician or family member has a financial relationship, unless the relationship meets one of a number of detailed exceptions. An improper referral is subject to a $15,000 civil money penalty. A separate penalty is imposed for the submission by the entity of a claim for the improperly referred service.

Contrary to popular belief, the Stark statute and the anti-kickback statute are two totally different laws. They are not even in the same titles

---

*From *AGG Notes,* published by Alice G. Gosfield, Esq. Copyright 1998 Alice G. Gosfield, Esq.

of the Social Security Act. There is no interrelationship between them. A Stark violation can exist regardless of the intent of the parties. The anti-kickback safe harbor regulations offer safety zones, but failure to conform with a safe harbor does not mean the statute is violated. On the other hand, because Stark is more restrictive, the fact that your circumstances do not violate the anti-kickback law does not mean you have no Stark problem. Consequently, in analyzing a transaction, one begins with Stark. If you flunk there, there is no need to look at the anti-kickback laws. In the Stark II proposed regulations preface, HCFA specifically asks for comments as to whether the Secretary should adopt a Stark exception which would say that if you fall into an anti-kickback safe harbor you are home free. That is *not* the case today.

Designated health services include clinical laboratory services; physical therapy services; occupational therapy services; radiology services including MRI, CT and ultrasound; radiation therapy and supplies; parenteral and enteral nutrients, equipment and supplies; prosthetics, orthotics and prosthetic devices and supplies; home health services; outpatient prescription drugs; and inpatient and outpatient hospital services.

The law provides numerous exceptions to the prohibition including referrals (1) for physician services within a group; (2) for in office ancillary services; (3) within a prepaid plan; with regard to investment interests, (4) to publicly traded investment entities, (5) to hospitals in Puerto Rico, (6) to rural providers, (7) to a hospital itself, (8) between lessor and lessee of office space or equipment; regarding compensation arrangements (9) for bona fide employment relationships, (10) personal services arrangements, (11) physician incentive plans, (12) remuneration unrelated to the provision of designated health care services; (13) physician recruitment payments, (14) isolated financial transactions, (15) group practice relationships with a hospital in place before December, 1989, and (16) payments by a physician to the referred to entity for items or services.

The statute defines and HCFA expansively views any economic benefit passing between the relevant parties as implicated by the law. This means that although Stark is limited only to Medicare and Medicaid physician referrals and then only where a financial relationship exists with the entity, far more transactions are included than common sense might dictate.

Details, Details

The basic problem with the Stark statute is not its breadth. The anti-kickback law is far broader in scope. Stark is focused only on physician referrals and then only for the designated services. The anti-kickback statute is for all federal programs and all who interact with them in providing services. Rather, the most difficult aspects of Stark lie in its extreme detail combined with the apparent ignorance of the drafters regarding Medicare's long standing approaches to a range of issues. For example, terms like "direct supervision", "incident to" and "personal supervision" are all used in the Stark statute. HCFA has now decided to explain its interpretation of these terms, emphasizing, however, that its position in these proposed rules is applicable only to Stark law issues and no other issues of the law.

The most dramatic manifestation of the fundamental problems with Stark is the length of the preface to these regulations: the typescript HCFA sent to the Federal Register to create the regulations was in excess of 400 pages in length. The preface encompasses more than 60 pages in the Federal Register. Given this complexity, this *AGG Note* deals ***selectively*** with those matters which have the broadest impact along with a few which are included for their entertainment value.

Good News

There is some good news to be found in HCFA's words, but even that characterization may vary for some. Where you stand on some of these matters depends on where you sit. Where HCFA is backing away from positions it took in the final Aug. 1995, regulations, those who have restructured to meet the last set of understandings may have less equanimity evaluating the dozen or so new liberalizations we identify here. (This characterization is ours alone. Others may view different provisions as good news.)

1. Prime among these issues is a change in the stance on the definition of a referral. In Aug. 1995, HCFA took the position that a referral by any member of a group which included a single physician with a financial relationship with an entity was just as tainted as the referral by the related physician himself. HCFA now sees that when the statute says a prohibited referral is one by "a physician who has a financial relationship," it literally means that physician and that physician only. The rest of the group is not affected (unless, of course, there is an explicit financial impact to them from their referrals or the referrals are a legal obligation imposed on them).
2. For the compensation issues, including calculation of productivity bonuses and rent, which may not take into account the volume or value of referrals between the parties, HCFA is willing to include *only* referrals for designated health services, and then only Medicare or Medicaid designated health services. Any other referrals may be rewarded and/or considered (barring of course, some other legislation like the anti-kickback statute which would otherwise impinge on the arrangement).
3. Invasive radiology procedures which are intended primarily to place a catheter or a needle are not included among the designated health services. This means cardiac catheterization is not a designated service implicated by Stark. Screening mammography is also excluded.
4. An optical shop in an ophthalmologist's office will not violate the law as long as the in-office ancillary services requirements are met. Please note: this does *not* protect orthopaedists offering crutches or collars in their offices.

5. A group practice may be owned by any kind of entity (e.g., a hospital, for-profit management company, integrated delivery system).
6. A group practice must be a single unified legal entity, but it may be composed of individual professional corporations which each employs its shareholder, provided all the other characteristics of a merged practice are present.
7. To refer for in-office ancillary services which are provided at a centralized location of the group practice, the group may have more than one centralized location, so that laboratory services can be in one building and physical therapy services in another.
8. De minimus items of economic value may be provided by an entity to which a physician refers, without risk of triggering the Stark statute, as long as they do not exceed $50 per item nor $300 in a year. (Whether this would pass muster under the anti-kickback rules is quite another issue, however.)
9. HCFA proposes a new and broad exception for any compensation arrangement which is in writing, covers all the relationships or refers to any other agreements regarding items or services passing between the parties, specifies a term of at least a year, specifies compensation which must be consistent with fair market value, involves an otherwise commercially reasonable transaction, and meets an anti-kickback safe harbor or otherwise complies with the anti-kickback statute.
10. Commercial reasonability is given its common sense meaning: an arrangement appears to be a sensible, prudent business agreement from the perspective of the particular parties involved, even in the absence of potential referrals. Note that this is not the same as fair market value.
11. Agreements which are required to have a term of at least one year may be terminated for cause prior to that point, as long as no new agreement is entered into until the original year has expired. On the other hand, an initial agreement must extend for full one year renewal terms and not convert to a month to month arrangement after the first year.
12. Where an entity arranges for personal services from a physician, the arrangement may be conducted through the physician's group.
13. For investment in a hospital, the physician may be invested in a hospital chain, provided that he still has clinical privileges at the facility to which he refers.
14. For the exceptions pertaining to services provided within a prepaid plan, HCFA would extend protection not only to referrals for services provided by the plan itself, but also services furnished to enrollees by outside physicians, providers, or suppliers under contract with these organizations, and those with whom contracted physicians have themselves contracted.

Definitions

Having identified the good news, we now move to the bulk of the discussion which is far more equivocal.

Designated Health Services

In defining the list of services, generally HCFA has chosen to adopt the definitions of services set forth in §1861 of the Social Security Act. Their views are expansive, except for the imaging issues addressed above. For example, establishment of a plan for maintenance physical therapy (which itself is not even a covered service under Medicare) counts as a designated service. Speech and language pathology are included, too. Moreover, for PT, OT and speech-pathology, the location of the service is irrelevant. If these services are provided in a skilled nursing facility with which the physician has a financial relationship, the law is triggered.

With regard to outpatient prescription drugs, HCFA says that drugs which could be bought by prescription in a drug store, such as oncology drugs, even if they ordinarily are only provided by physicians in their offices, count as designated services. They further extend this definition to include biologicals such as vaccines and blood clotting factors. As for prosthetics, HCFA includes intraocular lenses, although they ask for comments on whether implantable prosthetics should be counted.

Medicaid

Because the drafters of Stark did not address the nuance of health law and simply imposed on states the obligation to conform with this Medicare statute in order to get their federal financial participation for Medicaid, HCFA proposes to simply use the Medicare definitions of what is designated, even though the Medicare terms are not consistent with Medicaid's language.

Referral

Stark is unique in that the statute itself defines a referral—any request for an item or service payable under Part B (despite inclusion of home health and inpatient hospital services which are not paid under Part B). In addition, where the referral is for a consultation, the statute extends the referral chain from the requestor to any test or procedure which the consultant would order, perform or supervise. Radiology services ordered by a radiologist, radiation therapy ordered by a radiation oncologist and laboratory services ordered by a pathologist, when they are pursuant to a consultation request, are not referrals. Finally, the statutory definition also incorporates a physician's establishing a plan of care, which HCFA is interpreting to pertain only to a plan of care for designated health services (e.g, radiation therapy, home health, physical therapy).

HCFA takes the position that the form of the referral is irrelevant (in writing, oral, based on a completed prescription). Moreover, it does not matter whether the physician affirmatively directs the patient to the financially related entity. If the patient receives the service from the related entity, HCFA will presume the referral was made by the physician but will allow that presumption to be rebutted.

In this context, the definition of a consultation also is important. If there is no consultation, then the downstream test or procedure by the 'consultant' is not implicated for the referring physician. HCFA incorporates the general Medicare reimbursement principles on consultations. A Medicare consultation requires a specific request from a physician for a service and a written report back to the requesting physician. The hidden issue in this discussion, however, is that the Carrier's Manual states that if the requesting physician transfers care to the consultant with the initial request ("evaluate and treat"), then the services are visits and no consult is billed (CM §15506). It would seem, then, that tests or procedures in this context do not count as having been provided as a result of a consult.

Perhaps the most disturbing aspect of HCFA's views of a referral, though, lies in their extension of the scope of the practice referral rules to a **solo practitioner's office.** Since the request that ancillary personnel perform a service constitutes a referral, solo physicians would be swept under the ambit of the proposed regs.

GROUP PRACTICE

The group practice definition is a fundamental term. Physicians can refer to members of their own group practice and those supervised by such members. Members would be only employees and owners. A group practice must be legally created as such; and HCFA is liberal on this point. But virtual groups and some 'groups without walls' will not qualify since the proposed regs require that there must be centralized decision-making on expenses—loosely joined groups making their own overhead decisions, even if paid out of a joint checking account, apparently would not suffice. Profits must be distributed and overhead allocated in a manner determined by the group prior to the allocation period, so such judgments do not reflect volume or value of referrals. Location-specific and specialty or department-specific profit distributions would not qualify.

In response to industry complaints, HCFA has removed independent contractors from the definition of members of a group. This is very useful for purposes of meeting the infamous 75% rule (the average of clinical time spent with the group by all physicians in the group), but it also means that those independent contractors cannot supervise ancillary personnel performing designated health services. In addition, in calculating the 75% rule, no longer do only clinical services to the practice count. Physicians who spend time administratively for the group can include that time in the calculation of the 75% rule.

To qualify, the services of the group must be billed under a number assigned to the group. HCFA would now allow a group to have more than one billing number as long as the number is assigned to the group. This incorporates the Medicare reassignment rules too. (See *AGG Note,* March, 1997, "Physician Billing Under Part B: False Claims Revisited.")

Within the group practice definition, the statute refers to permissible compensation methodologies. Unlike the employment exception, members of a group may be paid a productivity bonus for services they provide themselves or which are *"incident to"* their services. On this point, HCFA has traveled through the looking glass and well beyond into another dimension altogether since they have determined that a physician request for a service by ancillary personnel qualifies as a referral. This, on its face, appears inconsistent with long-standing regulatory policies which describe "incident to" services as services which are an incidental although integral part of a physician's personal, professional service to a patient. Under those terms, there cannot be a referral in any ordinary sense since what the ancillary personnel are doing is part of the physician's service itself. Nevertheless, under this position a bizarre result emerges: The statute says that a group practice member may be compensated for incident to services, but not directly for the volume or value of his referrals. HCFA says: "Nor should a physician's compensation relate directly to the number of referrals for designated health services he or she has made to other group physicians, to the group's nonphysician staff, or to any other entity or individual. ... Thus, we believe a physician's compensation can reflect a bonus for designated health services the physician personally performs or 'incident to' services the physician directly supervises, *provided the services result from the referral of a physician other than the one performing or supervising the service."* (Emphasis added.) So, in a multispecialty group, when the family physician refers to the cardiologist who orders an echocardiogram he then interprets, neither the family physician who referred the patient initially, nor the cardiologist who "referred" the technical component of the echo he interpreted, could be given credit for the echo if he supervises it. Nor could oncologists be given credit within the group for any of the prescription drugs their nurses administer, if they supervise. All of these revenues must float up into an overall profit distribution.

In another demonstration of failed appreciation of technical Medicare rules, this approach does not take into account existing Carrier's Manual rules on physician supervision in a "physician directed clinic"—where (a) a physician or a number of physicians is present to perform medical services at all times the clinic is open; (b) each patient is under the care of a clinic physician and (c) the nonphysician services are under medical supervision. In these settings, "direct personal supervision may be the responsibility of several physicians as opposed to an individual attending physician. ...The physician ordering the service need not be the physician who is supervising the service." (CM §2050.3) Given this rule, then, who counts as the supervisor under HCFA's strange pronouncement? HCFA has solicited comments regarding its views of incident to compensation. They surely will get some.

Exceptions

Of the sixteen exceptions, many are relatively straightforward in their terms: investment in rural providers; investment in a hospital itself; bona fide employment relationships; physician incentive plans (but only because other regulations issued under the Medicare risk rules cover this issue). On the other hand, HCFA's consideration of managed care issues is particularly opaque and unaddressed in this newsletter. On the subject of remuneration from a hospital unrelated to the provision of designated health services, we had speculated this exception could only cover matters such as a referring physician being hired by the hospital to manage the on-premises Taco Bell. In fact, HCFA has clarified that a physician leasing his beach house to the hospital for a visiting professor could qualify. (The Taco Bell arrangement would also work under the terms of this exception, for those seeking additional revenue without going the Amway route.) We will not elaborate on all the exceptions. Several will be touched on briefly. In-office ancillary services, however, will be addressed more in depth.

Hospital Payment for Physician Recruitment

HCFA interprets this exception to pertain only where a new staff member must actually physically relocate into the geographic area. With regard to compensation to residents when they become staff members, HCFA opines that these financial relationships might qualify under the new general compensation exception they propose.

Rent of Equipment or Space

HCFA says little about these exceptions specifically except in clarifying commercial reasonability and taking the position that the requirement that the lessee use space exclusively means that when the lessee is in control of space, it may not sublease the space to anyone. "Per click" equipment leases are also disapproved when a hospital leases from a physician.

For Physician Services

In the statute, there is an exception for referral by a physician to another physician "in the same group practice". This exception is different from the requirement for referrals to another "member of the group" which applies to in-office ancillary services. So, for referrals for physician services, independent contractors ought to qualify. However, HCFA has overreached equating "in the group" with being "a member of the same group". As a result a physician may not refer to an affiliated independent contractor physician *unless* the nonmember physician services are provided "under the personal supervision" of another member of the group. "We would interpret 'personal supervision' to mean that the group practice physician is legally responsible for monitoring the results of any test or other designated health service and is available to assist the individual who is furnishing the service, even though the member physician need not be present while the service is being furnished." How such a supervisor would be "available" without being present is completely unexplained. Why the ancillary personnel need two physicians to deal with the service is equally unfathomable.

For In-Office Ancillary Services

This exception is of critical importance to any physician practice. Its component elements are absurdly complex. To meet this exception there are issues of (1) who may supervise and to what degree; (2) which services are eligible for inclusion; and (3) where the services are provided.

Supervision

As discussed, only a group member may supervise ancillary personnel. The statute requires direct, on premises supervision which requires the physician to be in the office suite although not necessarily in the same room as the technician. To compound the general confusion in these proposals, final regulations on diagnostic testing supervision were published with the updated Medicare fee schedule (on October 31, 1997). Here, HCFA refers to its proposed rules. Obviously the already adopted Medicare supervision rules for diagnostic tests are relevant. In general skeletal and abdominal films without the use of contrast media, do not require physician presence. Ultrasound, MRI, CT and all other diagnostic tests not identified as requiring personal supervision (continual presence of the physician in the room during the procedure) require standard direct supervision. The Stark proposed rules state that all in office ancillary services require direct supervision. The only leeway is in the physician's ability to leave the office for lunch or emergencies at the hospital. The interaction of the Stark statute with the already liberalized rules for x-ray ought to be taken into account in final Stark regs.

Within this issue also lies the metaphysical problem of what qualifies as the premises. Here, based on HCFA's approach, we might expect the carriers to hire real estate analysts since HCFA says that issues such as whether the office suite extends across a floor, or down the hall to non-contiguous rooms "is a decision that only the local carrier could make based on the layout of each group of offices."

In-office Services

To qualify for this exception the services must be furnished in the physician's office. "It is our view that a service is furnished wherever a procedure is actually performed upon a patient or in the location in which a patient receives and begins using an item." But, "any item that is given to a patient but is meant to be used at home or outside the physician's office, or any item that is delivered to the patient's home, has not been 'furnished' in the physician's office." DME is excluded from in-office ancillary services by statute. HCFA regards crutches as different from other DME, but since HCFA cannot override the statutory preclusion on this, they say that orthopedists can provide crutches, but only if they make no profit on them. The physician may bill only for the cost of acquiring and supplying the crutches. There is no insight into how these "costs" will be determined. HCFA only discusses crutches and no other similar items such as canes or collars.

Location

As discussed above, HCFA will allow more than one centralized location for in-office ancillary services, and allows any non-designated health services to be provided at a location claimed as the offices. But for purposes of determining whether these offices are in one building, the real estate analysts will have more work. "We are interpreting 'the same building' in which the physician practices to mean one physical structure, with one address, and not multiple structures that are connected by tunnels or walkways. In addition, we believe 'the building' consists of parts of the physical structure that are used as office or other commercial space. For example, a mobile x-ray van that is pulled into the garage of a building would not be part of that building."

The in-office ancillary services exception would, if adopted as drafted, provide a serious vein for analysis and scrutiny of many ordinary arrangements in the market.

Side Bar Issues

In its preamble, HCFA expounds on a range of questions it has received from the industry. Some of these are intriguing but little explicated.

Joint Ventures

"Just because a hospital or similar entity is affiliated with a physician or group of physicians does not automatically mean that the hospital or similar entity is compensating the physicians. Physicians and entities can have joint ventures and similar relationships in which the hospital or similar entity and the physicians share profits, but do not compensate each other." But if the only investment exceptions are those in hospitals, rural providers and publicly traded entities, then for whom is this meaningful? Radiologists, radiation oncologists and pathologists who do not "refer" when they order services pursuant to a consultation.

Integration and In Network Referrals

Where a hospital system employs physicians and makes in network referrals a condition of employment, HCFA believes the volume or value of referrals provision is violated. In a separate discussion of integrating systems, though, HCFA says that PHO arrangements which involve Medicare and Medicaid patients can require intra-network referrals as long as the payments meet the personal services exception. These positions seem inconsistent but since they are discussed in non-contiguous sections of the materials they are exceedingly difficult to reconcile.

Solicited Comments

Recognizing some of its limitations in addition to the issues noted in the text above, HCFA has solicited comments on a number of topics including: approaches to measuring dedication to a group other than on the basis of time spent there; services provided under a prepaid health plan under Medicaid; whether additional conditions should be imposed beyond those already identified.

Conclusion

The full flavor of these materials cannot be conveyed here. Not all of the blame is HCFA's. The statute remains both a drafting travesty and a policy debacle. When the most sophisticated health lawyers in the country think of Prozac and form 12 step support groups to understand the law and the regs, something is seriously wrong. To understand how this law motivates reasoned business relationships and improves health care in a fast changing world with vastly different incentives at work than in 1993 requires a toke on the Caterpillar's waterpipe. There is little to conclude today.

As a practical matter, whether to restructure and assume that HCFA's announced current thinking is enough protection to make it worthwhile to conform with this material will be an on-going challenge. Anyone contemplating any changes should get help. For the time being, we can only hope that final regulations save what is useful and take real world comments to heart. Repeal of the statute would be the best news yet.

Subject Index

A

ABCR
gene mutation in age-related macular degeneration, 264
Ablation
plume dynamics, effect on formation of central islands in excimer laser photorefractive keratectomy, 50
procedures, lash, anatomy and physiology of lash follicles related to, 155
profilometry, corneal, and steep central islands, 52
Abrasion
corneal, topical nonsteroidal anti-inflammatory drops without pressure patching for, 92
Academic
medical centers, carotid endarterectomy trends in patterns and outcomes of care at, 181
Acanthamoeba
keratitis coexistent with herpetic keratitis, 99
Acquired immunodeficiency syndrome (*see* AIDS)
Acrylic
foldable *vs.* silicone lens in primary glaucoma triple procedure, 15
Activity
-based costing management in private practice setting, 315
Acuity
visual
effect of removal of retained lens fragments after phacoemulsification on, 129
in optic nerve hypoplasia, bilateral, 183
Acyclovir
in retinitis, varicella-zoster virus, in AIDS, 116
Adenoid
cystic carcinoma
lacrimal gland, in childhood and adolescence, 261
neuroophthalmologic manifestations of, 223
Adenoma
pituitary, radiation optic neuropathy after stereotactic radiosurgery for, 185
Adenovirus
aerosolization by excimer laser, 96
Adolescents
adenoid cystic carcinoma of lacrimal gland in, 261
retinopathy incidence in insulin-dependent diabetes in, 119
Aerosolization
of infectious virus by excimer laser, 96
Age
corneal donor, 91
effect on refraction and corneal haze after photorefractive keratectomy, 46
-related macular degeneration (*see* Macula, degeneration, age-related)
AIDS
(*See also* HIV)
Pneumocystis carinii infection of conjunctiva in, 260
retinitis in, varicella-zoster virus, management of, 116
Air
as vitreous substitute, 109
Alcohol
-assisted corneal epithelium removal, 34
Allergan multifocal lens
discussion of, 3
Allergic
fungal sinusitis, orbital involvement in, 207
Amblyopia
treatment, ongoing, effect on surgical outcome in esotropia, 166
Aminocaproic acid
topical, for traumatic hyphema, 107
Amniotic
membrane transplantation for persistent epithelial defects with ulceration, 101
Amoils brush
for corneal epithelial removal, 34
Amyloidosis
corneal, familial subepithelial, 267
Anatomic
results after photocoagulation or radiation therapy for choroidal hemangiomas, 247
Anatomy
of eyelash follicles, 155
neurovascular orbital, high-resolution MRI of, 228
Ancillary
services, in-office, in Stark II proposed regulations, 353

Anesthesia
in cataract surgery, anterior chamber irrigation with unpreserved lidocaine 1% for, 11
parabulbar, for primary vitreoretinal surgery, 128
topical, in cataract surgery, 1
lidocaine during, unpreserved, 12
patient suitability for, indicators of, 14
Aneurysm
communicating artery, leaking anterior, pathogenesis of acute monocular blindness from, 183
Angiogenesis
inhibition by tissue inhibitor of metalloproteinase-3, 124
Anomalies
orbital venous, 199
Anterior chamber
irrigation with unpreserved lidocaine 1% for anesthesia during cataract surgery, 11
Antibiotic(s)
sensitivity testing, routine, in corneal ulcers, 94
topical postoperative, after strabismus surgery, 167
Antibody
antineutrophil cytoplasmic antibody testing in Wegener granulomatosis of orbit, 266
Anti-inflammatory
drops, topical nonsteroidal, without pressure patching for corneal abrasions, 92
drugs, nonsteroidal, in orbital myositis, 141
Antineutrophil
cytoplasmic antibody testing in Wegener granulomatosis of orbit, 266
Anti-transforming
growth factor-beta for corneal haze after excimer laser photorefractive keratectomy (in rabbit), 36
Antrostomies
maxillary, for orbital involvement in allergic fungal sinusitis, 209
Apnea
sleep, obstructive, and floppy eyelid syndrome, 147
Apoptosis
glaucoma and neuroprotection, 86
Applanation
tonometer, Goldmann, effect of excimer laser photorefractive keratectomy on intraocular pressure measurements using, 49
Aqueous
humor, polymerase chain reaction assays, in differential diagnosis of retinitis in HIV, 114
Argon
green laser photocoagulation for persistent central serous retinopathy, long-term follow-up results, 127
Arteritis
giant cell
diagnostic criteria, validity and reliability of, 179
pathogenesis, new concepts in, 258
Artery
carotid, optic nerve contact and compression by, in asymptomatic patients, 196
communicating, anterior, leaking aneurysms, pathogenesis of acute monocular blindness from, 183
Aspergillus flavus
sinusitis due to, allergic, orbital involvement in, 209
Aspiration
biopsy, fine-needle
in diagnosis of orbital metastases, 238
role in small melanocytic choroidal lesions, 235
Astigmatism
myopic, laser intrastromal keratomileusis for, 43
resolution after surgical resection of capillary hemangiomas, in infants, 175
Ataxia
after gabapentin in acquired nystagmus, 188
Autograft
patches, corneal, for covering exposed transscleral sutures, 28
Avulsion
optic nerve, 143
Axial
length in pseudophakic children, longitudinal changes in, 10
myopia, high, pseudophakic retinal detachment in, 27
Axonal
transection in lesions of multiple sclerosis, 188

B

Baclofen
in nystagmus, acquired, 187

Balloon
dacryocystoplasty for nasolacrimal duct system obstruction in epiphora, long-term results, 151
dacryoplasty for partial nasolacrimal duct obstruction, 137
water balloon slingshots causing ocular and orbital trauma, 170
Basal cell
carcinoma, superficial T1–T2, laser microsurgery for, 158
Basaloid
adenoid cystic carcinoma of lacrimal gland in childhood and adolescence, 261
Beta-blockade
topical, with intrinsic sympathomimetic activity, no advantage for respiratory and cardiovascular function of elderly, 74
Betaxolol
effect on respiratory and cardiovascular function of elderly, 74
Billing
balance, and private contracting by Medicare physicians, 336
Binkhorst formula
for intraocular lens power prediction after previous radial keratotomy, 6
Biopsy
aspiration, fine-needle
in diagnosis of orbital metastases, 238
role in small melanocytic choroidal lesions, 235
orbit, in Wegener's granulomatosis of orbit, 265
retino-choroidal, transvitreal, of suspected choroid malignant lesions, 246
Bipolaris spicifera
sinusitis due to, allergic, orbital involvement in, 209
Blebs
filtration, dissecting, clinicopathologic features and surgical management of, 79
Blindness
acute monocular, from leaking anterior communicating artery aneurysms, pathogenesis of, 183
Blow-out fracture
orbital, with restricted ocular movement, kinetic MRI of, 219
Brachytherapy
plaque, for choroidal hemangiomas, 244
visual and anatomic results of, 247
Brush
for corneal epithelium removal, 34
Business
side of group practice, evaluation of, 320

C

Caldwell-Luc maxillotomy
for orbital involvement in allergic fungal sinusitis, 209
Cancer
incidence after retinoblastoma, 248
Capillary
hemangioma
retinal, MRI in, in children, 214
surgical resection of, resolution of astigmatism after, in infants, 175
Capitated
payment for medical care, physicians' views on, 293
Capsule
posterior, opacification after cataract surgery in patients with uveitis, 25
tension ring, intraocular lens implantation using, and management of zonular dialysis in phacoemulsification, 17
Car
driving, impact of cataract surgery on, 5
Carbon dioxide
laser microsurgery for superficial T1–T2 basal cell carcinoma of eyelid margins, 158
Carcinoma
adenoid cystic
lacrimal gland, in childhood and adolescence, 261
neuroophthalmologic manifestations of, 223
basal cell, superficial T1–T2, laser microsurgery for, 158
squamous cell, cutaneous, perineural spread via orbit, 220
Cardiovascular
function of elderly, no advantage of topical beta-blockade with intrinsic sympathomimetic activity for, 74
Care
chiropractic, of pediatric glaucoma patient, 85
episode of, 331
health (*see* Health, care)
managed (*see* Managed care)
medical
commerce and professionalism in, 300

physicians' views on capitated payment for, 293
perioperative, of strabismus patient, 167
traditional, is gatekeeping better than? 292
Carotid
artery, optic nerve contact and compression by, in asymptomatic patients, 196
endarterectomy trends in patterns and outcomes of care at academic medical centers, 181
stenosis, critical, postprandial transient visual loss as symptom of, 180
Carteolol
effect on respiratory and cardiovascular function of elderly, 74
Carve-outs
specialty, and managed care, 330
Case
rate, and marketplace, 330
Caselaw
managed care liability, 326
Cataract, 1
effect on corneal topography results, 29
extraction *(see* surgery *below)*
/glaucoma procedures using temporal cataract surgery, 76
surgery, 1
(*See also* Phacoemulsification)
anesthesia in, anterior chamber irrigation with unpreserved lidocaine 1% for, 11
anesthesia in, topical, lidocaine during, unpreserved, 12
anesthesia in, topical, patient suitability for, indicators of, 14
capsule opacification after, posterior, in patients with uveitis, 25
in children, for pseudophakia, choice of lens and dioptric power after, 7
in children, for pseudophakia, longitudinal changes in axial length after, 10
in children, myopic shift after, 173
impact on car driving, 5
impact on low vision patients, 3
intraocular lens implantation after, multifocal, outcomes of, 2
after keratotomy, previous radial, and intraocular lens power prediction, 6
for maculopathy, postfiltration hypotony, 22
in patients undergoing primary glaucoma triple procedure, silicone *vs.* acrylic foldable lens implantation in, 15
rates, variation in Medicare prepaid and fee-for-service settings, 283
temporal, combined cataract and glaucoma procedures using, 76
after vitrectomy, gentamicin retinal toxicity after, 21
Cavernous
hemangioma, orbital, serial dynamic MRI of, 202
Cell(s)
basal cell carcinoma, superficial T1–T2, laser microsurgery for, 158
ganglion, TUNEL-positive, in primary open-angle glaucoma, 262
giant cell arteritis
diagnostic criteria, validity and reliability of, 179
pathogenesis, new concepts in, 258
squamous cell carcinoma, cutaneous, perineural spread via orbit, 220
type, prognostic value in uveal melanoma, 272
Cellulitis
periorbital and orbital, in *Haemophilus influenzae* vaccine era, 140
Central islands
formation in excimer laser photorefractive keratectomy, effect of ablation plume dynamics on, 50
steep, and corneal ablation profilometry (in animals), 52
Cerebral
swelling, diffuse, bilateral superior ophthalmic vein enlargement associated with, 185
C3F8
as vitreous substitute, 110
C4F8
as vitreous substitute, 110
C4F10
as vitreous substitute, 110
Chamber
anterior, irrigation with unpreserved lidocaine 1% for anesthesia during cataract surgery, 11
posterior, intraocular lens, low-power, implantation after clear lensectomy for high myopia, 4-year follow-up, 40
Charge
limits and private contracting by Medicare physicians, 336
Chemotherapy
for orbital metastases, 238
Children, 165
adenoid cystic carcinoma of lacrimal gland in, 261

amblyopia treatment in, ongoing, effect on surgical outcome in esotropia, 166
cataract surgery in (*see* Cataract, surgery, in children)
cellulitis in, periorbital and orbital, in *Haemophilus influenzae* vaccine era, 140
conjunctivitis in, ligneous, due to homozygous mutations in plasminogen gene, 275
glaucoma in, chiropractic care for, 85
glioma in, optic pathway, after previously negative neuroimaging, 212
infant (*see* Infant)
intraocular tumors and simulating lesions in, MRI in, 214
keratitis in, primary varicella-zoster, diagnosis by polymerase chain reaction, 100
lens in, intraocular, 1
current issues in, 165
ocular trauma in
sports-related, 3-year follow-up, 172
water balloon slingshots causing, 170
one-eyed, head turn during monocular viewing in, 174
optic nerve hypoplasia in, bilateral, clinical, neuroradiographic, and endocrinologic profile in, 183
orbital trauma from water balloon slingshots in, 170
pseudophakic
axial length in, longitudinal changes in, 10
choice of lens and dioptric power in, 7
retinal tumor in, melanogenic neuroectodermal, 279
retinoblastoma in (*see* Retinoblastoma)
retinopathy incidence in insulin-dependent diabetes in, 119
strabismus in (*see* Strabismus)
Chiron excimer laser
keratectomy, photorefractive, effect of ablation plume dynamics on central island formation after, 51
Chiropractic
care of pediatric glaucoma patient, 85
Cholesterol
sulfate in X-linked ichthyosis, 274
Choroid
hemangioma
irradiation for, low-dose ocular, long-term results, 243
photocoagulation or radiation therapy for, visual and anatomic results of, 247
lesions
melanocytic, small, role of fine-needle aspiration biopsy in, 235
suspected malignant, transvitreal retino-choroidal biopsy of, 246
melanoma, small, mortality in patients with, 238
neovascularization in age-related macular degeneration (*see* Macula, degeneration, age-related, choroidal neovascularization in)
Chromosome
1q21-q31, juvenile glaucoma locus on, exclusion of one pedigree affected by adult onset primary open-angle glaucoma from linkage to, 82
5q31-linked corneal dystrophies, kerato-epithelin mutations in, 274
6p25 region, familial glaucoma iridogoniodysplasia linked to, 83
Ciliary
body
leiomyoma, MRI of, in children, 214
medulloepithelioma, MRI of, in children, 214
Claudication
jaw, in giant cell arteritis, 179
Clinicopathologic
features of dissecting glaucoma filtering blebs, 79
study of cornea in X-linked ichthyosis, 273
Coats' disease
MRI in, in children, 214
Commerce
and professionalism in medical care, 300
Communicating artery
aneurysms, leaking anterior, pathogenesis of acute monocular blindness from, 183
Company
buyouts, physician practice-management, 321
Computed tomography
cerebral swelling on, diffuse, bilateral superior ophthalmic vein enlargement associated with, 185
of glioma, optic pathway, after previously negative neuroimaging, 212
helical *vs.* conventional axial, for steel intraocular foreign bodies, 204
in optic nerve avulsion, 143

of orbital involvement in allergic fungal sinusitis, 209
of orbital involvement in Wegener granulomatosis, 265
of orbital metastases, 237
of perineural spread of cutaneous squamous cell carcinoma via orbit, 221, 222
Computerized
analysis of slit lamp photographs in quantification of corneal haze after excimer laser photorefractive keratectomy, 33
Confidentiality
patient, under managed care, guarding, 316
Conjunctiva
infection, *Pneumocystis carinii,* in AIDS, 260
tumors, surgical management of, 239
Conjunctivitis
ligneous, due to homozygous mutations in plasminogen gene, 275
papillary, giant, after motility peg placement for hydroxyapatite orbital implant, 147
Connective tissue
disorders, heritable, ectopia lentis in, 255
Consultation
radiology, mandatory, effect on inpatient imaging use, 192
Contact lens
abrasions, treatment of, 94
Contamination
postoperative, after vancomycin and gentamicin use during phacoemulsification, 19
Contract
terms in managed care, 332
Contracting
private, by Medicare physicians (*see* Physicians, Medicare, private contracting by)
risk
global, and managed care, 328
making it work in specialty networks, 318
Corcoran v. Blue Cross of Louisiana, 327
Cornea, 91
ablation profilometry and steep central islands (in animals), 52
abrasions, topical nonsteroidal anti-inflammatory drops without pressure patching for, 92
amyloidosis, familial subepithelial, 267
donor age, 91
dystrophy
5q31-linked, kerato-epithelin mutations in, 274
Meesmann's, due to cornea-specific *K3* or *K12* gene mutations, 270
epithelium (*see* Epithelium, corneal)
erosion, recurrent, combined PRK and PTK in, 55
haze
definition of, 33
after excimer laser photorefractive keratectomy, effect of age on, 46
after excimer laser photorefractive keratectomy, management of, 33
in ichthyosis, X-linked, clinicopathologic study, 273
patches, autograft, for covering exposed transscleral sutures, 28
review of, 91
rim cultures
routine, value in penetrating keratoplasty, 103
value in corneal transplantation, 92
ring segments, intrastromal, for myopia, phase II results, 41
scar, definition of, 33
topography
effects of strabismus surgery on, 168
results, effect of cataract on, 29
transplantation (*see* Transplantation, cornea)
ulcers
antibiotic sensitivity testing in, routine, 94
epithelial defects with, persistent, amniotic membrane transplantation for, 101
Corpus callosum
optic nerve hypoplasia and, bilateral, 183
Corticosteroid(s)
-cyclophosphamide treatment of Wegener granulomatosis of orbit, 266
retrobulbar *vs.* sub-Tenon's, for cystoid macular edema refractory to topical medications, 24
topical, for corneal haze after excimer laser photorefractive keratectomy, 35
Cost
comparison of molecular *vs.* conventional screening of relatives at risk for retinoblastoma, 244
of corneal rim cultures, routine donor, in penetrating keratoplasty, 103
Costing
management, activity-based, in private practice setting, 315

C-reactive protein
in arteritis, giant cell, 179
Cryotherapy
in conjunctival tumors, 240
CT (*see* Computed tomography)
Cultures
corneal rim
routine, value in penetrating keratoplasty, 103
value in corneal transplantation, 92
Cupping
glaucomatous, methods to objectify reversibility of, 87
Cutaneous
eyelid lesions, accuracy of clinical diagnosis of, 156
squamous cell carcinoma, perineural spread via orbit, 220
Cyclophosphamide
-corticosteroid treatment of Wegener granulomatosis of orbit, 266
Cystic
carcinoma, adenoid
lacrimal gland, in childhood and adolescence, 261
neuroophthalmologic manifestations of, 223
Cystoid
macular edema refractory to topical medications, retrobulbar *vs.* sub-Tenon's corticosteroid therapy for, 24
Cytomegalovirus
human, eyes inoculated with, ganciclovir-loaded polymer microspheres in (in rabbit), 117
retinitis in HIV-infected patients, polymerase chain reaction assays of aqueous humor for, 114
Cytometry
flow, diagnosis of intraocular lymphoma by, 251
Cytoplasmic
antibody testing, antineutrophil, in Wegener granulomatosis of orbit, 266

D

Dacryocystoplasty
balloon, for obstructed nasolacrimal duct system in epiphora, long-term results, 151
Dacryocystorhinostomy
mitomycin C in, intraoperative, 150
revision, transcanalicular Nd:YAG laser for, 153
Dacryoplasty
balloon, for partial nasolacrimal duct obstruction, 137
Dapsone
in *Pneumocystis carinii* infection of conjunctiva in AIDS, 260
Debulking
tumor, for orbital metastases, 238
Decision-making
in treatment of subfoveal neovascularization in age-related macular degeneration, 135
Dexon
mesh wrapping and complications of hydroxyapatite orbital implants, 144
Diabetes mellitus
insulin-dependent, incidence of retinopathy and associated risk factors from time of diagnosis, 119
Dialysis
zonular, management in phacoemulsification and IOL implantation using capsular tension ring, 17
Diethylenetriamine pentaacetic acid
gadolinium-, MRI with
of perineural tumor infiltration of trigeminal nerve, occult, 226
serial dynamic, of orbital cavernous hemangioma, 202
Disc
optic
cupping, glaucomatous, methods to objectify reversibility of, 87
pallor, of untreated ocular hypertensives, rates of change of, 89
Diurnal
variation in vision, refraction, or keratometry after photorefractive keratectomy, lack of, 49
Doctor (*see* Physician)
Doppler
ultrasound, color, in optic nerve avulsion, 143
Driving
car, impact of cataract surgery on, 5
Drugs
anti-inflammatory, nonsteroidal, in orbital myositis, 141
Drusen
large, laser treatment for, short-term effects, 132
Dry eye
relation between signs and symptoms, in elderly, 138

DTPA
gadolinium-, MRI with
of perineural tumor infiltration of trigeminal nerve, occult, 226
serial dynamic, of orbital cavernous hemangioma, 202
Duke University
Private Sector Conference, 295
Dukes and after, 328
Dystrophy
corneal
5q31-linked, kerato-epithelin mutations in, 274
Meesmann's, due to cornea-specific *K3* or *K12* gene mutations, 270

E

Economics
social, 281
Ectopia
lentis in heritable disorders of connective tissue, 255
Edema
macular, cystoid, refractory to topical medications, retrobulbar *vs.* sub-Tenon's corticosteroid therapy for, 24
Ehlers-Danlos syndrome
ocular manifestations of, 257
Elderly
cardiovascular function of, no advantage of topical beta-blockade with intrinsic sympathomimetic activity for, 74
cataract extraction rates in Medicare prepaid and fee-for-service settings, variations in, 283
cataract surgery in, impact on car driving, 5
dry eye in, relation between signs and symptoms, 138
respiratory function of, no advantage of topical beta-blockade with intrinsic sympathomimetic activity for, 74
stroke outcomes in, in Medicare fee-for-service and managed care, 284
Electron
microscopy
in keratitis, primary varicella-zoster, 100
transmission, in X-linked ichthyosis, 274
Employee
Retirement Income Security Act and managed care liability, 327
unscrupulous office, how to spot, 307
Endarterectomy
carotid, trends in patterns and outcomes of care at academic medical centers, 181
Endocapsular
ring, 2
Endocrinologic
profile of patients with bilateral optic nerve hypoplasia, 182
Endophthalmitis
after corneal transplantation, 92
Endoscopic
polypectomies, for orbital involvement in allergic fungal sinusitis, 209
Endothelium
growth factor, vascular, effect of tissue inhibitor of metalloproteinase-3 on, 125
Entity liability
managed care, 326
Epiphora
nasolacrimal duct system obstruction in, balloon dacryocystoplasty in, long-term results, 151
Episode of care, 331
Epithelin
kerato-epithelin mutations in 5q31-linked corneal dystrophies, 274
Epithelium
corneal
defects, persistent, with ulceration, amniotic membrane transplantation for, 101
removal of, alcohol-assisted, 34
removal of, brush for, 34
growth within lamellar interface after laser in situ keratomileusis, 56
Equipment
rent of, in Stark II proposed regulations, 353
ERISA
managed care liability and, 327
Erythrocyte
sedimentation rate in giant cell arteritis, 179
Esotropia
surgical outcome in, effect of ongoing treatment of amblyopia on, 166
Ethmoidectomy
total, for orbital involvement in allergic fungal sinusitis, 209
Excimed UV 200 laser
plume, lack of virus transmission by, 58
Excimer
laser (*see* Laser, excimer)

Excision
pterygium, primary, intraoperative mitomycin in, 95
Exfoliation
glaucoma, clinical presentation and initial treatment patterns in, 73
Eye
(*See also* Ocular)
cytomegalovirus-inoculated, human, ganciclovir-loaded polymer microspheres in (in rabbit), 117
dry, relation between signs and symptoms, in elderly, 138
gene therapy for, 136
Eyelash
follicles, anatomy and physiology of, 155
Eyelid
floppy eyelid syndrome and obstructive sleep apnea, 147
lesions, cutaneous, accuracy of clinical diagnosis of, 156
margins, basal cell carcinoma of, superficial T1–T2, laser microsurgery for, 158
surgery, functional, 149

F

Fee-for-service
Medicare
cataract extraction rates in, 283
stroke outcomes in, 284
Fibrillin-1
in ectopia lentis, heritable, 255
Fibroblast
growth factor, basic, effect of tissue inhibitor of metalloproteinase-3 on, 125
Fibrovascular
loops, prognostic value in uveal melanoma, 272
Filtration
blebs, dissecting, clinicopathologic features and surgical management of, 79
surgery
criteria for success of, 87
maculopathy after, hypotony, cataract extraction for, 22
surgery (*see* Glaucoma, surgery)
Floppy eyelid syndrome
obstructive sleep apnea and, 147
Flow cytometry
diagnosis of intraocular lymphoma by, 251
Fluorometholone
topical, for corneal haze after excimer laser photorefractive keratectomy, 35
Follicles
eyelash, anatomy and physiology of, 155
Foreign bodies
steel intraocular, CT for, helical *vs.* conventional axial, 204
Foscarnet
/ganciclovir in varicella-zoster virus retinitis in AIDS, 116
Fox v. HealthNet, 327
Fracture
orbital, blow-out, with restricted ocular movement, kinetic MRI of, 219
Frontoethmoidectomy
for orbital involvement in allergic fungal sinusitis, 209
Functional
status after multifocal intraocular lens implantation, 2
Fungal
sinusitis, allergic, orbital involvement in, 207

G

Gabapentin
in nystagmus, acquired, 187
Gadolinium
-DTPA MRI
of perineural tumor infiltration of trigeminal nerve, occult, 226
serial dynamic, of orbital cavernous hemangioma, 202
Gallatin Medical
physician compensation in, 305
Ganciclovir
alone or combined with foscarnet in varicella-zoster virus retinitis in AIDS, 116
-loaded polymer microspheres in eyes inoculated with human cytomegalovirus (in rabbit), 117
Ganglion
cells, TUNEL-positive, in primary open-angle glaucoma, 262
Gases
intraocular, as vitreous substitutes, 109
perfluorocarbon, as vitreous substitutes, 110
Gatekeeping
is it better than traditional care? 292
Gene
glaucoma due to, primary open-angle, identification of, 81

βig-h3, mutation in 5q31-linked corneal dystrophies, 274
keratin *K3* or *K12,* cornea-specific, mutations causing Meesmann's corneal dystrophy, 270
Norrie disease, missense mutations in, in advanced retinopathy of prematurity, 271
plasminogen, homozygous mutations in ligneous conjunctivitis, 275
Stargardt disease, mutation in age-related macular degeneration, 264
therapy for the eye, 136
Genetic
characterization of retinoblastoma, routine, polymerase chain reaction in, 253
Gentamicin
during phacoemulsification, postoperative contamination after, 19
retinal toxicity after cataract surgery in eye that underwent vitrectomy, 21
Giant cell
arteritis
diagnostic criteria, validity and reliability of, 179
pathogenesis, new concepts in, 258
Glaucoma, 61
angle closure, acute, misdiagnosis of, 67
apoptosis and neuroprotection, 86
/cataract procedures using temporal cataract surgery, 76
definitions of, new, 87
exfoliation, clinical presentation and initial treatment patterns in, *vs.* primary open-angle glaucoma, 73
filtering blebs, dissecting, clinicopathologic features and surgical management of, 79
iridogoniodysplasia, familial, maps to 6p25 region implicated in primary congenital glaucoma and iridogoniodysgenesis anomaly, 83
juvenile, inverse, 256
normal tension, in patient with floppy eyelid syndrome and obstructive sleep apnea, 148
open-angle
chronic, topical beta-blockade with intrinsic sympathomimetic activity in, no advantage for respiratory and cardiovascular function in elderly with, 74
primary, adult onset, exclusion of one pedigree from linkage to juvenile glaucoma locus on chromosome 1q21-q31, 82
primary, gene causing, identification of, 81
primary, TUNEL-positive ganglion cells in, 262
primary, *vs.* exfoliation glaucoma, clinical presentation and initial treatment patterns in, 73
trabeculectomy outcome in, 76
visual field loss in, repeatable diffuse, 71
pediatric, chiropractic care for, 85
procedure, primary triple, silicone *vs.* acrylic foldable lens implantation in, 15
secondary, effect of removal of retained lens fragments after phacoemulsification on, 129
stage 1, 65
stage 2, 65
stage 3, 67
stages of, table relating to, 66–67
surgery
criteria for success of, 87
maculopathy after, hypotony, cataract extraction for, 22
in thyroid-associated orbitopathy, prevalence and implications of, 142
visual field damage in, variability in, reduction using size V stimuli, 72
Glaucomatous
cupping, methods to objectify reversibility of, 87
Glioma
optic pathway, after previously negative neuroimaging, 212
Gliosis
retinal, in children
massive, MRI in, 214
posttraumatic, MRI of, 214
Global risk contracting
managed care and, 328
Goldmann applanation tonometer
intraocular pressure measurements with, effect of excimer laser photorefractive keratectomy on, 49
Graft
autograft patches, corneal, for covering exposed transscleral sutures, 28
Granulomatosis
Wegener, of orbit, clinical and pathologic constellation of, 265
Graves' ophthalmopathy, 177
Group
practice

definition in Stark II regulations, 351
evaluation of business side of, 320
Growth
factor
anti-transforming growth factor-beta for corneal haze after excimer laser photorefractive keratectomy (in rabbit), 36
basic fibroblast, effect of tissue inhibitor of metalloproteinase-3 on, 125
vascular endothelial, effect of tissue inhibitor of metalloproteinase-3 on, 125
hormone deficiency and bilateral optic nerve hypoplasia, 183

H

Haemophilus influenzae
vaccine era, periorbital and orbital cellulitis in, 140
Half-moon syndrome
with magnetic resonance correlation, 233
Haze
corneal (*see* Cornea, haze)
HCFA clarifications
in private contracting by Medicare physicians (*see* Physicians, Medicare, private contracting by, HCFA clarifications)
Head
-turn in 1-eyed children during monocular viewing, 174
Healing
second-intention, role in periocular reconstruction, 161
Health
care
managed (*see* Managed care)
reform, medicolegal issues in era of, 323
revolution, and two cultures, 300
maintenance organization (*see* HMO)
Plan, Oregon, lessons for the nation, 288, 290
services, designated, definition in Stark II proposed regulations, 350
Hemangioma
capillary
retinal, MRI in, in children, 214
surgical resection of, resolution of astigmatism after, in infants, 175
choroid
irradiation for, low-dose ocular, long-term results, 243
photocoagulation or radiation therapy for, visual and anatomic results of, 247
orbital cavernous, serial MRI of, 202
Herpes
simplex virus
aerosolization by excimer laser, 96
in graft failure, primary, 106
keratitis coexistent with *Acanthamoeba* keratitis, 99
keratitis in HIV-positive *vs.* HIV-negative patients, 98
retinitis in HIV-infected patients, polymerase chain reaction assays of aqueous humor for, 114
HIV
(*See also* AIDS)
aerosolization by excimer laser, 97
-infected patients, differential diagnosis, polymerase chain reaction assays of aqueous humor in, 114
-positive *vs.* -negative patients, herpes simplex virus keratitis in, 98
HMO(s)
discussion of, 281
-Medicare revolving door, 286
profile, use to your advantage, 313
Holladay formula
for intraocular lens power prediction after previous radial keratotomy, 6
Homocystinuria
ectopia lentis due to, heritable, 256
Hormone
growth, deficiency, and bilateral optic nerve hypoplasia, 183
Hospital
payment for physician recruitment, in Stark II proposed regulations, 353
Human immunodeficiency virus (*see* HIV)
Humphrey Field Analyzer
for repeatable diffuse visual field loss in open-angle glaucoma, 71
Hydroxyapatite
implant, 138
orbital, complications of, 144
orbital, motility peg placement for, complications of, 146
Hydroxychloroquine
retinopathy, incidence of, 113
visual screening and, in rheumatology outpatient clinic, 112
Hyperlysinemia
ectopia lentis due to, heritable, 257
Hyperopia
keratectomy for, excimer laser photorefractive, 44

Hyperplastic
persistent vitreous, primary, MRI in, in children, 214
Hypertension
ocular, in thyroid-associated orbitopathy, prevalence and implications of, 142
systemic, as risk factor for choroidal neovascularization in second eye of patients with juxtafoveal or subfoveal choroidal neovascularization secondary to age-related macular degeneration, 123
Hypertensives
ocular, untreated, rates of change of optic disc pallor of, 89
Hyphema
traumatic, topical aminocaproic acid for, 107
Hypoplasia
optic nerve, bilateral, clinical, neuroradiographic, and endocrinologic profile of patients with, 182
Hypotony
maculopathy, postfiltration, cataract surgery for, 22

I

Ibuprofen
in myositis, orbital, 141
Ichthyosis
X-linked, clinicopathologic study of cornea in, 273
βig-h3
gene mutation in 5q31-linked corneal dystrophies, 274
Imaging, 191
inpatient, effect of mandatory radiology consultation on use of, 192
magnetic resonance (*see* Magnetic resonance imaging)
neuroimaging
in optic nerve avulsion, 143
previously negative, optic pathway glioma after, 212
Imbalance
after gabapentin in acquired nystagmus, 188
Immunodeficiency
syndrome, acquired (*see* AIDS)
virus, human (*see* HIV)
Implant
hydroxyapatite (*see* Hydroxyapatite, implant)
polypropylene, porous, 138
Infant
glaucoma in, chiropractic care for, 85
hemangioma in, capillary, resolution of astigmatism after surgical resection of, 175
premature, retinopathy in
advanced, missense mutations in Norrie gene in, 271
with total retinal detachment, MRI of, 214
Infectious
virus aerosolization by excimer laser, 96
Inflammatory
syndrome, orbital, differentiated from orbital lymphoma by MRI, 160
In-office
ancillary services in Stark II proposed regulations, 353
Inpatient
imaging use, effect of mandatory radiology consultation on, 192
Insulin
-dependent diabetes, incidence of retinopathy and associated risk factors from time of diagnosis, 119
Integration
in Stark II proposed regulations, 355
Interferon
alfa-2a, no effect on choroidal neovascularization in age-related macular degeneration, 126
alfa-2b, topical, for corneal haze after excimer laser photorefractive keratectomy, 36
Intraocular
foreign bodies, steel, CT for, helical *vs.* conventional axial, 204
gases as vitreous substitutes, 109
lens (*see* Lens, intraocular)
lymphoma, flow cytometric diagnosis, 251
pressure
measurements using Goldmann applanation tonometer, effect of excimer laser photorefractive keratectomy on, 49
reduction after excimer laser photorefractive keratectomy, 69
tumors, MRI in, in children, 214
Intrastromal
corneal ring segments for myopia, phase II results, 41
keratomileusis, laser, for high myopia and myopic astigmatism, 43

Iridogoniodysplasia
familial glaucoma, maps to 6p25 region implicated in primary congenital glaucoma and iridogoniodysgenesis anomaly, 83
Irradiation (*see* Radiation)
Islands
central
formation in excimer laser photorefractive keratectomy, effect of ablation plume dynamics on, 50
steep, and corneal ablation profilometry, 52
Itraconazole
for orbital involvement in allergic fungal sinusitis, 209

J

Jaw
claudication in giant cell arteritis, 179
Joint
ventures in Stark II proposed regulations, 355
Juvenile
(*See also* Children)
glaucoma
inverse, 256
locus on chromosome 1q21-q31, exclusion of one pedigree affected by adult onset primary open-glaucoma glaucoma from linkage to, 82
Juxtafoveal
choroidal neovascularization secondary to age-related macular degeneration, and risk factors for choroidal neovascularization in second eye, 122

K

K3
gene mutation, cornea-specific, causing Meesmann's corneal dystrophy, 270
K12
gene mutation, cornea-specific, causing Meesmann's corneal dystrophy, 270
Keratectomy
photorefractive
excimer laser *(see below)*
pain relief after, dilute topical proparacaine for, 57
photorefractive, excimer laser
age effect on refraction and corneal haze after, 46
central island formation after, effect of ablation plume dynamics on, 50
combined with phototherapeutic keratectomy for recurrent corneal erosion, 55
corneal ablation profilometry and steep central islands after, 52
corneal haze after, management of, 33
effect on intraocular pressure measurements using Goldmann applanation tonometer, 49
for hyperopia, 44
intraocular pressure reduction after, 68
lack of diurnal variation in vision, refraction, or keratometry after, 49
outcomes, effect of variations in surgical technique and patient management on, 47
repeat, 54
phototherapeutic, 36
excimer laser, combined with photorefractive keratectomy for recurrent corneal erosion, 55
Keratin
K3 or *K12* gene mutations, cornea-specific, causing Meesmann's corneal dystrophy, 270
Keratitis
Acanthamoeba, coexistent with herpetic keratitis, 99
herpes simplex virus, in HIV-positive *vs.* HIV-negative patients, 98
herpetic, coexistent with *Acanthamoeba* keratitis, 99
varicella-zoster, primary, diagnosis by polymerase chain reaction, 100
Keratoconus
keratoplasty in, deep lamellar, 105
Kerato-epithelin
mutations in 5q31-linked corneal dystrophies, 274
Keratometry
lack of diurnal variation in, after photorefractive keratectomy, 49
Keratomileusis
laser
in situ, epithelial growth within lamellar interface after, 56
intrastromal, for high myopia and myopic astigmatism, 43
Keratoplasty
(*See also* Transplantation, corneal)
lamellar, deep, with complete removal of pathological stroma for vision improvement, 104
penetrating, value of routine corneal rim cultures in, 103
Keratotomy
radial

previous, cataract surgery after, and intraocular lens power prediction, 6
refractive outcome after, 37
Ketorolac
drops, topical, without pressure patching for corneal abrasions, 92
Kuhl v. Lincoln National, 327

L

Lacrimal
gland carcinoma, adenoid cystic, in childhood and adolescence, 261
Lactoferrin
in corneal amyloidosis, familial subepithelial, 267
Lamella
interface, epithelial growth within, after laser in situ keratomileusis, 56
keratoplasty, deep, with complete removal of pathological stroma for vision improvement, 104
Lamp
slit, in quantification of corneal haze after excimer laser photorefractive keratectomy, 33
Laser
excimer
ablation, do intact viral particles survive? 59
aerosolization of infectious virus by, 96
keratectomy with, phototherapeutic, combined with photorefractive keratectomy for recurrent corneal erosion, 55
keratectomy with (*see* Keratectomy, photorefractive, excimer laser)
plume, lack of virus transmission by, 58
reablation, 54
keratomileusis
in situ, epithelial growth within lamellar interface after, 56
intrastromal, for high myopia and myopic astigmatism, 43
microsurgery for superficial T1–T2 basal cell carcinoma of eyelid margins, 158
Nd:YAG, transcanalicular, for revision dacryocystorhinostomy, 153
photocoagulation
for choroidal hemangiomas, visual and anatomic results of, 247
for retinopathy, persistent central serous, long-term follow-up results, 127
treatment for large drusen, short-term effects, 132
Lash
follicles, anatomy and physiology of, 155
LASIK
epithelial growth within lamellar interface after, 56
Law
private contracting by Medicare physicians and, 339
Legal
issues
in era of health care reform, 323
for ophthalmologists, 323
Leiomyoma
ciliary body, MRI of, in children, 214
Lens
contact, abrasions, treatment of, 94
dislocation, spontaneous, in heritable disorders of connective tissue, 255
fragments, retained, removal after phacoemulsification, effect on secondary glaucoma and visual acuity, 129
Lens, intraocular
acrylic foldable *vs.* silicone, in primary glaucoma triple procedure, 15
in children, 1
axial length changes after, longitudinal, 10
current issues in, 165
for pseudophakia, choice of lens and dioptric power, 7
implantation using capsular tension ring in patient with zonular dialysis, 17
multifocal, 1
outcomes, 2
posterior chamber, low-power, implantation after clear lensectomy for high myopia, 4-year follow-up, 40
power prediction, after cataract surgery following previous radial keratotomy, 6
silicone *vs.* acrylic foldable, in primary glaucoma triple procedure, 15
Lensectomy
clear, and implantation of low-power posterior chamber intraocular lens for correction of high myopia, 4-year follow-up, 40
Liability
managed care (*see* Managed care, liability)

Lid (*see* Eyelid)
Lidocaine
  unpreserved 1%, during cataract surgery
    anterior chamber irrigation with, 11
    with topical anesthesia, 12
Light
  microscopy of melanogenic neuroectodermal retinal tumor, 279
Ligneous
  conjunctivitis due to homozygous mutations in plasminogen gene, 275
Location
  in Stark II proposed regulations, 354
Lubrication
  for corneal haze after excimer laser photorefractive keratectomy, 35
Lymphoma
  intraocular, flow cytometric diagnosis, 251
  non-Hodgkin's, ocular, clinical study, 242
  orbital, MRI differentiation from orbital inflammatory syndrome, 160

M

Macula
  degeneration, age-related
    ABCR gene mutation in, 264
    choroidal neovascularization in, interferon alfa-2a ineffective in, 126
    choroidal neovascularization in, juxtafoveal or subfoveal, and risk factors for choroidal neovascularization in second eye, 122
    choroidal neovascularization in, occult, 121
    choroidal neovascularization in, subfoveal, decision-making in treatment of, 135
  edema, cystoid, refractory to topical medications, retrobulbar *vs.* sub-Tenon's corticosteroid therapy for, 24
Maculopathy
  postfiltration hypotony, cataract surgery for, 22
Magnetic resonance imaging
  in children with intraocular tumors and simulating lesions, 214
  in differentiation of orbital lymphoma from orbital inflammatory syndrome, 160
  dynamic, serial, of orbital cavernous hemangioma, 202
  of glioma, optic pathway, after previously negative neuroimaging, 212
  high-resolution, of neurovascular orbital anatomy, 228
  kinetic, of orbital blow-out fracture with restricted ocular movement, 219
  of neuroophthalmologic manifestations of adenoid cystic carcinoma, 223
  in optic nerve avulsion, 143
  of optic nerve contact and compression by carotid artery in asymptomatic patients, 196
  of orbital involvement in allergic fungal sinusitis, 208, 209
  of orbital metastases, 237
  of orbital venous anomalies, 200
  of perineural spread of cutaneous squamous cell carcinoma via orbit, 220, 221
  of perineural tumor infiltration of trigeminal nerve, occult, 226
  in strabismus, posttraumatic, 217
  in temporal crescent syndrome, 233
Malignant
  lesions, suspected choroidal, transvitreal retino-choroidal biopsy of, 246
Managed care
  contract terms in, 332
  disclosing incentives and limits of, 296
  episode of care, 331
  global risk contracting and, 328
  guarding patient confidentiality under, 316
  how fast can things change? 308
  liability, 325
    caselaw, 326
    Dukes and after, 328
    entity, 326
    ERISA and, 327
    negligent selection and, 326
    tradition and, 325
    utilization management and, 327
  marketplace and case rate, 330
  marketplace trends and, 328
  Medicare, stroke outcomes in, 284
  specialty carve-outs and, 330
Management
  office (*see* Office, management)
  physician practice-management company buyouts, 321
  practice (*see* Office, management)
Marfan's syndrome
  ocular manifestations of, 256

Marketplace
case rate and, 330
trends in, and managed care, 328
Maxillary
antrostomies for orbital involvement in allergic fungal sinusitis, 209
Maxillotomy
Caldwell-Luc, for orbital involvement in allergic fungal sinusitis, 209
Medicaid
definition in Stark II proposed regulations, 350
Medical
care
commerce and professionalism in, 300
physicians' views on capitated payment for, 293
centers, academic, carotid endarterectomy trends in patterns and outcomes of care at, 181
Medicare
fee-for-service, stroke outcomes in, 284
-HMO revolving door, 286
physician (*see* Physician, Medicare)
prepaid and fee-for-service settings, variation in cataract extraction rates in, 283
Medications
topical, cystoid macular edema refractory to, retrobulbar *vs.* sub-Tenon's corticosteroid therapy for, 24
Medicolegal
issues in era of health care reform, 323
Medulloepithelioma
ciliary body, MRI of, in children, 214
Meesmann's corneal dystrophy
cornea-specific *K3* or *K12* gene mutations causing, 270
Melanocytic
choroidal lesions, small, role of fine-needle aspiration biopsy in, 235
Melanogenic
neuroectodermal tumor of retina, 279
Melanoma
choroidal, small, mortality in patients with, 238
retinal, primary malignant, 279
uveal
fibrovascular loops in, prognostic value of, 272
MRI of, in children, 214
PAS patterns in, reassessment of, 277
radiation therapy for, metastatic risk for distinct patterns of local recurrence after, 249
Membrane
amniotic, transplantation for persistent epithelial defects with ulceration, 101
Meningioma
radiation optic neuropathy after stereotactic radiosurgery for, 185
Mesh
wrapping, Dexon, and complications of hydroxyapatite orbital implants, 144
Metalloproteinase-3
tissue inhibitor of, inhibition of angiogenesis by, 124
Metastases
orbital, diagnosis and course, 237
Metastatic
risk for distinct patterns of postirradiation local recurrence of posterior uveal melanoma, 249
Methylprednisolone
IV, for orbital involvement in allergic fungal sinusitis, 209
Microscopy
confocal, in quantification of corneal haze after excimer laser photorefractive keratectomy, 33
electron
in keratitis, primary varicella-zoster, 100
transmission, in X-linked ichthyosis, 274
light, of melanogenic neuroectodermal retinal tumor, 279
Microsurgery
laser, for superficial T1–T2 basal cell carcinoma of eyelid margins, 158
Mitomycin C
-associated blebs, 79
intraoperative
in dacryocystorhinostomy, 150
in pterygium excision, primary, 95
Molecular
vs. conventional screening of relatives at risk for retinoblastoma, cost comparison of, 244
Monocular
blindness, acute, from leaking anterior communicating artery aneurysms, pathogenesis of, 183
viewing, head turn in 1-eyed children during, 174
Mortality
in patients with small choroidal melanoma, 238
Motility
peg
advances with, 145

placement for hydroxyapatite orbital implant, complications of, 146
MRI (*see* Magnetic resonance imaging)
Multiple sclerosis
lesions, axonal transection in, 188
optic neuritis in, visual function 5 years after, 195
Myopia
astigmatism due to, laser intrastromal keratomileusis for, 43
corneal ring segments for, intrastromal, phase II results, 41
high
axial, pseudophakic retinal detachment in, 27
keratomileusis for, laser intrastromal keratomileusis, 43
lensectomy for, clear, and implantation of low-power posterior chamber intraocular lens, 40
keratectomy for, photorefractive, excimer laser (*see* Keratectomy, photorefractive, excimer laser)
Myopic
shift after cataract removal in childhood, 173
Myositis
orbital, outcome, 141

N

Nasolacrimal
duct obstruction
in epiphora, long-term results of balloon dacryocystoplasty in, 151
partial, balloon dacryoplasty for, 137
Nd:YAG
laser, transcanalicular, for revision dacryocystorhinostomy, 153
Neck
pain in giant cell arteritis, 179
Necrosis
retinal, progressive outer, management in AIDS, 116
Neodymium:YAG laser
transcanalicular, for revision dacryocystorhinostomy, 153
Neovascularization
choroidal, in age-related macular degeneration (*see* Macula, degeneration, age-related, choroidal neovascularization in)
Nerve
optic
avulsion, 143
contact and compression by carotid artery in asymptomatic patients, 196
hypoplasia, bilateral, clinical, neuroradiographic, and endocrinologic profile of patients with, 182
trigeminal, occult perineural tumor infiltration of, diagnostic considerations, 226
Networks
in network referrals in Stark II proposed regulations, 355
specialty
making risk contracting work in, 318
risk based, success factors of, 317
Neuritis
optic, visual function 5 years after, 194
Neuroectodermal
tumor of retina, melanogenic, 279
Neurofibromatosis
type 1, with optic gliomas after previously negative neuroimaging, 212
Neuroimaging
in optic nerve avulsion, 143
previously negative, optic pathway glioma after, 212
Neuro-ophthalmologic
manifestations of adenoid cystic carcinoma, 223
Neuro-ophthalmology, 177
Neuropathy
optic, radiation, after stereotactic radiosurgery, 184
Neuroprotection
glaucoma and apoptosis, 86
Neuroradiographic
profile of patients with bilateral optic nerve hypoplasia, 182
Neurovascular
orbital anatomy, high-resolution MRI of, 228
Nidek NT-1000 automated noncontact tonometer
for intraocular pressure measurement after excimer laser photorefractive keratectomy, 69
Norrie disease
gene mutations, missense, in advanced retinopathy of prematurity, 271
Nucleoli
mean of ten largest, prognostic value in uveal melanoma, 272
Nystagmus
acquired, gabapentin *vs.* baclofen in, 187
in optic nerve hypoplasia, bilateral, 183

O

Occlusion
retinal vein, central, natural history and clinical management of, 120
Octa fluorocyclobutane
as vitreous substitute, 110
Ocular
(*See also* Eye)
hypertension in thyroid-associated orbitopathy, prevalence and implications of, 142
hypertensives, untreated, rates of change of optic disc pallor of, 89
intraocular (*see* Intraocular)
irradiation, low-dose, for choroidal hemangiomas, long-term results, 243
lymphoma, non-Hodgkin's, clinical study, 242
movement, restricted, orbital blow-out fracture with, kinetic MRI of, 219
trauma
sports-related, 3-year follow-up, 172
water balloon slingshots causing, 170
Oculoplastic
surgery, 137
adopting new technology, 137
Office
employee, unscrupulous, how to spot, 307
in-office ancillary services in Stark II proposed regulations, 353
management, 303
getting patients to pay, 311
use HMO profile to your advantage, 313
staff productivity, how to increase, 306
Oil
silicone, as vitreous substitute, 110
Oncology, 235
Opacification
posterior capsule, after cataract surgery in patients with uveitis, 25
Ophthalmic
vein enlargement, bilateral superior, associated with diffuse cerebral swelling, 185
Ophthalmologists
legal issues for, 323
Ophthalmopathy
Graves', 177
Optic
disc
cupping, glaucomatous, methods to objectify reversibility of, 87
pallor, of untreated ocular hypertensives, rates of change of, 89
nerve (*see* Nerve, optic)
neuritis, visual function 5 years after, 194
neuropathy, radiation, after stereotactic radiosurgery, 184
pathway gliomas after previously negative neuroimaging, 212
Orbit
anatomy, neurovascular, high-resolution MRI of, 228
cellulitis in *Haemophilus influenzae* vaccine era, 140
fracture, blow-out, with restricted ocular movement, kinetic MRI of, 219
hemangioma, cavernous, serial MRI of, 202
implant, hydroxyapatite
complications of, 144
motility peg placement for, complications of, 146
inflammatory syndrome differentiated from orbital lymphoma by MRI, 160
involvement in allergic fungal sinusitis, 207
lymphoma, MRI differentiation from orbital inflammatory syndrome, 160
metastases, diagnosis and course, 237
myositis, outcome, 141
perineural spread of cutaneous squamous cell carcinoma via, 220
periorbital cellulitis in *Haemophilus influenzae* vaccine era, 140
trauma from water balloon slingshots, 170
venous anomalies, 199
Wegener granulomatosis of, clinical and pathologic constellation of, 265
Orbitopathy
thyroid-associated, prevalence and implications of ocular hypertension and glaucoma in, 142
Orbitotomy
anterior, for orbital involvement in allergic fungal sinusitis, 209
Oregon Health Plan
lessons for the nation, 288, 290
Osteotomy
site size after dacryocystorhinostomy, effects of intraoperative mitomycin C on, 150

P

Pain
  neck, in giant cell arteritis, 179
  relief after photorefractive keratectomy, dilute topical proparacaine for, 57
Pallikaris brush
  for corneal epithelial removal, 34
Panhypopituitarism
  optic nerve hypoplasia and, bilateral, 183
Panretinal
  photocoagulation in central retinal vein occlusion, 120
Papillary
  conjunctivitis, giant, after motility peg placement for hydroxyapatite orbital implant, 147
Parabulbar
  anesthesia for primary vitreoretinal surgery, 128
Pars plana
  vitrectomy
    anesthesia for, parabulbar, 128
    for removal of retained lens fragments after phacoemulsification, effect on secondary glaucoma and visual acuity outcomes, 129
PAS
  patterns in uveal melanoma, reassessment of, 277
Patches
  corneal autograft, for covering exposed transscleral sutures, 28
Pathologic
  study of Wegener granulomatosis of orbit, 265
Pathology, 255
Patient
  confidentiality under managed care, guarding, 316
  getting patients to pay, 311
  putting patients first, 298
  suitability for topical anesthesia in cataract surgery, indicators of, 14
Payment
  capitated, for medical care, physicians' views on, 293
  getting patients to pay, 311
  hospital, for physician recruitment in Stark II proposed regulations, 353
Pediatric (*see* Children)
Peg
  motility
    advances with, 145
    placement for hydroxyapatite orbital implant, complications of, 146
Pentamidine
  aerosolized, prophylactic, in AIDS, and *Pneumocystis carinii* infection of conjunctiva, 260
Perfluoro-butane
  as vitreous substitute, 110
Perfluorocarbon
  gases as vitreous substitutes, 110
  liquids as vitreous substitutes, 111
Perfluoroperhydrophenanthrene
  in retinal tears, giant, 131
Perfluoropropane
  as vitreous substitute, 110
Perineural
  spread of cutaneous squamous cell carcinoma via orbit, 220
  tumor infiltration, occult, of trigeminal nerve, diagnostic considerations, 226
Periocular
  reconstruction, role of second-intention healing in, 161
Periodic acid Schiff
  patterns in uveal melanoma, reassessment of, 277
Perioperative
  care of strabismus patient, 167
Periorbital
  cellulitis in *Haemophilus influenzae* vaccine era, 140
Phacoemulsification
  (*See also* Cataract, surgery)
  capsular tension ring for zonular dialysis in, 17
  lens fragments after, retained, removal of, effect on secondary glaucoma and visual acuity, 129
  vancomycin and gentamicin during, postoperative contamination after, 19
Philadelphia
  experience with managed care, 308
Photocoagulation
  for choroidal hemangiomas, visual and anatomic results of, 247
  laser, for retinopathy, persistent central serous, long-term follow-up results, 127
  panretinal, in central retinal vein occlusion, 120
Photography
  Scheimpflug anterior segment, in quantification of corneal haze after excimer laser photorefractive keratectomy, 33
  slit lamp, in quantification of corneal haze after excimer laser photorefractive keratectomy, 33

Photorefractive
keratectomy (*see* Keratectomy, photorefractive)
Phototherapeutic
keratectomy, 36
excimer laser, combined with photorefractive keratectomy for recurrent corneal erosion, 55
Physician(s)
attitudes toward gatekeeping, 292
getting patients to pay, 311
Medicare, private contracting by, 335
assignment and participation, 336
charge limits and balance billing, 336
future, 343
HCFA clarifications, 340
HCFA clarifications, non-covered services, 342
HCFA clarifications, physician issues, 342
HCFA clarifications, scope of private contract, 341
HCFA clarifications, to whom the law pertains, 340
historical background, 335
law and, 339
original proposal, 338
practice-management company buyouts, 321
quality, as pay yardstick, 305
recruitment, hospital payment for, in Stark II proposed regulations, 353
services, in Stark II proposed regulations, 353
specialty networks, making risk contracting work in, 318
surplus, impending, 301
tool to help physicians review each other, 310
views on capitated payment for medical care, 293
Physiology
of eyelash follicles, 155
Pituitary
adenoma, radiation optic neuropathy after stereotactic radiosurgery for, 185
Plasminogen
gene in ligneous conjunctivitis, homozygous mutations in, 275
Plume
ablation, dynamics, effect on formation of central islands in excimer laser photorefractive keratectomy, 50
laser excimer, lack of virus transmission by, 58
Pneumocystis carinii
infection of conjunctiva in AIDS, 260
Polymer
microspheres, ganciclovir, in eyes inoculated with human cytomegalovirus (in rabbit), 117
Polymerase chain reaction
analysis for viral particles after excimer laser ablation, 59
assays of aqueous humor in differential diagnosis of retinitis in HIV, 114
keratitis diagnosis by, primary varicella-zoster, 100
in routine genetic characterization of retinoblastoma, 253
Polymethylmethacrylate
capsular tension rings in phacoemulsification and intraocular lens implantation with zonular dialysis, 17
Polypectomies
endoscopic, for orbital involvement in allergic fungal sinusitis, 209
Polypropylene
implant, porous, 138
Posterior chamber
intraocular lens, low-power, implantation after clear lensectomy for high myopia, 4-year follow-up, 40
Postoperative
contamination after vancomycin and gentamicin during phacoemulsification, 19
Postprandial
vision loss, transient, as symptom of critical carotid stenosis, 180
Practice
group
business side of, evaluation of, 320
definition in Stark II regulations, 351
management (*see* Office, management)
physician practice-management company buyouts, 321
private, activity-based costing management in, 315
Prairie Medical Group
physician compensation in, 305
Prednisone
in myositis, orbital, 141
in optic neuritis, visual function 5 years after, 195
Prematurity
retinopathy of
advanced, missense mutations in Norrie disease gene in, 271
with total retinal detachment, MRI of, 214
Pressure
intraocular

measurements using Goldmann applanation tonometer, effect of excimer laser photorefractive keratectomy on, 49
reduction after excimer laser photorefractive keratectomy, 69
Private contracting
by Medicare physicians (*see* Physicians, Medicare, private contracting by)
Private practice
setting, activity-based costing management in, 315
Private Sector
Conference, Duke University, 295
Productivity
staff, how to increase, 306
Professionalism
and commerce in medical care, 300
Profilometry
corneal ablation, and steep central islands (in animals), 52
Proparacaine
dilute topical, for pain relief after photorefractive keratectomy, 57
Protein
C-reactive, in giant cell arteritis, 179
Pseudophakia
in children
axial length in, longitudinal changes in, 10
choice of lens and dioptric power in, 7
Pseudophakic
retinal detachment in high axial myopia, 27
Psychosocial
implications of strabismus surgery, in adults, 169
Pterygium
excision, primary, intraoperative mitomycin in, 95
Pupil
screening examination, routine dilated, value of, 282

Q

Quality
of life after intraocular lens implantation, multifocal, 2
your new pay yardstick, 305

R

Radial
keratotomy
previous, cataract surgery after, and intraocular lens power prediction, 6
refractive outcome after, 37
Radiation
dose and cancer incidence after retinoblastoma, 248
optic neuropathy after stereotactic radiosurgery, 184
therapy
for choroidal hemangiomas, visual and anatomic results of, 247
ocular, low-dose, for choroidal hemangiomas, long-term results, 243
photon or heavy charged particle, for orbital metastases, 238
for uveal melanoma, metastatic risk for distinct patterns of local recurrence after, 249
Radioactive
plaque brachytherapy for choroidal hemangiomas, 244
Radiology
consultation, mandatory, effect on inpatient imaging use, 192
Radiosurgery
stereotactic, radiation optic neuropathy after, 184
Radiotherapy (*see* Radiation, therapy)
Rationing
by any other name, 302
Reablation
excimer laser, 54
Reconstruction
periocular, role of second-intention healing in, 161
Referral
definition in Stark II proposed regulations, 350
Reform
health care, medicolegal issues in era of, 323
Refraction
after keratectomy, photorefractive, effect of age on, 46
lack of diurnal variation in, after photorefractive keratectomy, 49
Refractive
outcome after radial keratotomy, 37
surgery, 33
Reis-Bückler's dystrophy
corneal, kerato-epithelin mutations in, 274
Relatives
at risk for retinoblastoma, cost comparison of molecular *vs.* conventional screening for, 244
Rent
of equipment or space in Stark II proposed regulations, 353

Respiratory
function of elderly, no advantage of topical beta-blockade with intrinsic sympathomimetic activity for, 74
Retina, 109
detachment
pseudophakic, in high axial myopia, 27
total, retinopathy of prematurity with, MRI of, 214
gliosis in children
massive, MRI in, 214
posttraumatic, MRI of, 214
hemangioma, capillary, MRI in, in children, 214
necrosis, progressive outer, management in AIDS, 116
tears, giant, perfluoroperhydrophenanthrene for, 131
toxicity, gentamicin, after cataract surgery in eye that underwent vitrectomy, 21
tumor, melanogenic neuroectodermal, 279
vein, central, occlusion, natural history and clinical management of, 120
Retinitis
in HIV, differential diagnosis, polymerase chain reaction assays of aqueous humor in, 114
varicella-zoster virus, in AIDS, management of, 116
Retinoblastoma
cancer risk after, 248
genetic characterization of, routine, polymerase chain reaction in, 253
MRI of, in children, 214
relatives at risk for, cost comparison of molecular *vs.* conventional screening of, 244
Retino-choroidal
biopsy, transvitreal, of suspected choroid malignant lesions, 246
Retinopathy
hydroxychloroquine, incidence of, 113
incidence in insulin-dependent diabetes, 119
of prematurity
advanced, missense mutations in Norrie disease gene in, 271
with total retinal detachment, MRI of, 214
serous, persistent central, laser photocoagulation for, long-term follow-up results, 127
Retrobulbar
vs. sub-Tenon's corticosteroid therapy for cystoid macular edema refractory to topical medications, 24
Review
tool to help doctors review each other, 310
Rheumatoid
outpatient clinic, hydroxychloroquine and visual screening in, 112
Ring
capsular tension, in phacoemulsification and intraocular lens implantation with zonular dialysis, 17
endocapsular, 2
Risk
based specialty networks, success factors of, 317
contracting
global, and managed care, 328
making it work in specialty networks, 318
Roferon-A
no effect on choroidal neovascularization in age-related macular degeneration, 126
Rose bengal testing
for dry eye, in elderly, 138

S

Sarcoma
risk after retinoblastoma, 248
Scar
corneal, definition of, 33
Scatterometer
in quantification of corneal haze after excimer laser photorefractive keratectomy, 33
Scheimpflug anterior segment photography
in quantification of corneal haze after excimer laser photorefractive keratectomy, 33
Schirmer test
for dry eye, in elderly, 138
Scleral
dissection in surgical management of conjunctival tumors, 240
wrapping and complications of hydroxyapatite orbital implants, 144
Sclerosis
multiple
lesions of, axonal transection in, 188
optic neuritis in, visual function 5 years after, 195

Sentara Medical Group
physician compensation in, 305
Septum pellucidum
optic nerve hypoplasia and, bilateral, 183
Serous
retinopathy, persistent central, laser photocoagulation for, long-term follow-up results, 127
SF-6
as vitreous substitute, 110
Silicone
intraocular lens *vs.* acrylic foldable lens in primary glaucoma triple procedure, 15
oil as vitreous substitute, 110
Sinusitis
allergic fungal, orbital involvement in, 207
Sjögren's syndrome
dry eye in, relation between signs and symptoms of, in elderly, 138
Sleep
apnea, obstructive, and floppy eyelid syndrome, 147
Slingshots
water balloon, causing ocular and orbital trauma, 170
Slit lamp
in quantification of corneal haze after excimer laser photorefractive keratectomy, 33
Soccer
-related ocular injuries, 3-year follow-up, 172
Social
economics, 281
Sodium
hyaluronate, effect on trabeculectomy outcome in open-angle glaucoma, 76
Space
rent of, in Stark II proposed regulations, 353
Specialty
carve-outs and managed care, 330
networks
making risk contracting work in, 318
risk based, success factors of, 317
Sphenoidotomy
for orbital involvement in allergic fungal sinusitis, 209
Sports
-related ocular injuries, 3-year follow-up, 172
Squamous cell
carcinoma, cutaneous, perineural spread via orbit, 220
SRK II formula
for intraocular lens power prediction after previous radial keratotomy, 6
Staff
productivity, how to increase, 306
Stargardt disease
gene mutation in age-related macular degeneration, 264
Stark II proposed regulations, 346
background and context, 346
definitions, 350
designated health services, 350
group practice, 351
Medicaid, 350
referral, 350
details, details, 347
essence of, 346
exceptions, 352
hospital payment for physician recruitment, 353
for in-office ancillary services, 353
for in-office services, 354
location, 354
for physician services, 353
rent of equipment or space, 353
supervision, 354
good news, 348
side bar issues
integration and in network referrals, 355
joint ventures, 355
solicited comments, 355
Steel
intraocular foreign bodies, CT for, helical *vs.* conventional axial, 204
Stenosis
carotid, critical, postprandial transient visual loss as symptom of, 180
Stereotactic
radiosurgery, radiation optic neuropathy after, 184
Strabismus
in optic nerve hypoplasia, bilateral, 183
patient, perioperative care of, 167
posttraumatic, MRI in, 217
surgery
effects on corneal topography, 168
psychosocial implications of, in adults, 169
Stroke
outcomes in Medicare fee-for-service and managed care, 284
Stroma
intrastromal
corneal ring segments for myopia, phase II results, 41
keratomileusis, laser, for high myopia and myopic astigmatism, 43

pathological, deep lamellar keratoplasty with complete removal of, for vision improvement, 104
Sturge-Weber syndrome
choroidal hemangioma and, low-dose ocular irradiation for, 243
Subepithelial
corneal amyloidosis, familial, 267
Subfoveal
choroidal neovascularization in age-related macular degeneration
decision-making in treatment of, 135
risk factors for choroidal neovascularization in second eye and, 122
Sub-Tenon
anesthesia for vitreoretinal surgery, primary, 128
vs. retrobulbar corticosteroid therapy for cystoid macular edema refractory to topical medications, 24
Sulfite oxidase
deficiency causing heritable ectopia lentis, 257
Sulfur
hexafluoride as vitreous substitute, 110
Supervision
in Stark II proposed regulations, 353
Surgery
eyelid, functional, 149
filtration
criteria for success of, 87
maculopathy after, hypotony, cataract extraction for, 22
oculoplastic, 137
adopting new technology, 137
radiosurgery, stereotactic, radiation optic neuropathy after, 184
strabismus
effects on corneal topography, 168
psychosocial implications of, in adults, 169
vitreoretinal, primary, parabulbar anesthesia for, 128
Sutures
transscleral, exposed, corneal autograft patches for covering, 28
Swelling
cerebral, diffuse, bilateral superior ophthalmic vein enlargement associated with, 185
Sympathomimetic
activity, intrinsic, topical beta-blockade with, no advantage for respiratory and cardiovascular function of elderly, 74

T

Technology
new, adoption in oculoplastic surgery, 137
Telemedicine
discussion of, 191
Temporal
crescent syndrome with magnetic resonance correlation, 233
Thyroid
-associated orbitopathy, prevalence and implications of ocular hypertension and glaucoma in, 142
Tissue
connective tissue disorders, heritable, ectopia lentis in, 255
inhibitor of metalloproteinase-3, inhibition of angiogenesis by, 124
Tomography
computed (*see* Computed tomography)
Tonometer
Goldmann applanation, effect of excimer laser photorefractive keratectomy on intraocular pressure measurements using, 49
Nidek NT-1000 automated noncontact, for intraocular pressure measurement after excimer laser photorefractive keratectomy, 69
Topography
corneal
effects of strabismus surgery on, 168
results, effect of cataract on, 29
Toxicity
gentamicin retinal, after cataract surgery in eye that underwent vitrectomy, 21
Toxoplasma
gondii retinitis in HIV-infected patients, polymerase chain reaction assays of aqueous humor for, 114
Trabeculectomy
in glaucoma, open-angle, outcome, 76
Tradition
managed care liability and, 325
Transcanalicular
Nd:YAG laser for revision dacryocystorhinostomy, 153
Transplantation
amniotic membrane, for persistent epithelial defects with ulceration, 101
cornea
(*See also* Keratoplasty)
corneal rim cultures in, value of, 92
donor age and, 91

graft failure after, primary, herpes simplex virus in, 106
Transscleral
sutures, exposed, corneal autograft patches for covering, 28
Transvitreal
retino-choroidal biopsy of suspected choroid malignant lesions, 246
Trauma
hyphema due to, topical aminocaproic acid for, 107
ocular
sports-related, 3-year follow-up, 172
water balloon slingshots causing, 170
orbital, from water balloon slingshots, 170
retinal gliosis due to, MRI of, in children, 214
strabismus due to, MRI in, 217
Triamcinolone
retrobulbar *vs.* sub-Tenon's, for cystoid macular edema refractory to topical medications, 24
Trigeminal
nerve, occult perineural tumor infiltration of, diagnostic considerations, 226
Trimethoprim
in *Pneumocystis carinii* infection of conjunctiva in AIDS, 260
Tumor
conjunctiva, surgical management of, 239
debulking for orbital metastases, 238
intraocular, MRI in, in children, 214
perineural, occult, infiltration of trigeminal nerve, diagnostic considerations, 226
retinal, melanogenic neuroectodermal, 279
size, prognostic value in uveal melanoma, 272
TUNEL
-positive ganglion cells in primary open-angle glaucoma, 262

U

Ulcers
corneal
antibiotic sensitivity testing in, routine, 94
persistent epithelial defects with, amniotic membrane transplantation for, 101
Ultrasound
B-scan, in optic nerve avulsion, 143
Doppler, color, in optic nerve avulsion, 143
Utilization
management and managed care liability, 327
Uvea
melanoma (*see* Melanoma, uveal)
Uveitis
patients, posterior capsule opacification after cataract surgery in, 25

V

Vaccine
Haemophilus influenzae, periorbital and orbital cellulitis in era of, 140
Vancomycin
during phacoemulsification, postoperative contamination after, 19
Varicella
-zoster virus
keratitis, primary, diagnosis by polymerase chain reaction, 100
particles, intact, do they survive excimer laser ablation? 59
retinitis in AIDS, management of, 116
retinitis in HIV-infected patients, polymerase chain reaction assays of aqueous humor for, 114
Vascular
cardiovascular function of elderly, no advantage of topical beta-blockade with intrinsic sympathomimetic activity for, 74
endothelial growth factor, effect of tissue inhibitor of metalloproteinase-3 on, 125
fibrovascular loops, prognostic value in uveal melanoma, 272
neurovascular orbital anatomy, high-resolution MRI of, 228
Vein
ophthalmic, enlarged bilateral superior, association with diffuse cerebral swelling, 185
orbital, anomalies, 199
retinal, central, occlusion, natural history and clinical management of, 120
Virus
cytomegalovirus
human, eyes inoculated with, ganciclovir-loaded polymer microspheres in (in rabbit), 117
retinitis in HIV-infected patients, polymerase chain reaction assays of aqueous humor for, 114

herpes simplex (*see* Herpes, simplex virus)
immunodeficiency, human (*see* HIV)
infectious, aerosolization by excimer laser, 96
particles, intact, do they survive excimer laser ablation? 59
transmission by excimer laser plume, lack of, 58
varicella-zoster (*see* Varicella, -zoster virus)

Vision
improvement, deep lamellar keratoplasty with complete removal of pathological stroma for, 104
after keratectomy, photorefractive, lack of diurnal variation in, 49
low, impact of cataract surgery on patients with, 3

Visual
acuity
effect of removal of retained lens fragments after phacoemulsification on, 129
in optic nerve hypoplasia, bilateral, 183
field
damage, glaucomatous, variability reduced using size V stimuli, 72
loss, repeatable diffuse, in open-angle glaucoma, 71
function 5 years after optic neuritis, 194
loss, postprandial transient, as symptom of critical carotid stenosis, 180
results after photocoagulation or radiation therapy for choroidal hemangiomas, 247
screening and hydroxychloroquine in rheumatoid outpatient clinic, 112

VISX Twenty Twenty B excimer laser system
for keratectomy, photorefractive, corneal ablation profilometry and steep central islands after, 52

VISX Twenty Twenty excimer laser
photorefractive keratectomy, outcomes, effect of variations in surgical technique and patient management on, 47

Vitrectomy
cataract surgery after, gentamicin retinal toxicity after, 21
pars plana
anesthesia for, parabulbar, 128
for retained lens fragments after phacoemulsification, effect on secondary glaucoma and visual acuity outcomes, 129

Vitreon
in retinal tears, giant, 131

Vitreoretinal
surgery, primary, parabulbar anesthesia for, 128

Vitreous
hyperplastic persistent, primary, MRI in, in children, 214
substitute(s), 109
air as, 109
intraocular gases as, 109
perfluorocarbon gases as, 110
perfluorocarbon liquids as, 111
silicone oil as, 110
sulfur hexafluoride as, 110

W

Water
balloon slingshots causing ocular and orbital trauma, 170

Wegener granulomatosis
orbit, clinical and pathologic constellation of, 265

Weill-Marchesani syndrome
ocular manifestations of, 256

X

X-linked
ichthyosis, clinicopathologic study of, 273

Y

YAG
neodymium:YAG laser, transcanalicular, for revision dacryocystorhinostomy, 153

Z

Zonular
dialysis management in phacoemulsification and IOL implantation using capsular tension ring, 17

Zoster
varicella-zoster virus (*see* Varicella, -zoster virus)

Author Index

A

Abramson DH, 248
Aiuto LT, 140
Akiba H, 202
Alexander RA, 277
Al-Hazmi A, 233
Allen C, 119
Allikmets R, 264
Alward WLM, 81
Anand-Apte B, 124
Andrade R, 182
Aprecio RM, 58
Arora AK, 67
Asbell PA, 41
Averbuch-Heller L, 187
Avramopoulos D, 82
Awner S, 167

B

Ballal DR, 170
Bandieramonte G, 158
Barone SR, 140
Barros H, 172
Bartley GB, 161, 258
Batchelder TJ, 282
Batra VN, 37
Beck RW, 194
Benger R, 220
Berkowitz M, 144
Bernstein PS, 135
Bessant DA, 69
Blackburn P, 59
Blumenthal D, 292
Blumenthal M, 55
Bodenheimer T, 288, 290
Boice JD Jr, 248
Bos JJ, 151
Bree RL, 192
Bressler NM, 121
Broste SK, 196
Brown RS, 284
Bruni S, 253
Bullock JD, 170
Burke JP, 169
Burnier MN, 272
Burris TE, 41
Burumcek E, 127

C

Carlomagno M, 315
Carter GM, 283
Cassels-Brown A, 74
Castro-Correia J, 172
Causino N, 292
Chacko JG, 204
Chan JW, 183
Char DH, 237, 249
Chatterjee A, 69
Chatzistefanou K, 25
Chauhan BC, 71, 72
Chavis PS, 233
Cherchio M, 12
Chesanow N, 308
Chung SM, 212
Cinque P, 114
Clarkson JC, 120
Clunie D, 233
Cockerham GC, 106
Cockerham KP, 142
Colin J, 40
Comey CH, 184
Condon PI, 43
Conway CM, 85
Corden LD, 270
Crouch ER Jr, 107
Cytryn AS, 160

D

Dahan E, 7
Dana MR, 25
Danise A, 114
Dausch D, 45
Davis H, 169
Davis JL, 251
Daxer A, 228
de la Cruz Z, 273
de-Pablos M, 19
De Potter P, 146, 239
DeVito CA, 286
Diaz MD, 95
Diggory P, 74
Djemaï A, 274
Dolan KP , 311
Domnitz Y, 46
Dorr DA, 49
Draper V, 315
Drusedau MUH, 7
Dugel PU, 24

E

Eagle RC Jr, 279
Ebenezer N, 83
Economou-Petersen E, 82
Edelstein C, 146
Elder MJ, 155
Ellis WG, 183
Ettl A, 228
Ewing-Chow D, 156

F

Fernandez C, 74
Ferro JF, 19
Figueroa RE, 204
Filipe JAC, 172
Finger AL, 321
Fingert JH, 81
Fireman B, 282
Flindall RJ, 24
Flynn HW, 129
Foss AJE, 277
Foster BS, 143
Francis IC, 220
Fraser SG, 14, 67
Freitag SK, 279
Friedman GD, 282
Fuhry L, 187
Fulcher T, 43
Fulmer JG Jr, 320

G

Gallie BL, 174, 244
Garner A, 199
Garrity JA, 161
Gayton JL, 76
Gills JP, 12
Gimbel HV, 17
Girkin CA, 184
Glaser JS, 226
Goldberg MA, 49, 99
Goldzweig CL, 283
Goltz HC, 174
Gopal L, 128
Grandinetti D, 305, 313
Gray MK, 107
Grierson DJ, 112
Guyer DR, 126

H

Hagen KB, 58
Halm EA, 292
Hanssens M, 242
Harbour JW, 249
Hartzer MK, 271
Hashimoto M, 202
Haviv D, 46

Hayreh SS, 179
Hefetz L, 46
Helena MC, 56
Herrero-Vanrell R, 117
Hessemer V, 27
Heston JP, 17
Hirst LW, 273
Hodge WG, 98
Hogan RN, 100
Hohla K, 50
Holland DR, 166
Holloway RG Jr, 181
Hoyt WF, 183
Hu S, 100
Hungerford JL, 247, 277

I

Igarashi S, 22
Iglehart JK, 295
Irvine AD, 270

J

Jacobi FK, 27
Jacobson DM, 196
Jager RD, 57
Jain S, 57
Jamieson H, 14
Jani B, 142
Janssen AG, 151
Javitt JC, 2
Jensen OA, 246
Jin GJC, 6
Johnson DA, 170
Johnson MH, 204
Jordan T, 83

K

Kaiser PK, 92
Kao SCS, 150
Karacorlu S, 127
Kasahara N, 22
Katz SJ, 192
Kazerooni EA, 192
Keefe KS, 272
Kempster RC, 273
Kerrigan LA, 262
Kersten RC, 156
Kertes PJ, 131
Kettering JD, 58
Khan HN, 244
Khanna RK, 185
Kielar RA, 267
Kitsos G, 82
Klapper SR, 207
Klein R, 45, 119
Klintworth GK, 267
Kloess PM, 95
Koch PS, 11
Koide R, 219
Kondo J, 104
Konstas AGP, 73
Korvatska E, 274
Kowal VO, 94
Krafft AE, 106
Kramer J, 228
Kremer I, 55
Krohn RW, 317, 318
Kroll S, 237, 249
Krumholz DM, 21
Kulwin DR, 156
Kutzko KE, 72

L

Laibson PR, 94
Lambert SR, 10
Lapid-Gortzak R, 28
Leach CM, 169
LeBlanc RP, 71
Lee AG, 207, 223
Lee S-H, 101
Lemon LC, 15
Lepera P, 158
Levey SB, 94
Levin LA, 180
Levy GD, 113
Liao CL, 150
Lichter PR, 298
Lifshitz T, 28
Lipshitz I, 54
Liu E, 144
Loewenstein A, 54
Logroño MJ, 19
Lommatzsch A, 243
Lowry JC, 161
Lübeck, 50
Lucarelli MJ, 143
Lunsford LD, 184
Lyle WA, 6

M

Madigan WP Jr, 217
Madreperla SA, 247
Maguire LJ, 103
Maguire MG, 121, 122
Malik GM, 185
Maloney RK, 37
Manners R, 83
Manning CA, 95
Mannor GE, 141
Mansour K, 151
March GA, 143
Mardelli PG, 49
Margolis TP, 98
Massry GG, 212
Mastrangelo D, 253
Mathers WD, 99
McArthur JH, 300
McCarty CA, 47
McClatchey SK, 173
McLean IW, 106, 261, 272
McLeish WM, 153
McNab AA, 147, 220
Meisler D, 56
Melia BM, 238
Messmer EP, 260
Metz DM, 21
Meyer DR, 149
Miller T, 237
Mingers A-M, 275
Mittman BS, 283
Moglia D, 158
Mönestam E, 3, 5
Moore FD, 300
Moorthy RS, 116
Mootha VV, 180
Moreira LB, 96
Morgan CF, 212
Morgan RO, 286
Morreim EH, 296
Moseley IF, 141
Mudun A, 127
Mulhern M, 43
Munier FL, 274
Munnerlyn CR, 52
Munõz B, 138
Munz SJ, 113
Mushlin AI, 181

N

Nardi M, 168
Newman NJ, 223
Noack J, 50
Norrani HZ, 244

O

Oestreicher JH, 144
Ohtsuka K, 202
Olitsky SE, 167

P

Pal C, 142
Palta M, 119

Parikh S, 128
Parks MM, 173
Paschal J, 113
Patel BCK, 153
Patrinely JR, 207
Pellegrini G, 168
Pendergast SD, 271
Pepose JS, 49
Pepper MS, 124
Perry SR, 265
Peterson J, 188
Pham CJ, 185
Phillips B, 153
Phillips PH, 223
Picken HA, 293
Piebenga LW, 49
Pineda R II, 92
Plager DA, 175
Plowman PN, 247
Podhajsky PA, 179
Potter P, 214
Power WJ, 100
Prause JU, 246
Priem H, 242
Proia AD, 79
Putterman AM, 160

Q

Quigley HA, 262

R

Raanan MG, 12
Raitta C, 75
Raman R, 179
Ransohoff RM, 188
Reinhardt U, 301
Retchin SM, 284
Reynolds JD, 167
Rizzo S, 168
Robinet A, 40
Rootman J, 265
Rose GE, 141
Rosenbaum JD, 21
Ruggli GM, 260
Ruiz P, 251

S

Sanchez D, 96
Sanchez JC, 182
Sanders V, 76
Sauerwein W, 243
Schanzlin DJ, 41
Schatz NJ, 226
Schaumberg DA, 25
Schein OD, 138
Scherfig E, 246
Schilling H, 243
Schneck GL, 160
Schuster V, 275
Seddon JM, 135
Seidenspinner S, 275
Selker HP, 293
Shah S, 69
Shahinian L Jr, 57
Sharma T, 128
Shastry BS, 271
Shaw AM, 71
Shields CL, 146, 214, 239
Shields JA, 214, 239, 279
Shields MB, 79
Shimmick JK, 52
Shin DH, 15
Shroyer NF, 264
Siatkowski RM, 182
Sibayan SAB, 22
Singh D, 29
Singh N, 264
Siriwadena D, 14
Siriwardena D, 67
Smecka Z, 45
Smiddy WE, 129
Snyder SK, 175
Song MS, 15
Sorkin JA, 10
Specht CS, 261
Squitieri N, 253
Steinbach MJ, 174
Sternberg P, 132
Stevens TS, 121
Stewart WC, 73
Stone EM, 81
Stroman GA, 73
Sugita J, 104
Sullivan TJ, 199
Sun R, 17
Sutphin JE, 99
Swensson O, 270

T

Taravella MJ, 59
Teich SA, 116
Telfair WB, 52
Tellado MV, 261
ten Hove MW, 266
Thach AB, 24, 217
Tielsch JM, 138
Tönnies R, 50
Totsuka N, 219
Trapp BD, 188
Trentacost DJ, 2
Trousdale MD, 96
Tseng JHS, 150
Tseng SCG, 101
Tusa RJ, 187

U

Ulrich GG, 79

V

Valancy J, 307
Valnickova Z, 267
Van Der Karr MA, 76
Varssano D, 54
Veloso AAS Jr, 117
Verbraeken HE, 242
Vergani S, 114
Vesti E, 75
Viciana AL, 251
Vilar NF, 129
Virnig BA, 286
Voest E, 124

W

Wachtmeister L, 3, 5
Walker LM , 316
Wall M, 72
Wang F, 2
Ward TP, 217
Warner JJ, 196
Weakley DR Jr, 166
Weber R, 260
Weekly KJ, 320
Weinberg A, 59
Weinberg DV, 116
Wender A, 28
Weston BC, 103
Weyand CM, 258
Whitacre MM, 49
White VA, 265
Wiffen SJ, 103
Wiley MJ, 310
Williams PB, 107
Wilson SE, 56

Witter DM Jr, 181
Wong FL, 248
Wright JE, 199
Wynia MK, 293

Y

Yeh S-CJ, 284
Yerkes LA, 306

Z

Zack DJ, 262
Zhu Q, 117